Kentro® Body Balance

The Secret Pleasures of Posture

May you move with vitality and joy
Angelika Thusius

Kentro® Body Balance

The Secret Pleasures of Posture

Angelika Thusius

RiverWood Books
Ashland, Oregon

RiverWood Books, P.O. Box 3400, Ashland, Oregon, 97520.
Web site: www.riverwoodbooks.com

FIRST EDITION 2005
08 07 06 05 5 4 3 2 1

Cover photographs of the author at age of 60 by Robert Frost
Cover design by David Ruppe
All movement photographs by Robert Frost
All illustrations and poems by Angelika Thusius

Printed in Korea

LIBRARY OF CONGRESS CATALOGING-IN-PUBLICATION DATA

Thusius, Angelika.
Kentro body balance : the secret pleasures of posture / by Angelika Thusius.
p. cm.
ISBN 1-883991-90-0 (pbk.-illustrations)
1. Posture. 2. Health. 3. Mind and body. 4. Exercise. 5. Human mechanics. I. Title.
RA781.5.T48 2004
613.7'8—dc22
2004001944

Table of Contents

To my mother, Gela,
who showed me the way
to the wonder in nature
and all its creatures.

Preface: My Story

IN 1972, WHEN I WAS THIRTY YEARS OF AGE, my life changed in an instant. On my way to teach an art class in Paris, I fell down two flights of marble stairs. The next day, in the hospital, I discovered I had fractured my sacrum and coccyx; twisted my sacrum, back, and neck; and compressed the nerves around my left hip. In time, the fractures healed, but I continued to be in severe pain. I was uncomfortable sitting in any kind of chair, nor could I find any comfort lying down. My occupation, painting, had become almost impossible.

For the next nine years, I sought help from orthopedic doctors, acupuncturists, massage therapists, homeopaths, kinesiologists, and chiropractors, but all to no avail. I attended orthopedic exercise programs, along with yoga and water therapy classes. Although I found relief in osteopathy, after two to three weeks the old crippling aches would return. I was given eleven different diagnoses—from specialists in France, Germany, and England. They concluded that the symptoms from my fall would worsen with age due to frailty, blocked energy, and my "body type."

Despite these discouraging prognoses, I had a strong desire to recuperate.

I was born in Bremen, Germany, in 1942. My early years were characterized by feelings of immobility and a fear of moving spontaneously. When I was seven years old, I traveled with my family to Honduras, where my parents had lived before the war. The agreeable surroundings helped me to relax and I began to feel a new agility when I danced to tropical rhythms.

Twenty-three years later, trying to recover from my accident, the memory of this shift in my motion and visions of resilient Hondurans told me that I, too, was part of the flowing movements I loved to paint. I believed that if I could find a way to remobilize my pelvis and back, I would surely be on the road to recovery.

Ten years later, at the age of forty, I found some help by taking classes at the Iyengar Yoga Institute and the Institut Superieur D'Aplomb in Paris. Four years later, I was certified to teach yoga and body balance. However, even after all the years of studying and practicing exercises, yoga postures, balancing stretches, and body-oriented visualizations, I was still in pain, and I still felt separated from my body. Almost in despair, I embarked on a road less traveled.

I had always disliked my looks and how I moved, yet I did not want to look or move like someone else. I wished to be comfortable in my own skin—in my own body—I wished to fully embody *me*. I longed for a joyful, freeing sense of posture. I became committed to letting the beauty of moving freely and gleefully unfold for me, and as it did, I wanted to share this experience with others. I gave up my goal of achieving a straight back and *changing* my posture.

The more I focused on reshaping myself into *unique* postural expression, the more cautious I became of glorifying people with balanced movement. Thanks to growing up in Honduras, and living in many other cultures, I knew people could be *physically flexible while still being mentally inflexible and emotionally stressed.* Likewise, *a positive mental attitude does not automatically create enduring physical mobility.*

I began to develop an alternative approach. I started listening more to my body and how it responded to various stretches. I gravitated toward simple movements. Practicing such discernment had positive results. Now, I encourage my students to trust their senses, to avoid idealizing people with attractive stances, to dissolve any notions of being stuck in their postural habits, and to practice at their own rhythm. I take each student's particular back and body history, range of movement, and lifestyle into consideration, and I listen carefully to how they respond to the movements I teach them.

Descriptions in *Gray's Anatomy* became the structural inspiration of my research. My enthusiasm for learning and teaching how to move with ease and to enjoy our daily gestures led me to develop a movement method that is beneficial for everyone—KENTRO Body Balance.[1]

I knew I needed a pedagogical approach that would merge physical function with sensing and feeling movements. Innovative physiological observations alone are a far cry from the creation of practical, effective movements that stem from compassion toward ourselves. I believe that fostering an affectionate relationship with our bodies is essential if we are to have *comfortable* balance in our movements and that centering *ease* is fundamental to the resolution of physical strain. Sparked by my transformations and testimonials from students, this caring attitude toward posture has become the central tenet of my teaching.

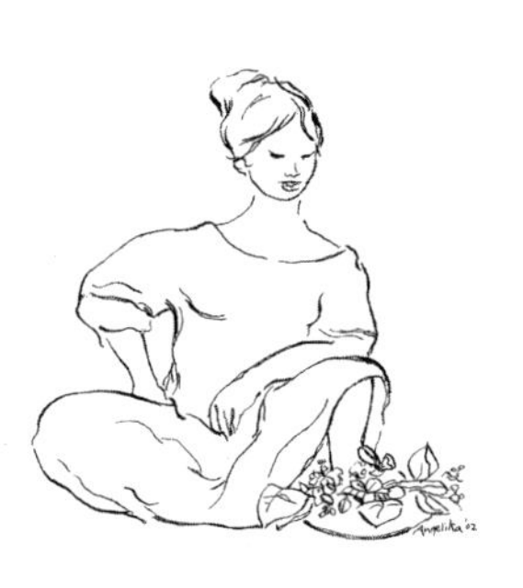

I hope to convey harmonious movement in this drawing of a Honduran woman.

My artistic background served as excellent preparation for teaching movement. In Greece, Honduras, Mexico, Spain, Brazil, Morocco, and Italy, I had painted women and men who moved in flowing connection to their environment. Twenty years of sensing and painting such physical plasticity helped me to sense and guide my own body into smooth motion.

Linking my artistic experiences with ordinary gestures helped me to avoid putting myself—and future students—into a physical, psychic, or ethnic mold of any kind. Images of people with optimal bearing became illustrations of our bodies' potential for mobility. Photographs of people with supple bodies carrying heavy baskets on their heads demonstrated to me the importance of bodily weight distribution for upright comfort—even if we carry only our own body weight. But these images told me nothing about how the people felt inside their skin or, more importantly, by what process students with strained balance could regain elasticity. To avoid moving in a mechanical way (imitating these flexible women and men), I replaced any *should*s with an aesthetic approach to posture, sensing and honing my own gestures.

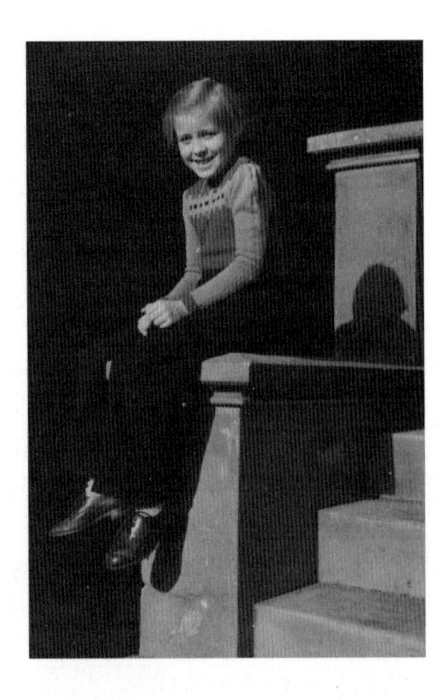

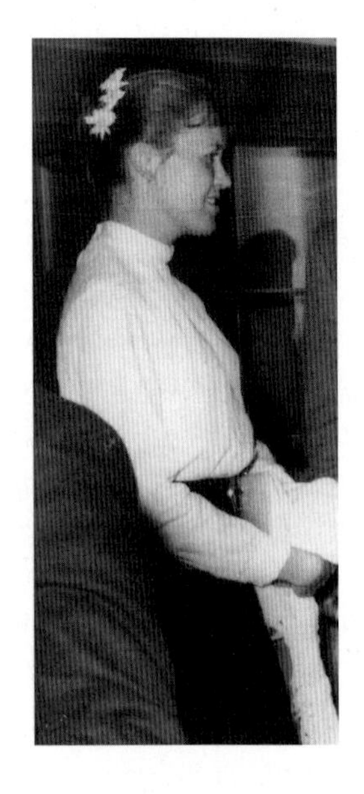

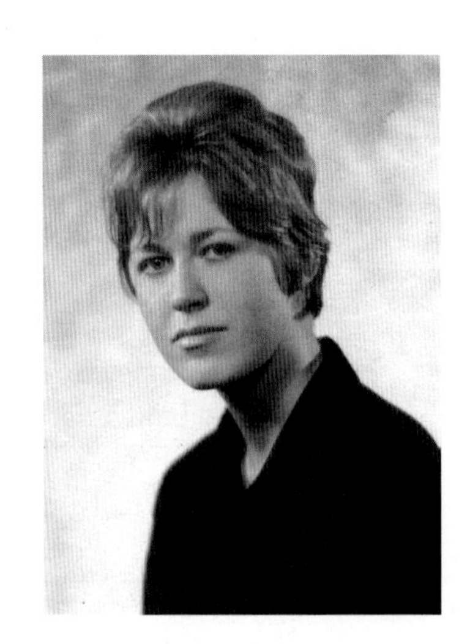

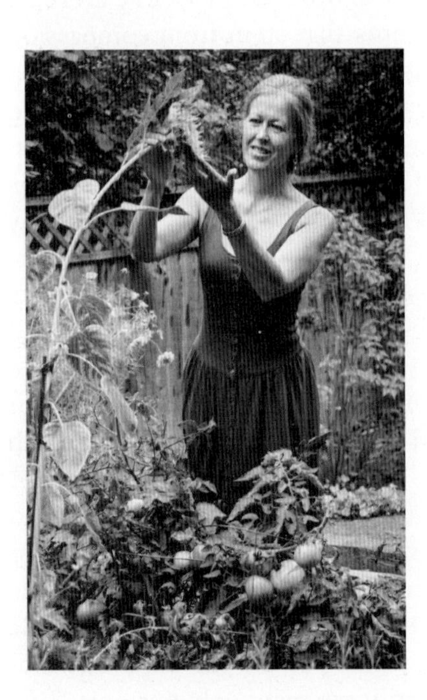

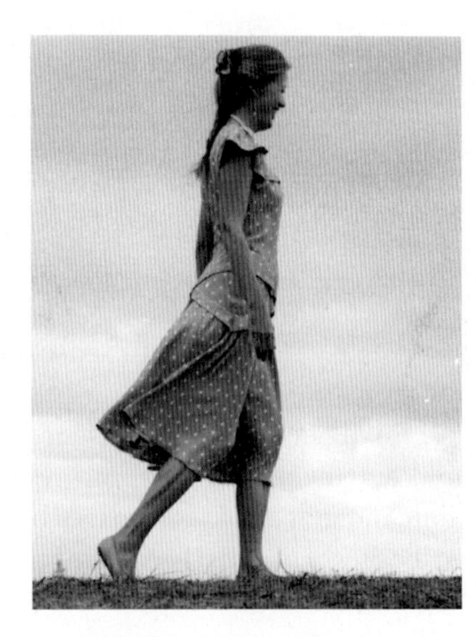

Clockwise from top left:
Angelika Thusius at seven years old: a rounded back and stressed shoulders.

Thusius at sixteen years old: a rounded back and general stiffness.

Thusius at nineteen years old: general tiredness, neck and hip pain.

Thusius at forty-eight years old: a straighter back, improved energy, and general flexibility.

Thusius at fifty-four years old: relaxed shoulders and increasing resiliency.

My personal history has helped me empathize with the challenges that confront my students. Nine years of seeking relief from injuries through conventional medicine gave me extensive, firsthand experience of the emotional and mental discouragement that comes from hearing many negative prognoses. These statements had reinforced the criticism I received as a child and young adult about my posture, and served only to depress me further. For example, during a high school dance class, the teacher pushed me into a corner of the room because I was unable to stretch. Later, my college fencing teacher said I was too weak for that sport. Yet once I began seeing posture as fluid movement, I found ways to add a relaxing, centering approach to practicing KENTRO guidelines. The quality of my thoughts and feelings shifted. Little by little, my limiting beliefs dissolved as I moved with more ease.

My accident served as a catalyst, constantly turning my attention to the quality of my habitual movements. Above all, I focused on appreciating my bearing, recalling how my best paintings had emerged from "falling in love" with a subject. This loving attention to my body carried me from restriction to resilience [See photograph series on p. x].

Helping people to regain harmonious expression through movement became my life's work. I developed a comprehensive body-centering and body-balancing program of simple movements that shift our bodies into suppleness without struggle. Practicing the movements fosters beneficial qualities of the heart: confidence, cheer, and tranquility.

Since my very first year of teaching KENTRO movements in the mid-eighties, I was able to stop the seemingly endless (and expensive) cycle of consulting chiropractors, naturopaths, and medical doctors. My hip, back, neck, and sciatic nerve pain resolved. Although my back still has compensations, my spine has lengthened as my tissues have become more elastic. I now measure 5'9 1/2" instead of my earlier height of 5'8".

At sixty-three years of age, my shoulders are broad and relaxed, and my neck, pelvic, back, and leg muscles are supple. My whole body is more flexible and stronger than it was before my accident thirty-three years ago.

According to my massage therapist, I have no "knots" in my back muscles. And a physical therapist who measured my muscle tone told me I was more toned than she was—a twenty-five-year-old who exercises daily.

Regaining enjoyable physical mobility did not require reforming my diet or changing my lifestyle; I simply shifted *how* I moved by sensing my way into centered-balanced movement. This principle is essential to my continuous inquiry into the close relationship between form, feeling, rhythm, and movement—as I experience it myself, and as I observe it in students who are progressively reshaping their bodies, and in people who move with natural ease.

Many of the KENTRO movements are inspired by people who look for the most comfortable way to do things. For example, I had often seen Honduran gardeners who lean their pelvis against a tree trunk and bend forward to peel fruits or to put on or take off their sandals (instead of hopping around awkwardly on one leg); Italian women who lean their pelvis against a wall (instead of sitting on a bench) while they bend over to peruse some photos; and Greek dancers who simply bend forward as much as possible, staying in that placement for a while (instead of doing a stretch routine), as their only "warm up."

It dawned on me that in these situations, the Hondurans, Italians, and Greeks were stretching, stabilizing, and relaxing their pelvis easily, as in the KENTRO movement *Grounding*, with level hips and a straight back, even when their weight was just on one leg.

I had already sensed a stretch in my hamstring (back of the thigh), sacral, and back muscles by bending forward in smooth balance. I tried out steadying my buttocks against a tree, or desk. I found that by placing a chair in front of me as I stood with my back close to a wall, bending forward and lifting up my buttocks as high as possible, I could "glue" the base of the buttocks (the ischial area) on the wall. I then rested my crossed forearms on the top of the chair for counter-weight, with my forehead on my forearms. This passive placement yielded thorough yet gentle stretching throughout the hamstring, buttocks, and back muscles. Soon, this placement became the KENTRO movement *Pelvis Up the Wall*.

When I started teaching in Paris and London in 1986, my first classes were filled with people who represented a cross-section of ordinary life: bank administrators, students from a Greek dance class, midwives, pregnant women, and nursing mothers from a birthing center. In 1987, I went to teach in Honduras and several U.S. cities, and in 1988, my husband and I moved back to the United States. By the mid-nineties, a full program of KENTRO movements had evolved. Each movement has become both an exercise and a form of grace—a delightful sense of physical belonging. On the cover of this book I move freely, with joy, at sixty years of age.

Teaching a variety of individuals in such a range of occupations and surroundings convinced me that anyone can increase flexibility. Practicing KENTRO guidelines enables us to move in pleasurable connection with our ordinary occupations.

Notes

1. KENTRO is the Greek word for 'center.' KENTRO® is trademarked by Angelika Thusius.

Mapping Your Journey: How to Use This Book

IF YOU FOCUS SOLELY ON THE MOVEMENTS in this book, you will probably come to view the KENTRO method as just another eccentric exercise system. Likewise, if you only skim the inspirational chapters in this book, your imagination may be tickled, but you will risk developing an unattainable, idealized image of your self. Let the inspirational and practical guidelines intertwine smoothly with your KENTRO practice.

This book encompasses subtle inner body feelings (our sense of space, grounding, proportion, motion, and rhythm), as well as anatomical structure and function. Balancing your movements while neglecting what you *feel* (centering) can reshape your posture, but it is a little like body motion without heart.

Eclectic, Practical, and Inspirational Use of This Book

You can begin at any point in this book. Be liberal yet selective in your approach to the KENTRO program of twelve basic movements or all thirty-three movements; there is no linear progression in the practice of the movements (once you have incorporated the principles outlined in *Elemental Placement*). However, since much of the content is innovative, I urge you to read a few sections *before* trying out the movements outlined in Part II so you avoid confusion and fruitless motions. For beneficial practice, peruse the following sections: *Preface, Introduction, Setting the Stage*, chapters 1-5, 7-8, and vignettes 10 and 29.

How to Assimilate the Information, Images, and Metaphors in This Book

You may be surprised by the frequent reminders that the practice of centering-balancing movements is essential for supple motion. Pedagogically speaking, information that offers us an optimistic vision of reality is worth repeating, because we learn by repetition—especially when the information is new. This reframing of basic KENTRO notions, combined with KENTRO practice will awaken your sensory nature, develop a playful attitude, and help you trust that your body is indeed reshapeable. Little by little, as you read and absorb the similar yet multifaceted passages, you will realize all the chapters offer interchangeable KENTRO observations. The images are not "models" to imitate; they only depict our bodies' potential for free motion. While everyone's joints function similarly, individual posture is shaped by particular musculature. Practice KENTRO for personal centered balance. Combine KENTRO guidelines for sensing your movements with structural guidelines (found in *Gray's Anatomy*) as well as pragmatic observations of people with physical ease. Be practical. Immediately integrate centered-balanced movements with your ordinary gestures. Refer often to chapter 2, 3, and chapter 9, vignettes *Sense and Sensibility, Blissful Aches*, and *Stages of Freedom*. Consult chapter 11, *Combining KENTRO Movements* frequently to sense how to move with limberness in a variety of activities. It is ineffective to rush through the Practice section of this book. Consider spreading your practice over a period of at least eight months—regard this time as similar to the time required to learn a new sport, martial art, or meditation. Be patient with your soft tissues, they need many months to become resilient. Eight months is not very long when you realize you are creating genuine shifts in your postural expression.

KENTRO CONCEPTS

Since every chapter repeats certain keywords, here is a KENTRO lexicon that describes how these words apply to KENTRO centering-balancing guidelines:

Balancing. Comfortable weight distribution in the body, thanks to bone support.
Centering. A profound letting go and ease, thanks to supple flesh and a caring attitude.
Comfort. An energizing relaxation and a sense of weightlessness.
Ease. Fluid movement and a feeling of spaciousness enabled by centered balance.
Exercise. Invigorating movements that create resilient muscular function.
Grounding. A feeling of contentment, comfort, and ease.
Inner Artist. A deep place within.
Posture. Flowing movement, personal expression.
Stretching. A gentle, harmonious extension/expansion of tissues, similar to a yawn.
Secret. Intimate experience of comfort and ease—unique to centered balance.
Soulful. Personal, sensed, and felt movements, as opposed to dulled movements.
Spirited. Vital, full of life.

Introduction: Bright Possibilities

WE ARE A NATION OF UNCOMFORTABLE PEOPLE. Many of us feel inflexible and physically vulnerable. Even if we jog, play sports, or use gyms, we may feel stiff and dislike our looks. We often experience pain and fatigue, even after simply bending, sitting, or standing for moderate periods of time. One half of all working Americans have back problems each year.[1]

When we get spinal pain, we tend to rely on therapies and medications that reduce symptoms but that do not necessarily result in enduring relief. We try to get by with our chronic pain. We may purchase ergonomic furniture, change our jobs, or relinquish some of our favorite activities, but we may continue to hurt. Ordinary activities, like getting into the car or picking up a package, sometimes flare up our symptoms.

Most of us can regain flexibility.

The ability to move freely and confidently is within our reach, regardless of occupation, culture, history of injury, age, body weight, lifestyle, or constitution. We can again experience resiliency and stamina in our daily living. KENTRO Body Balance provides the guidelines for moving with ease. KENTRO movements are inspired by people who are supple, whether they sit at desks or work in physically demanding occupations.

KENTRO Body Balance offers a series of gentle movements that stretch, release, exercise, and invigorate every area of our bodies, *during* both rest and activity. These movements dissolve joint, back, and neuromuscular problems, and they can be practiced anywhere, anytime. The innovative KENTRO method is based on optimal body mechanics. It is the culmination of thirty years of my sensing movements from within as well as from observing children and adults who move with lasting limberness. Students of KENTRO report fuller respiration and increased poise as well as remarkable improvements in the mobility of their necks, back, hips, and shoulders.

KENTRO guidelines blend balancing and centering the body. Body *balancing* allows us to move with our weight appropriately distributed throughout the body. Physical *centering* moves us beyond measurable balance; it involves an affectionate attitude toward our bodies, an attitude that enlivens our sensory system and is essential to generating suppleness and grounding. As a result, posture is no longer "right" or "wrong;" it becomes a fluid part of us that soothes and strengthens us in our habitual gestures.

This interconnectedness may sound unfamiliar. We tend to separate the shape and stance of our body from its anatomical functioning, just as we separate balancing from centering. We may think of centering only as a visualization or meditation technique. But when we integrate centering with balance in our repetitive motions, preconceptions

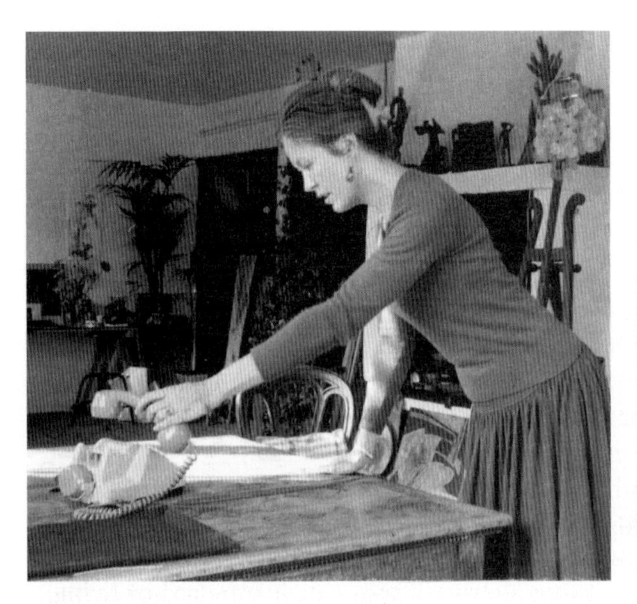
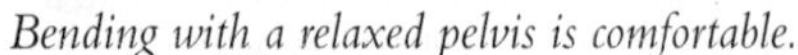
Bending with a relaxed pelvis is comfortable.

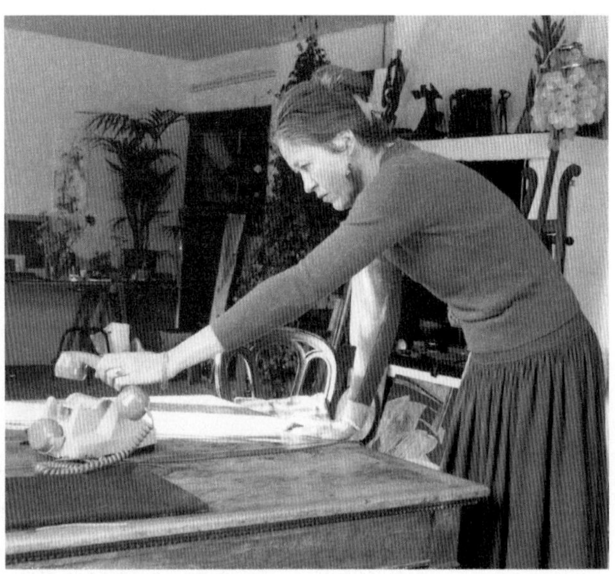
Bending with a tucked pelvis is uncomfortable.

about our bodies can finally disappear. The *activity itself* will limber and tone us. We become part of an organic process that relieves us from rigid, judgmental, mechanistic concepts about our carriage and appearance.

The KENTRO program merges physiology and psyche, anatomy and art, structure and soul, and bridges the gap between vibrant physical expression and vitalizing feelings. Activities that once seemed like chores become pleasurable as we incorporate KENTRO movements into our lives. Our bodies adapt lightly to our daily needs.

This book is intended to help you cultivate an exquisitely simple way of moving joyfully and energetically through centering-balancing your actions. It offers a heartening way of engaging with your body and provides practical tools for well-being. Gardening and lifting groceries will strengthen and straighten your back. You will be able to sit without discomfort at the computer for hours on end. Your abdomen will become strong without doing abdominal crunches. And your body will feel broad, tall, and expansive. You will find yourself in a refreshing relationship with your body and your world because you are comfortable.

NOTES

1. B. Vallfors, "Acute, Subacute and Chronic Lower Back Pain: Clinical Symptoms, Absenteeism and Working Environment," *Scandinavian Journal of Rehabilitation Medicine* (II, 1985): 1-98.

Setting the Stage: Postural Movement in Highly Industrialized Countries

IN OUR HIGHLY INDUSTRIALIZED and technologically advanced culture, we possess an extensive healthcare system, efficient medical treatment, refined surgical procedures, a variety of exercise programs, and worthwhile integrative therapies that complement conventional medicine. Yet many of us suffer from physical discomfort (e.g., stiffness, aches, or chronic pain) during our everyday occupations. We may tire or develop a backache after standing, bending, or sitting for as little as an hour. We twist our bodies slightly and experience muscular distress. As a result of our paradoxical cultural situation, comprehensive healing methods, and a high standard of living, juxtaposed with precarious motion—we have adopted a fearful, restrictive view of our bodies. We do not *expect* to be physically comfortable in our daily living.

Viewing our bodily expression as a facet of our cultural makeup can free us from postural dictates. Our *culture* reflects our behavior and its products, our improvement, refinement or development by study or training, and our concepts and habits. We can assume that repetitive gestures—whether habitual or learned—can reflect specific postural habits in specific cultural environments. In highly industrialized societies, we attempt to achieve "correct" posture by constantly tightening the outer muscles and pushing our bodies into shape, and as a result, we industrialized our movements. How did we arrive at this predicament?

In the 1920s and 30s, there was a significant change in the ideas and aesthetics of posture in highly industrialized countries. This shift points to the seductive appeal of the fast, sophisticated, and urban way of doing things, which included a novel definition of attractive posture (i.e., controlled, "good" bearing). Out of this notion emerged the mechanistic idea of forcefully fixing our looks.

Modernity was accompanied by a disregard for slow, seemingly monotonous physical labor and many activities came to be viewed as chores. The popular and preferred body stance required people to flatten and "hold in" their muscles in the pelvic area—the very area central to moving freely and in smooth balance. This lean, taut look has turned out to be both mentally and physically stressful. It demands the constant contraction (shortening) of muscles in the abdomen and the overstretching (tucking) of the buttock muscles to straighten the pelvis. This causes the legs to go forward and the pelvis to tilt into a posterior angle, resulting in the continuous strain of thigh ligaments because the strong thighbones are out of optimal (vertical) alignment. Such tilting pushes us out of limbering equilibrium: When the weight is no longer centered over the leg bones and the leg bones are no longer vertical, there is strain on muscles and

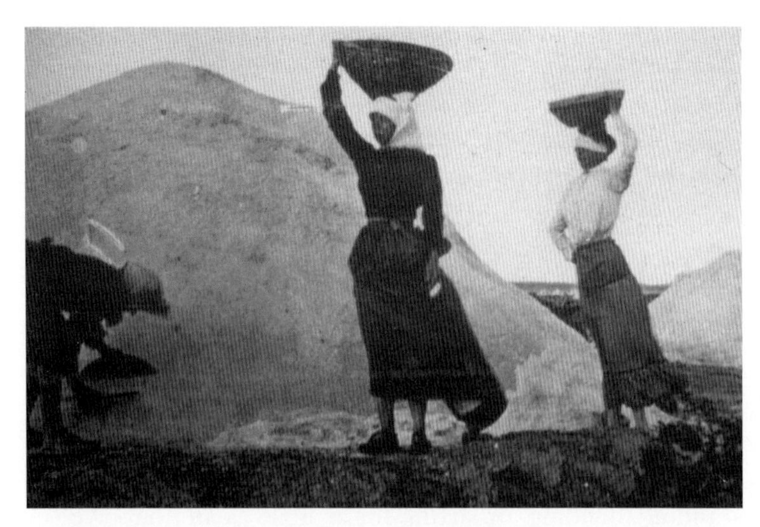

These early-twentieth-century French women transporting salt illustrate comfortable upright posture—they are not slouched or round-shouldered. Notice the woman on the far left bending from her hips with a straight back and bent knees. The third woman from the left has a visibly supple, straight back.

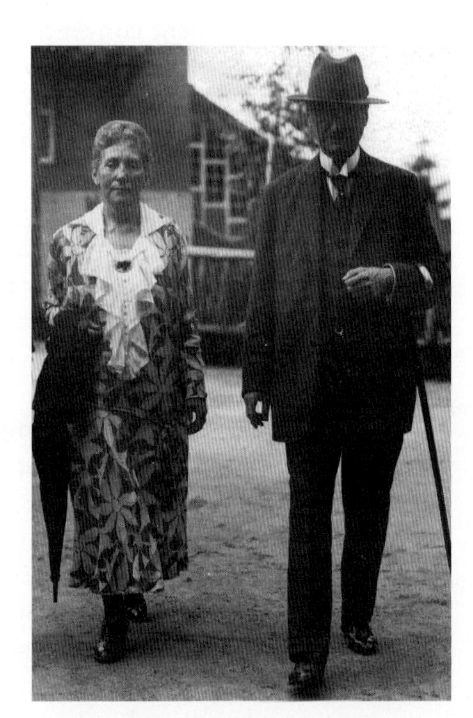

My German paternal grandparents habitually moved with comfortable, upright postural expression. Their backs are straight; their shoulders broad and dropped.

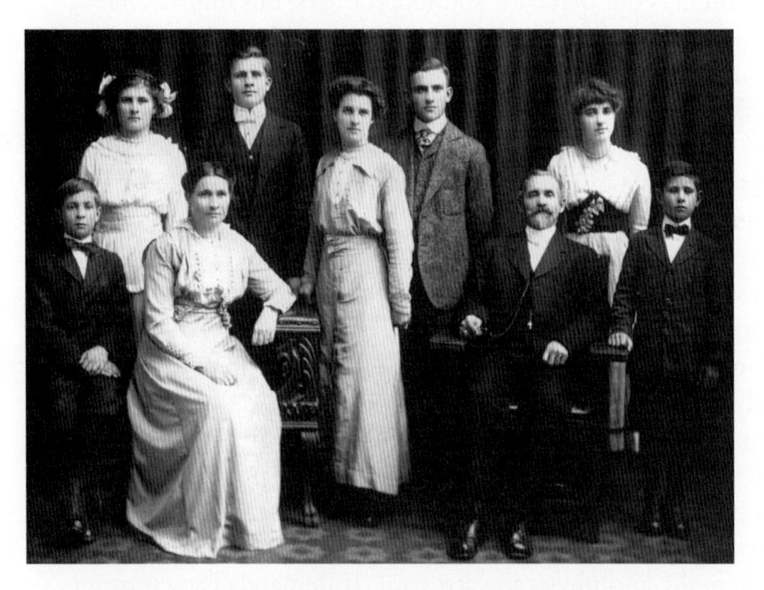

My American father-in-law (the child on the right) and his family. Notice their dropped shoulders, broad torsos, and comfortable upright posture.

ligaments. The body compensates by shortening and arching the lower back muscles and over-curving, rounding, and over-stretching the upper back muscles. Further up, the head and neck jut forward [Figs. A-D]. We may feel weighted down and hope that flattening and tightening our pelvis and abdomen into the posterior tilt will lighten our distress. Yet forcing our bodies to "fit" into a postural form will not increase mobility. This striving for "good" posture remains fashionable today and has influenced all of us, from doctors to dancers.

The goal of modernism was to develop machines, gadgets, and timesaving devices that would do our work for us and relieve us of our routine occupations, allowing us to live a more relaxed lifestyle. Ironically, increased leisure time has coincided with growing discomfort in our actions due to the overtaxing, modern way of moving. We have invented special furniture that is supposed to alleviate postural strain, but this is only a temporary, palliative aid.

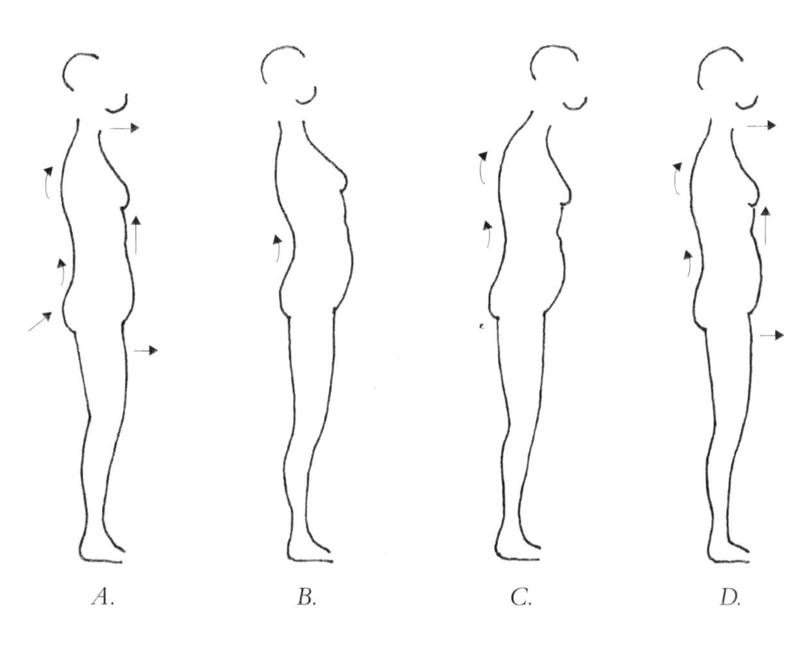

The Problem:
Modern "correct" posture pushes your body into stressful compensations.

A. Tucking the buttocks and tightening the abdomen pushes the legs out front, out of vertical alignment.

B. With reduced leg and pelvic support, the weight moves out front and the lower back over-arches to prevent the upper back from falling forward.

C. With the lower back over-arching, the upper back compensates by over-rounding to prevent the upper body from falling backward.

D. When we stop tucking and tightening our bodies, we are still distressed because our bodies are still compensating.

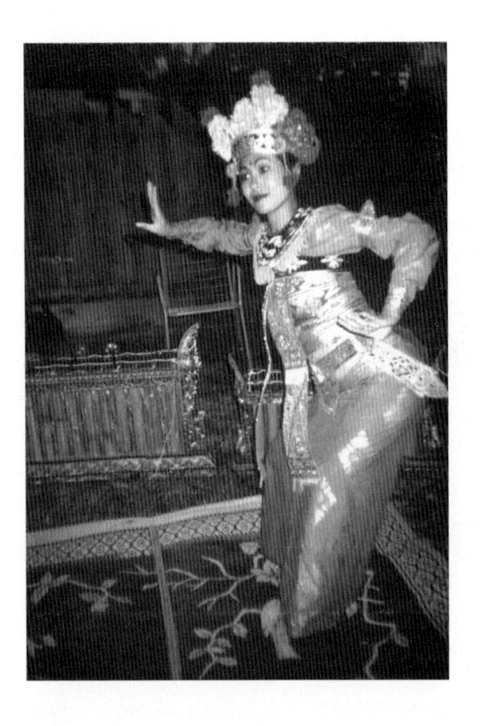

This Balinese dancer bends easily from the hips; her back straightens and her shoulders relax.

During the early twentieth century, people came to identify success with the avoidance of situations that involve bending, lifting, or carrying. This emphasis on inactivity, combined with our attempts to mirror the conventional body form, hindered our physical dynamics. When abdominal, neck, back, thigh, and buttock muscles lose their natural elasticity due to unnecessary physical effort or disuse, we tend to feel weak and unhappy with our shape. We may believe our anatomical structure is wrong for us. We may *intellectualize* the body instead of *sensing* our movements. Yet this approach disconnects us from our bodies, veering us in the direction of a Roman bust where only the head and shoulders are acknowledged. Or we may sign up for programs that "fix" us by hardening the outer muscles, which grow disproportionately larger than the internal musculature.

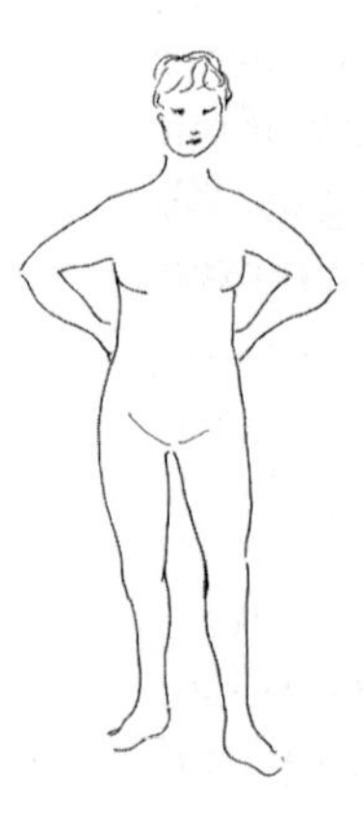

Based on one of French artist E. Degas' small sculptures of ballet dancers (1878), the sturdy dancer illustrates smooth balance—no tucking or tightening in her body.

Our bodies very capably compensate for constrained kinetics, but when tissues are unable to function in harmonious relation to one another, we lose our sense of ease. It becomes increasingly difficult to distinguish tension from relaxation.

A brief aesthetic and ethnological look at historical changes in posture can broaden our views. Fashion is one example of a cultural phenomenon that can hinder or enhance motion. The word *waist* is a fashion term. Over the centuries, the waist has moved up (e.g., ancient Greek and French empire styles) and down (e.g., the last sixty years). The waist has been corseted, as in the Victorian era, or left alone. Some fashions, like the Japanese obi or the Indonesian wraparound sash, cover a good portion of the back, making it easy to bend from the hips. In these fashions there is no "waist" at all. American blue jeans possess a broad, triangular insert on the upper back of the pants that accommodates the natural angle of the pelvis.

In recent decades, we have also become aware of a variety of aesthetics surrounding body weight. Presently, in the United States, a thin body with a flattened pelvis and developed arm and leg muscles is considered the most attractive and most physically fit. These cultural messages have led to grave eating disorders (e.g., bulimia and anorexia) where already slender women strive obsessively to avoid gaining weight.

We see different models of beauty and health in other societies. In some Mediterranean cultures "body," or voluptuous fleshiness, is desirable in women. When I visit

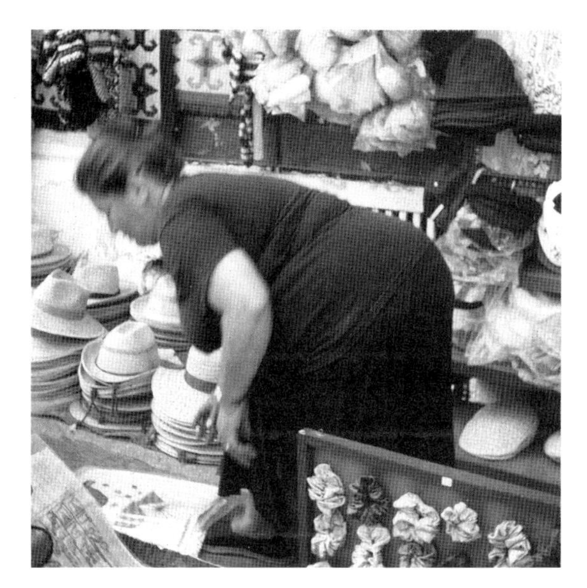

Smooth balance refers to comfortable body weight-distribution, not to body shape. Notice the limber motion of this Greek woman.

Honduras—where thinness is considered slightly unhealthy—friends often greet me with the compliment,"*Parece que ya engordaste*," or "It looks like you have gained some weight," even though my weight has not changed.

We can avoid this struggle of trying to fit our bodies into idealized postural forms influenced by images of modern, muscled models, or exotic-looking people from other countries. By practicing KENTRO guidelines, we encourage an affectionate view of our bodies and come to see our bearing not as a fixed form but as tissues reshaping us. We can assist this process by combining structurally sound balanced actions with the powerful poetics of centering relaxation. Our bodies can regain plasticity [Figs. E-H, p. xxii].

Just as we enjoy choosing our food, clothing, art, and healing methods, regardless of what the culture deems desirable or correct, we can choose to let go of limiting movement patterns, instead moving as we wish.

My parents, who were originally from Germany, exemplified the modern posture, suffering chronic shoulder and back pain. As I grew up, I reflected their distress. When I was a teenager, I consciously tried to sit up straight by pushing up my rib cage and tightening my stomach. Even though the Honduran women and men around us were strong and relaxed, my family did not assimilate their buoyant movements.

Only when my body regained limberness could I really see and *sense* the difference between strained and resilient motion. After a few more years of practicing centering-balancing guidelines, I recognized in myself certain strained gestures that were typical of my parents and I was able to release them totally. At the same time, I became more aware of fluid ways of moving, such as the rhythmic actions of Honduran friends and Greek dance teachers, which inspired my personal expression.

KENTRO movements are liberating. We can free ourselves from culturally diminishing views of the body, and we can move with pleasurable ease in our ordinary activities.

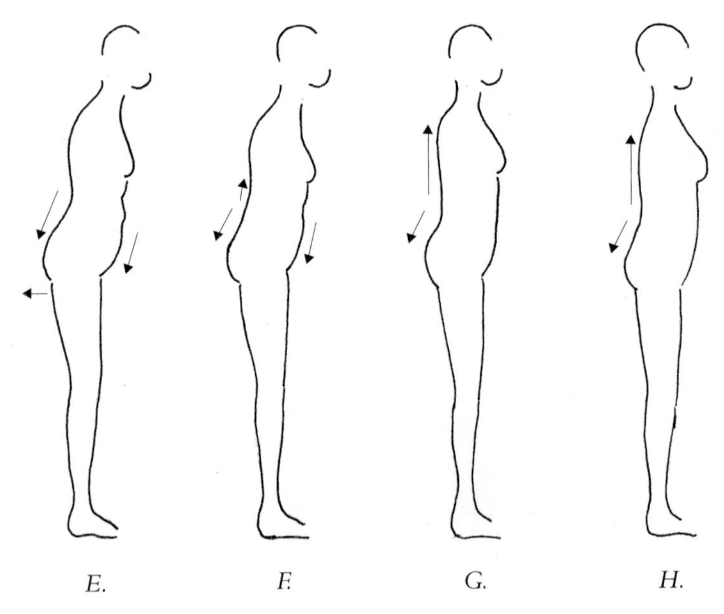

The Solution: Letting your body reshape you into comfort and ease. (*See* Part II, Elemental Placement and Elemental Movements).

E. Relaxing your body and letting your legs move back while you shift most weight into the heels, as well as letting your pelvis shift into a more anterior angle (which happens easily when you bend slightly forward from the hips).

F. Relaxing your body and letting your lower back straighten (with your diaphragm and abdomen stretching down) while your legs rotate slightly outward.

G. Relaxing your body and letting your upper back straighten while your shoulders soften and drop.

H. Relaxing your body and letting your neck straighten while your head moves slightly back and up.

PART I

Common Sense

The body is the angel of the soul

JOHN O'DONOHUE

CHAPTER 1:

The Kentro Body Balance Method

Defining KENTRO

KENTRO BODY BALANCE is a unique program of simple movements designed to teach comfort and ease in everyday life. Based on three decades of observations within industrialized and developing societies around the world, the KENTRO method integrates motions that are natural to all young children and people who move with limberness throughout their lives. This natural, fluid expression is sharply contrasted with the habits of individuals from highly industrialized societies—people who feel discomfort, who put great effort into their daily activities, who lack mobility, and who experience a high incidence of muscular and joint problems. The Practice of KENTRO (Greek for 'center') movements can reshape us into supple, robust beings, capable of moving with balanced and centered postural expression.

We can practice these spirited movements at our own pace and rhythm, at any age and in any place or occupation. Slight shifts in our gestures, combined with a compassionate sense of our bodies, provide harmonious and efficient ways to develop lasting flexibility and strength in each area of our bodies.

As caretakers of our bodies, we can ground ourselves into optimal bone support and relaxed, toned flesh. We can let go of limiting beliefs and unnecessary physical effort.

Any ordinary activity, such as gardening, vacuuming, sitting, or lifting a child, can stretch and move us into pleasurable resiliency. We will better enjoy our looks and our actions.

What Makes KENTRO Unique

KENTRO Body Balance interweaves the following core elements to create a method of practice for reshaping and rediscovering our bodies:

- A caring attitude toward your body.
- Descriptions of optimal anatomical structure and function.
- Observations of men, women, and children who are physically supple and strong.
- Comprehensive guidelines for reshaping yourself into enduring comfort and ease.
- Your body's adaptive abilities—both past and future—are cause for gratitude.
- There are no *shoulds* in your practice; there is only the *process*.
- You are released from all culturally determined, idealized, pathological, and

Maja, a Swiss KENTRO student, sits comfortably while she draws.

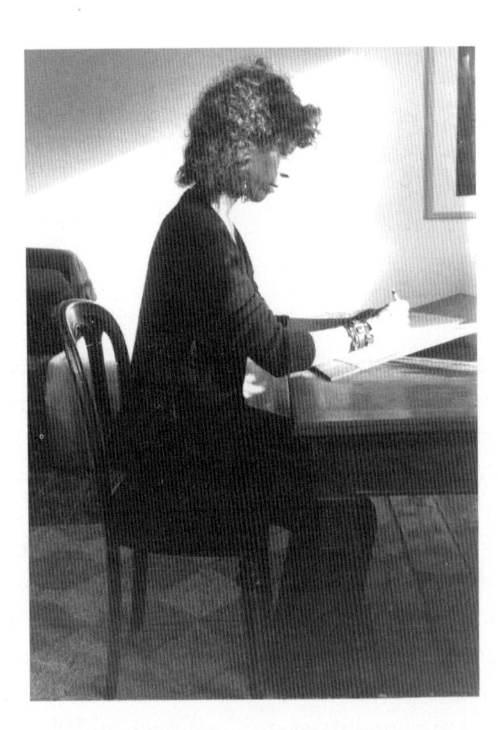

This Greek teenager moves with ease.

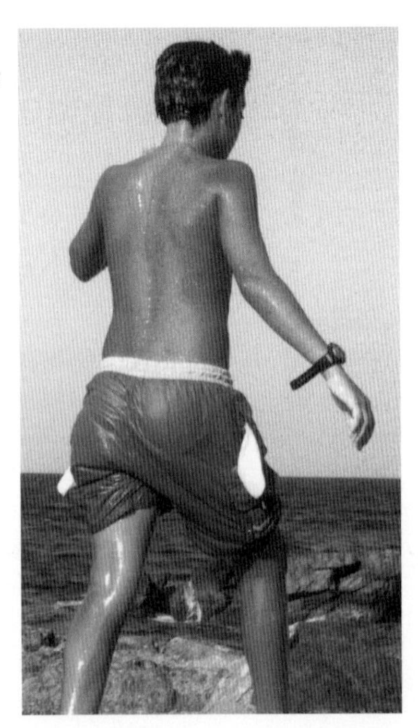

controlling models of "correct" postural movement; you are freed to love your body.

- You develop a natural aesthetics of sensing; you learn to distinguish resiliency from strain, flexibility from stiffness.
- Conventional definitions of terms are broadened. For example, *comfort* is no longer experienced as passive collapse, but as vibrant ease in the body.
- You needn't fix or change your posture; you simply practice balancing and centering movements that *result* in lasting change.
- You combine comfortable balance (body mechanics) with relaxing centering (grounding feelings).
- You are empowered by doing your own fieldwork. You read *Gray's Anatomy*, and you observe people who move with smooth balance.
- You trust in the inherent potential of your body to reshape itself into resiliency.

Common Benefits

For those who practice KENTRO centering-balancing guidelines at least three times a day—slowly, playfully, and gently—there are radical benefits. Below are some of the many advantages you will receive.

- You will experience increased bone support and elastic flesh irrespective of your weight or shape.
- You can reshape your body into increased flexibility at any age.
- You will not have to buy specialized chairs or pillows to be comfortable.

- Over time, centered-balance movements will happen on their own.
- You will resolve long-lasting joint, nerve, and muscular strain into resiliency.
- You can strengthen and make limber your most physically vulnerable areas—your lower back, pelvis, and shoulders.
- You will know how to relax, stretch and tone your body through everyday activity—ironing, building a shed, or cleaning the oven.
- You can improve basic life-support systems—sensory, circulatory, nervous, respiratory, and digestive.
- You will know which KENTRO movements best prepare your body for standing, bending, or sitting for an extended period of time, whether it be for a sport, domestic activity, or work.
- Acupuncture, chiropractic adjustments, and physical therapy will be enhanced by centered balance.
- You will cease to worry about posture when you experience increased ease of movement.
- You will sense how to sit comfortably in any seat (sofa, armchair, or airplane).
- You will be able to sense the difference between straining and relaxing your body during rest and activity.
- You will *feel* physically grounded, at home in your body and your everyday activities.
- You will discover an affectionate connectedness to your body; you delight in your posture, enjoy your appearance, and relish how alive you feel during your activities.
- You will find repetitive and ordinary movements, like typing or cooking, pleasurable and refreshing.
- Kentro practice will deepen the benefits of healing visualizations, meditation, yoga, or breathing techniques.
- Your body will reshape you into *your* unique spirited posture and movements.
- You will not have to change your lifestyle, posture, or furniture; instead, small centering, balancing movements will shift your body into harmonious gestures.
- You will feel safe as you move from the inside out and feel the links between your body and its subtle ramifications.
- Your everyday actions will be filled with simplicity.

A NOTE TO DOCTORS: Due to the anatomically sound principles of the KENTRO method, doctors can confidently recommend the centering and balancing movements to their patients. These movements can enhance medical treatments and improve muscular, nervous, skeletal, respiratory, and circulatory functions. By practicing KENTRO movements, patients will regain an unusually limber lower back; a straightened, broadened upper back; surprising pelvic resiliency (without a tightened abdomen or tucked sacrum); and comfort and mobility throughout the body.

CHAPTER 2:
A Compassionate Sense of Our Bodies

Body Voice

See me
in all my beauty and imperfection
to reshape and free you

Hear me
as I yawn, sigh
and shake you with belly laughs

Touch me
my toned, soft flesh
and the flower of my skin

Feel me
relaxing, contracting
and filling you with ease

Hold me
at the center
where we move as one

KENTRO BODY BALANCE guidelines foster the idea that *we are gifted with postural expression that is naturally joyous and resilient.* Merging this paradigm with our movements frees us into welcoming, noticing, and feeling our bodies, which can then reshape our tissues with ease. This process of deliberately choosing to bring fluidity into our daily activities begins to generate a compassionate image of our bodies. We focus on what feels right and relaxed to us.

In the *Endorphin Effect*, William Bloom mentions that we are "more like waves and currents than we are like solid bricks."[1] Yet, many of us hold a mechanistic mindset of our body and struggle to "fix" and "maintain" our posture as we would a solid object, such as a car. Hardening our flesh into a specific shape is stressful and goes against the grain of our pliable physicality. Most of the time we feel disconnected from our repetitive physical motions. We are used to straining our bodies; it feels normal. With our tissues tight, it is more difficult to sense our movements.

During my years of studying exercises, yoga, and balance, I tried to "do it right" and, for a while I imitated certain people who were "in balance". When I followed these notions, my movements remained strained and were accompanied by self-defeating thoughts such as: "I still have poor posture."

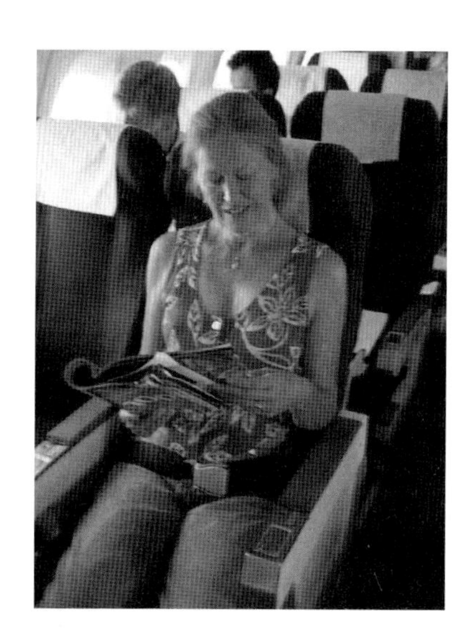

We can remain comfortable and limber while we travel. Placing a flat wedge in the upper back allows the shoulders to relax and the back to straighten without effort (see Chapter 9, #7, The Art of Wedge-Making).

Alternatively, whenever I began with a more loving attitude toward my body, listening to what it was telling me, I witnessed a small yet dramatic shift in my perceptions and movements. I stopped struggling to control my posture during a stretch or exercise. I was receptive to my senses and feelings. Instead of dwelling on the recommended outer body-shape goal, I forgot about *doing* or *achieving* anything. I found a source within that gradually became more familiar, a place of warmth that imbued my gestures with restfulness. I practiced moving without effort, at my own pace and rhythm.

Before I started teaching the KENTRO method, I could hardly sit back due to sharp pain in my upper back. After centering and balancing my movements, I became aware of a definite shift in the quality of my feelings. Once, while sobbing, I felt at ease as I was sitting back in the chair. My sobs did not overwhelm me. I noticed that instead of my back slouching forward, it remained straight yet comfortable, and my shoulders were not taut. The draining feelings receded soon, softly. Despite my vulnerability, I felt strengthened, soothed and protected by my body. Tension flowed out of me and I was physically tranquil.

Prior to practicing a gentle, receptive approach to my movements, I used to have to force myself to sit upright during meditation. Bending to lift groceries was a chore. By integrating KENTRO movements with my activities, all this exertion and back pain gradually dissolved. Now I can sit in airplanes for ten hours at a time, my back limber the entire flight. It is no longer tiring to write at my desk for hours without interruption because I take brief breaks to turn my pelvis, stretch my legs, rotate my arms and bend forward with KENTRO movements. Bending now feels like a dance movement. And I look forward to lifting groceries because I feel this action strengthening my back, arms, and pelvis.

Students of the KENTRO program report similar experiences of feeling more confidence and pleasure in ordinary activities as they become more limber.

Our bodies thrive on gentle care.

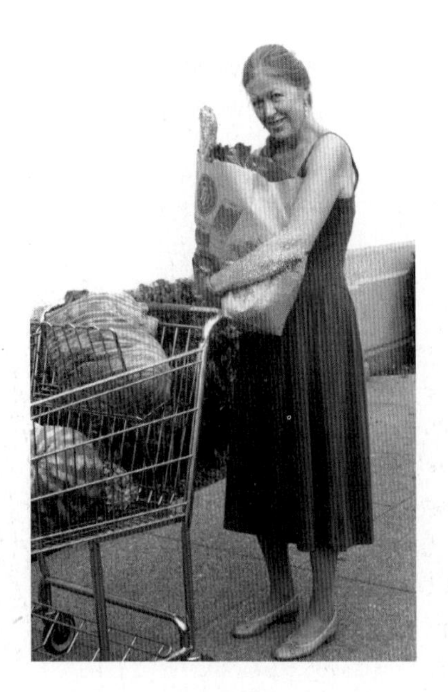

Discomfort. Tucking the pelvis and carrying groceries from the shoulder muscles weakens the abdomen and upper back.

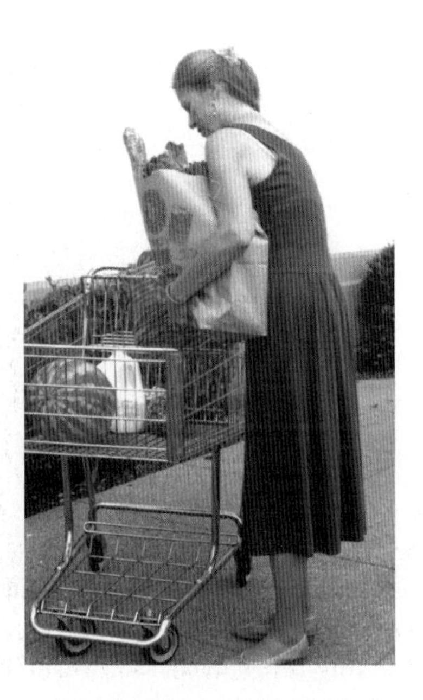

Discomfort. Bending with a tucked pelvis tightens the buttocks, rounds the back, and shifts the weight of the grocery bag toward the front of the body.

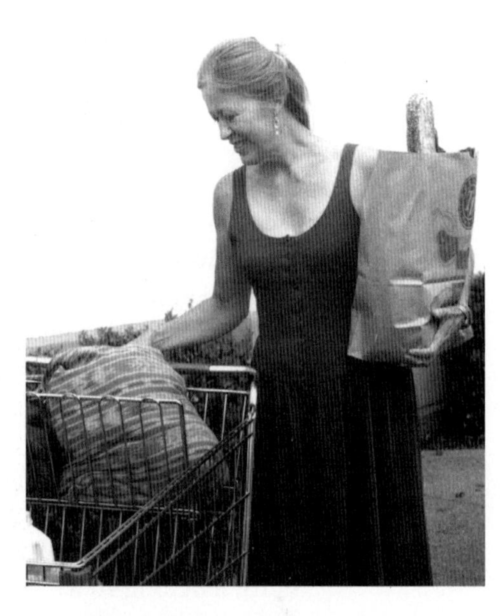

Comfort. With centering, balancing movements, the weight of the grocery bag shifts toward the thigh and sacrum; the hips can stay level, the back straight, and the shoulders relaxed.

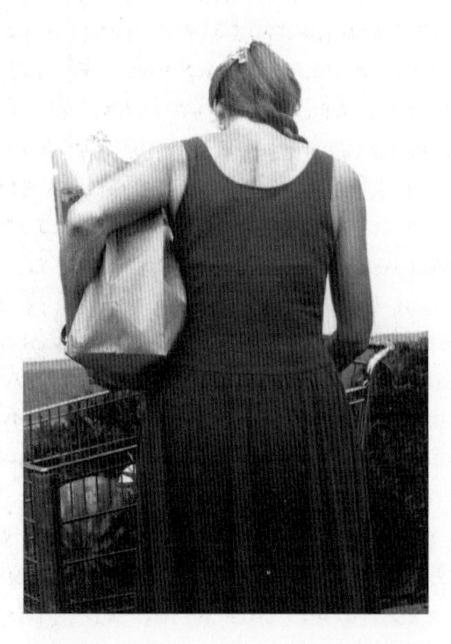

Comfort. The back remains straight (notice the even groove in the back); the buttocks, upper back, and upper arm muscles contract to carry the groceries.

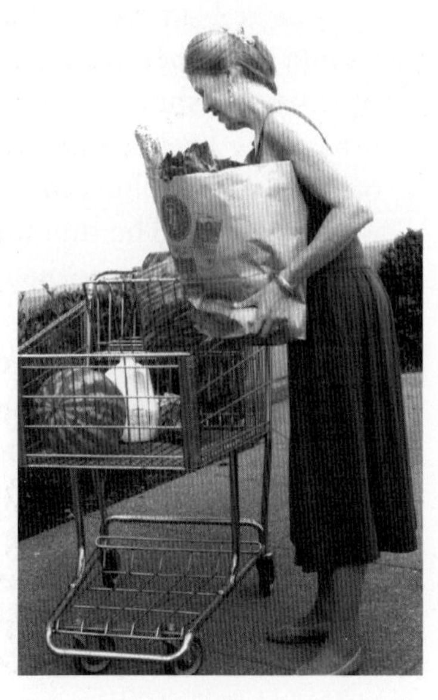

Comfort. Bending from the hips with a flexible pelvis stretches and strengthens the back and buttocks; the weight of the groceries is transferred to the sacral area, hips, and thighs.

It is refreshingly easy and requires no skills to incorporate centering and balancing our gestures with a lighthearted sense of our bearing, compared to the hard work of "correcting" our posture. In a playful manner, we can:

- *Acknowledge* our body — saying "hello" to it while we image ourself as supple and cheerful (as a child, or, the last time we danced); remembering such a situation will immediately energize us because it distances us from a depleting view of ourselves.
- *Allow* our body to let go of strain, and allow our mind to forget about *changing* our posture; this non-doing clears the way for our movements to reshape us into plasticity that extends beyond bodily shifts.
- *Appreciate* our spirited body for having continuously and faithfully adapted in a remarkable fashion to our overtaxing it, or not exercising it. Instead of being stressed over what is wrong with our posture, we can spontaneously tell our body how gorgeous it is, or admire our stronger back; such endearments create endorphins (enhancing feelings) and increase physical well-being.
- *Affectionately* pamper and treat our body with gentleness and tender thoughts as if it were a very young child who responds best to cuddles and compliments. Instead of venting dislike, denial, or impatience onto our body, we are now actively participating in its renewal.

As we embody these four "A's" while we practice KENTRO movements, we will be able to discern strain from flexibility, and perceive which movements feel appropriate and vitalizing for us.

When we add an affectionate attitude toward comfortable balance of our movements, we can move into expansive expression of ourselves. Only through leisurely movements and affinity with our bodies do we experience the suppleness and relaxation that extends beyond physical change. As we move through the day, we appreciate how our bodies feel, and we find pleasure in our appearance, gestures, and activities.

Posture no longer represents a problem that we must "fix." Posture becomes flowing movement.

A compassionate approach to KENTRO practice is our most powerful resource for an abundance of benefits. A happy kinesthetic memory, willingness to be transformed, feeling gratitude and kindness all merge to free our body into smooth action. With practice, we can savor delightful feelings that move us while we walk or cook a meal, like a sweet secret that reveals itself slowly, progressively, in our everyday lives.

CHAPTER 3:
A Passionate View of Physiology

Muscles and Bones

A feeling in my muscles
of toned, fluid flesh –
shaped by a passionate sculptor
with an eye for ease
and a hand that longs to form
free movement.

A feeling in my bones
of solid support
of bearing weight, in comfort.
Arches, promontories, joints
by a subtle architect
designed.

WE CAN INFUSE OUR EVERYDAY actions with enthusiasm and passion because our bodies are designed to function as a harmonious work of art in motion [Figs. 3.1– 3.5]. As children, we experienced moving to our heart's content. Indeed, our bodies have the capacity to vitalize us while we stand, sit, bend, or walk. Following KENTRO balancing-centering guidelines animates our musculoskeletal, nervous, and sensory systems to restore us with youthful mobility.

Using our mind as a muscle, we can stretch our understanding of "body" and "movement" toward the essence of our postural expression, and thus re-view our body in a potent way. The French word for mind is *esprit*. Our spirited mind desires suppleness. With a little prompting, it will gladly journey beyond mechanistic, dehydrated, and static postural models to view our body as a vessel for living our nature and discovering our humanness. We can be bold: Trying on a lovable image of our bearing may at first feel foolish, or unrealistic. However, focusing on images of smooth balanced centering of our actions will generate unexpected ease of movement. Instead

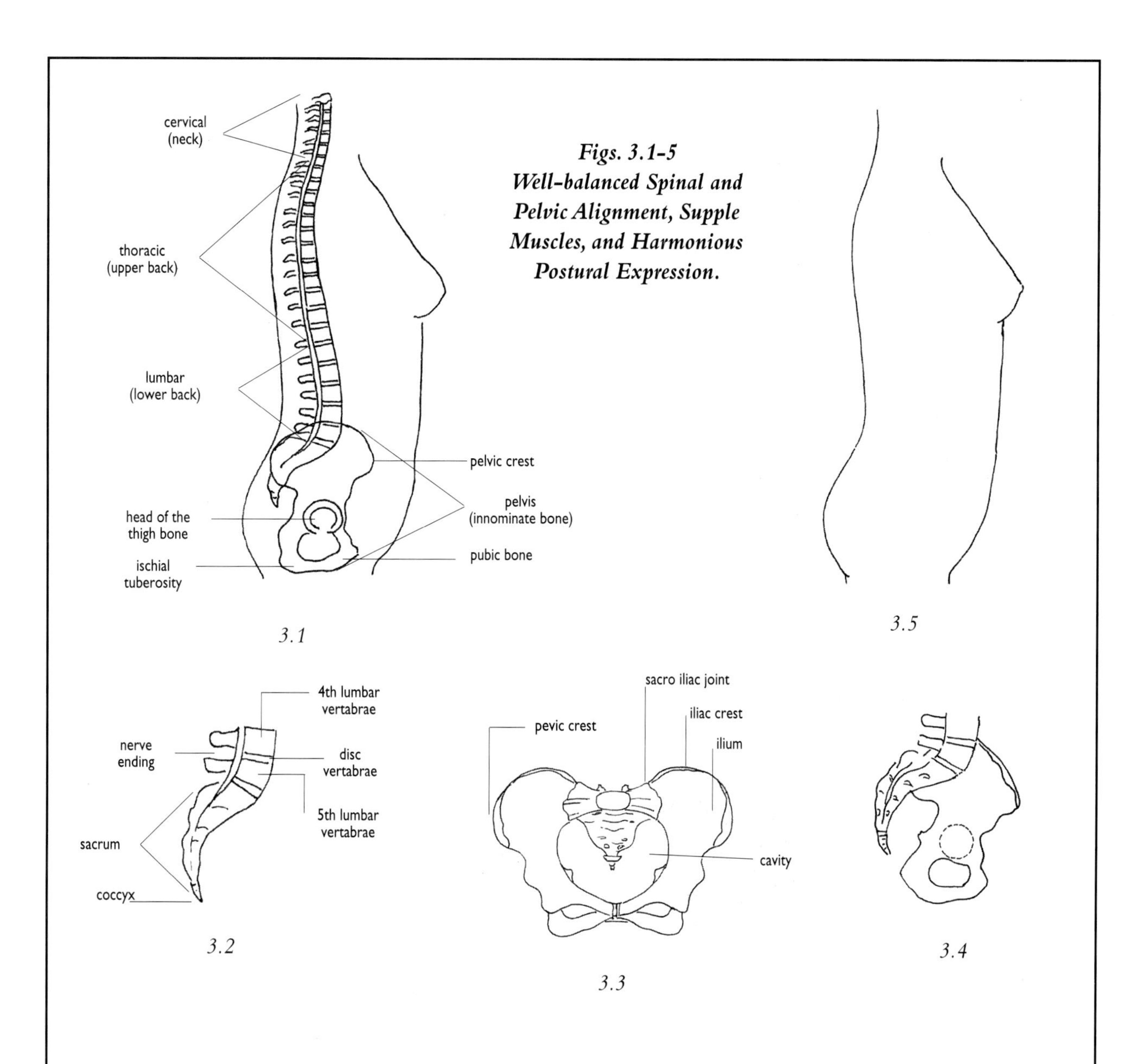

Figs. 3.1-5
Well-balanced Spinal and Pelvic Alignment, Supple Muscles, and Harmonious Postural Expression.

The body is a work of art in motion. In Figure 3.1, the supple spine is supported by the gently angled pelvis and the flesh is soft yet firm. This is an outer view of the pelvis (innominate bone and hip socket). The close-up of an angled sacrum in Figure 3.2 depicts the generous rounding of the sacrum. Figure 3.3 is a frontal view of the spacious, anteriorly-rotated pelvis. This naturally angled sacrum and obliquely, optimally placed pelvis combines Gray's illustration of the pelvis with the same pelvic angle as shown in photos of real bones in contemporary English and Greek anatomy textbooks. Figure 3.4 shows the inner side of the pelvis (innominate bone and sacrum). This drawing smoothly balanced pelvis is based on the pelvis and spine I use in my classes, as well as [1934, 1938, 1989, 1990, and 1997] American and English medical photos and illustrations. The dotted lines indicate the location of the hip socket (clearly visible in the outer view of the pelvis, in 3.1). Figure 3.5 shows an outline of a body with resilient, soft yet firm tissues, as well as upright comfort.

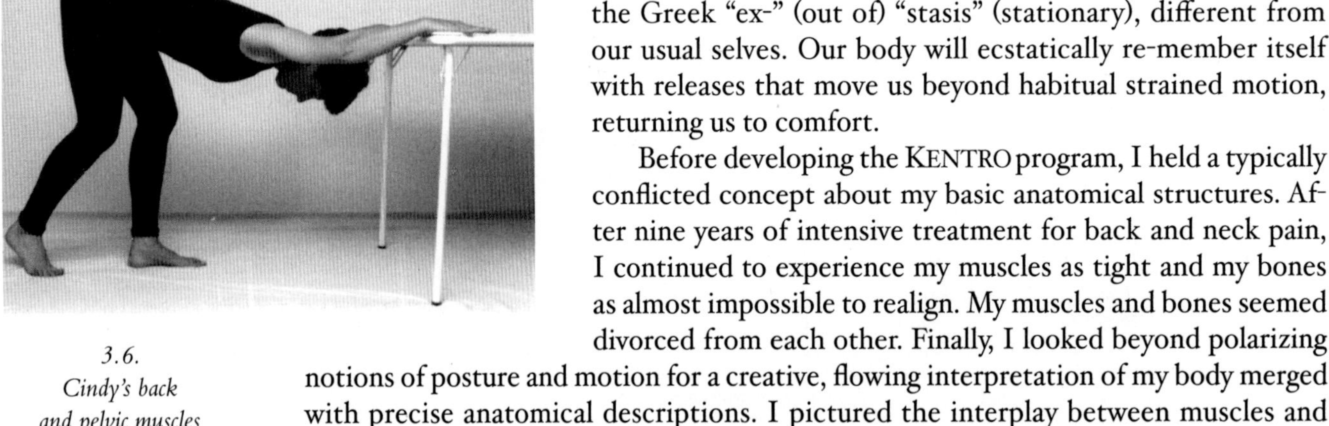

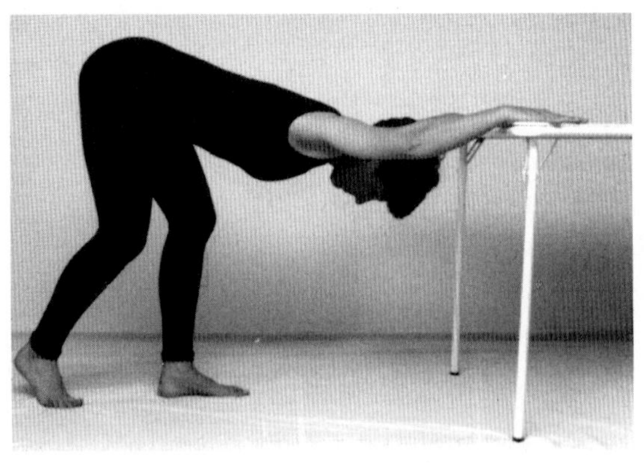

3.6.
Cindy's back and pelvic muscles have regained elasticity.

of feeling stuck in our body, our gestures become spiced with vibrant, child-like energy. The word "ecstasy" derives from the Greek "ex-" (out of) "stasis" (stationary), different from our usual selves. Our body will ecstatically re-member itself with releases that move us beyond habitual strained motion, returning us to comfort.

Before developing the KENTRO program, I held a typically conflicted concept about my basic anatomical structures. After nine years of intensive treatment for back and neck pain, I continued to experience my muscles as tight and my bones as almost impossible to realign. My muscles and bones seemed divorced from each other. Finally, I looked beyond polarizing notions of posture and motion for a creative, flowing interpretation of my body merged with precise anatomical descriptions. I pictured the interplay between muscles and bones in a labor of love, while they knit together relaxation and renewal:

Muscles came to represent soft, expressive, reshaping energy that aids our freedom of movement.

Bones came to embody the solid, stabilizing, constant inner support system.

I felt riveted to discovering how our bodies can resolve chronic pain and regain resiliency in an effortless way ... so I left behind my life as a visual artist to teach smooth postural expression. Now with every new student I have the adventure of noticing physical form with fresh eyes: instead of focusing on students' holding patterns or restrictions, I see their bodies as broad, fully relaxed, expansive, and vital. While I teach, I encourage students to infuse their practice with the same imaging. Later, the students see their bodies expressing their charismatic selves.

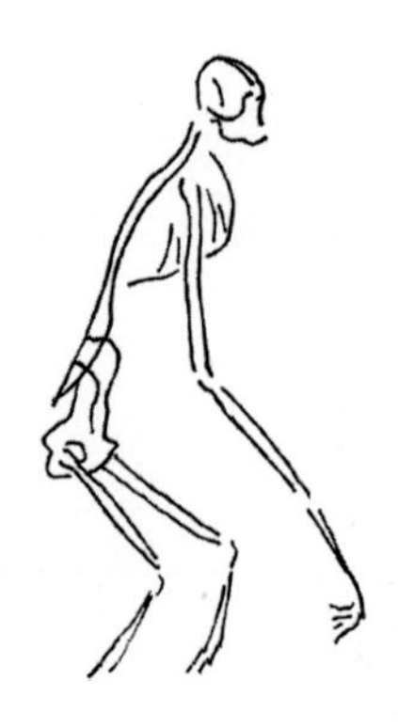

3.7
This drawing of an ape depicts the flat pelvis of apes, as well as the "angled" hips and knees, which indicate cumbersome upright motion.

As we center and balance our actions, our tissues begin to function according to nature's blueprint [Fig. 3.6]. Our mind feels stimulated by the sensuous motion and engages in an aesthetic image of the body. In turn, our musculoskeletal and sensory systems energize us into pleasurable actions.

Yet, whenever we move with stressful posture, these synchronized physiological systems are hampered. We may feel stiff or sluggish. Even standing, bending, or sitting down may feel cumbersome for us. Many of us conclude that we inherited a weak back, or that we should push our bodies into fitness. We develop a limited view of our anatomy.

We can broaden our perception of our physiology by perusing anatomically sound load-bearing structural systems, which are essential for comfortable bipedal (upright) motion. In natural history museums, we can observe the naturally straight sacrums and posteriorly (backward) rotated pelvises of higher apes, who have to bend-"angle" their knees when they try to be upright [Fig. 3.7]. In contrast to the apes, the human pelvis is characterized by an angled sacrum, and the pelvis is more anteriorly (forward) rotated—more box-like, providing better muscular attachment for upright standing, walking, and general weight-bearing. These inner architectural constructs suggest fine

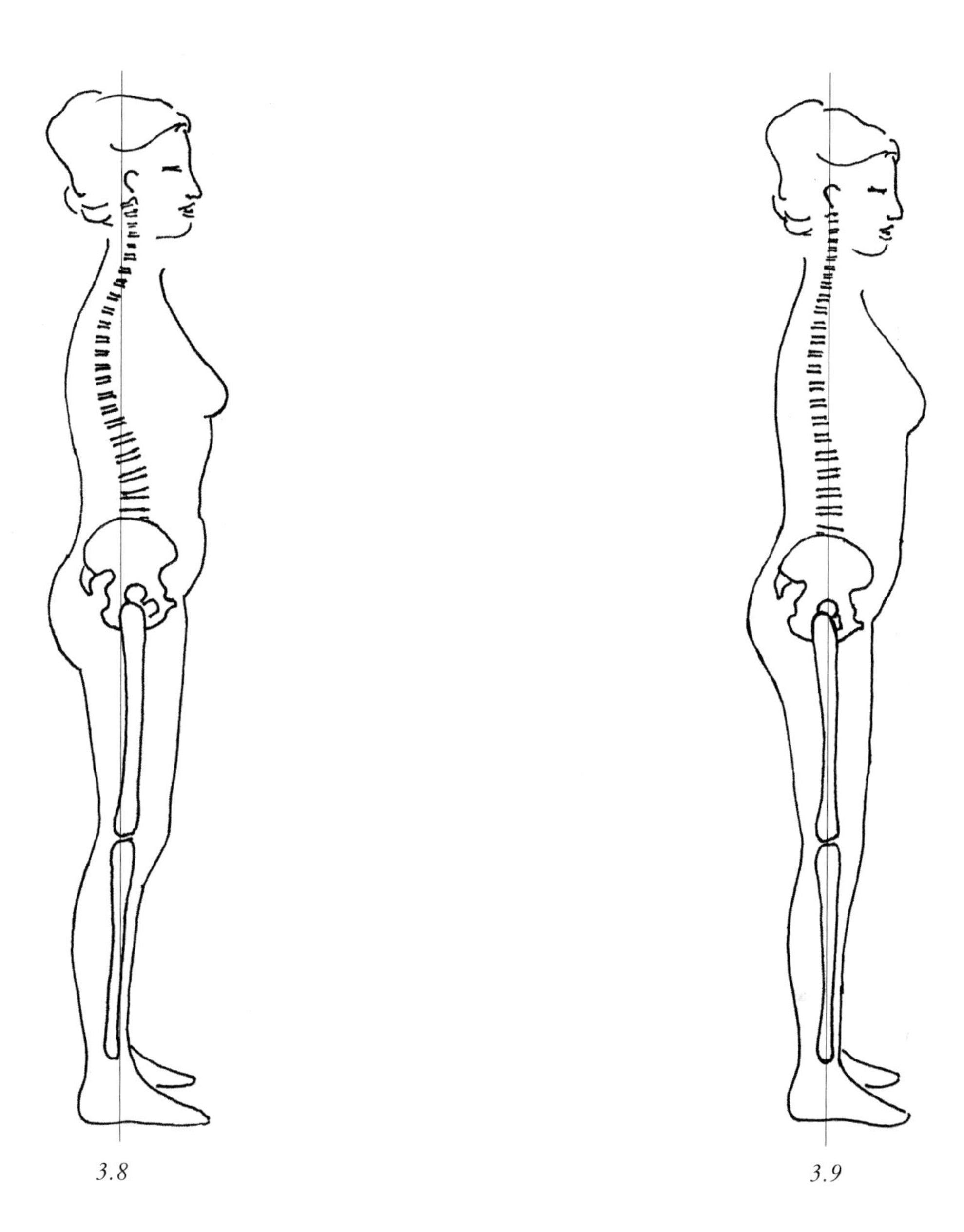

3.8 **Stressfully Balanced Weight Distribution in Conventional Spinal Alignment.**
The tucked pelvis is at the posteriorly angled and the line of gravity descends behind the hip sockets.

3.9. **The KENTRO Approach to Comfortably Balanced Weight Distribution and Spinal Alignment:**
The relaxed pelvis is at a more anterior angle, only about 5 degrees more than in Figure 3.8. This small shift in pelvic placement makes a vast difference: It moves us toward optimal postural expression. The legs are slightly farther back and the line of gravity goes through the middle of the head of the thigh bones (femurs), corresponding with Gray's recommendations. Notice that the line of gravity descends through the center of the ears, vertebrae, hip bones, and ankle joints. There is more vertical alignment of the spine and through the length of the strong leg bones, providing more weight support. Increased bone support reduces tightening (compensations) of the muscles to support body weight.

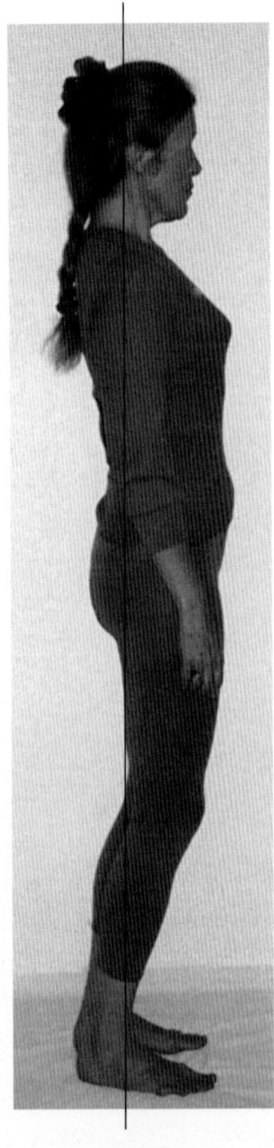

3.10

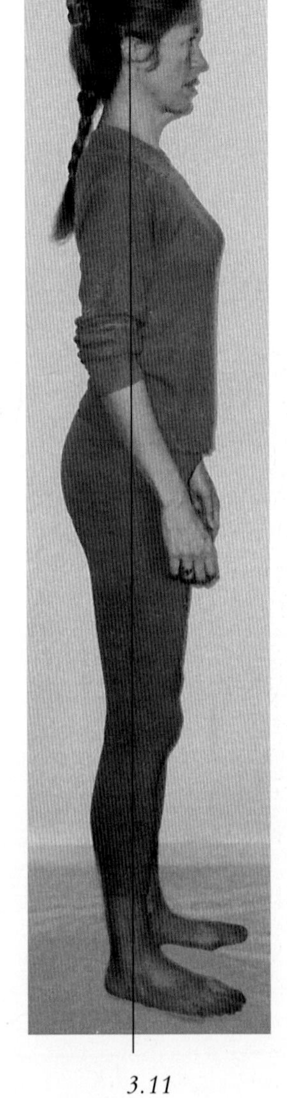

3.11

3.10. **Strained Musculature.**

This stance illustrates various common postural compensations. As a result of insufficient bone support, the musculature and other tissues tighten and remain in "holding patterns:" The pelvis and the legs are pushed out front; the knees are bent; the abdomen is tightened, the lumbar area is shortened; the rib cage is raised up; and the shoulders and the head are pulled back. Likewise, when the knees are pulled back (locked) instead of bent (as in Fig. 3.8), the plumb line misses the center of the legs. There is too much weight (pressure) on the front of the legs and feet (as in Fig. 3.8).

3.11. **Centering Relaxation.**

Increased bone support fosters ease of movement and decreases "holding" in tissues: The plumbline indicates that weight is comfortably distributed through the center of the legs, hip joints, shoulders, and ears. When muscles do not have to compensate anymore, they can become supple.

skeletal/muscular function. We can find clear descriptions of the naturally anteriorly-slanted pelvis in *Gray's Anatomy* and in English and Greek contemporary medical photos and textbooks. This optimally placed pelvis is defined by the forward, downward slant of the pelvic crests. The platform-like sacrum then easily transmits upper body weight to the femurs (thighs)—the strongest, longest bones in the body. [Fig. 3.3].[1] In contrast, conventional, modern postural images generally exemplify a more posteriorly, backward and upward slanted pelvis [Fig. 3.8]. Gray states, "the weight passes through the sacro-vertebral angle and then bisects a line drawn transversely through the middle of the heads of the thighbones."[2] This centered weight distribution resulting from an anteriorly placed pelvis is evident in the medical drawings of outstanding, contemporary English and American anatomy textbooks, as well as images in American anatomy books before the appearance of modern "correct" posture [Figs. 3.1, 3.4, 3.9].[3] In contrast, the weight descends behind the heads of the thighbones with the posteriorly slanted pelvis [Fig. 3.8].

Conventional "correct" posture proposes a posterior tilt with a base lumbo-sacral angle of thirty degrees, which is often stated to be optimal.[4] Yet studies indicate that men with sacral angles under thirty-five degrees are more prone to osteoarthritis at the lumbo-sacral joints.[5] Tucking the buttocks and holding in the belly straightens the sacrum and shifts the pelvis into a posterior tilt [Fig. 3.8].

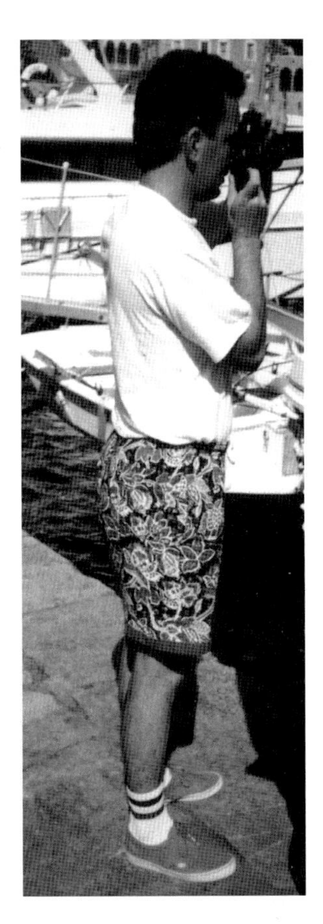

3.12. **Smoothly Balanced Weight Distribution and Relaxed Stances.**
The Greek man illustrates smoothly balanced weight distribution and a relaxed stance (no muscular strain). His pelvis is anteriorly rotated, his legs and spine are vertically aligned, his back is straight, and his shoulders are dropped.

Practicing KENTRO movements keeps us from pushing our bodies into the stressful posteriorly angled pelvis [Fig. 3.10]. Centered balance guides our bodies toward the comfortable more anterior pelvic angle, in proportion to the angle of our particular sacrum. Thus upright comfort is natural for us [Figs. 3.11 and 3.12].

Our skeletal alignment is closely linked to our postural expression [Figs. 3.13–3.3.16, next page].[6] When we move with poorly balanced weight distribution, our gestures reflect stressful spinal and joint adaptations.[7] Our muscles continue to be strained. For example, a pronounced curve in the upper back indicates over-compressed vertebrae on the front side of the spine. The muscles and other soft tissues are also over-compressed (i.e., shortened, tight) in the same area, while the muscles on the back of the spine are over-stretched. Likewise, a pronounced arch in the lower back indicates a spinal compensation—when the discs and tissues are over-compressed on the back of the spine, they are over-stretched on the front of the spine [Figs. 3.17–3.19, p. 17].

Being attentive to and sensing our bearing and movements is rewarding: Awareness precedes function and function influences our structure and form.[8] How sensitive

Figs. 3.13–3.16

Striking differences and similarities in models of "standard" vertebral columns.

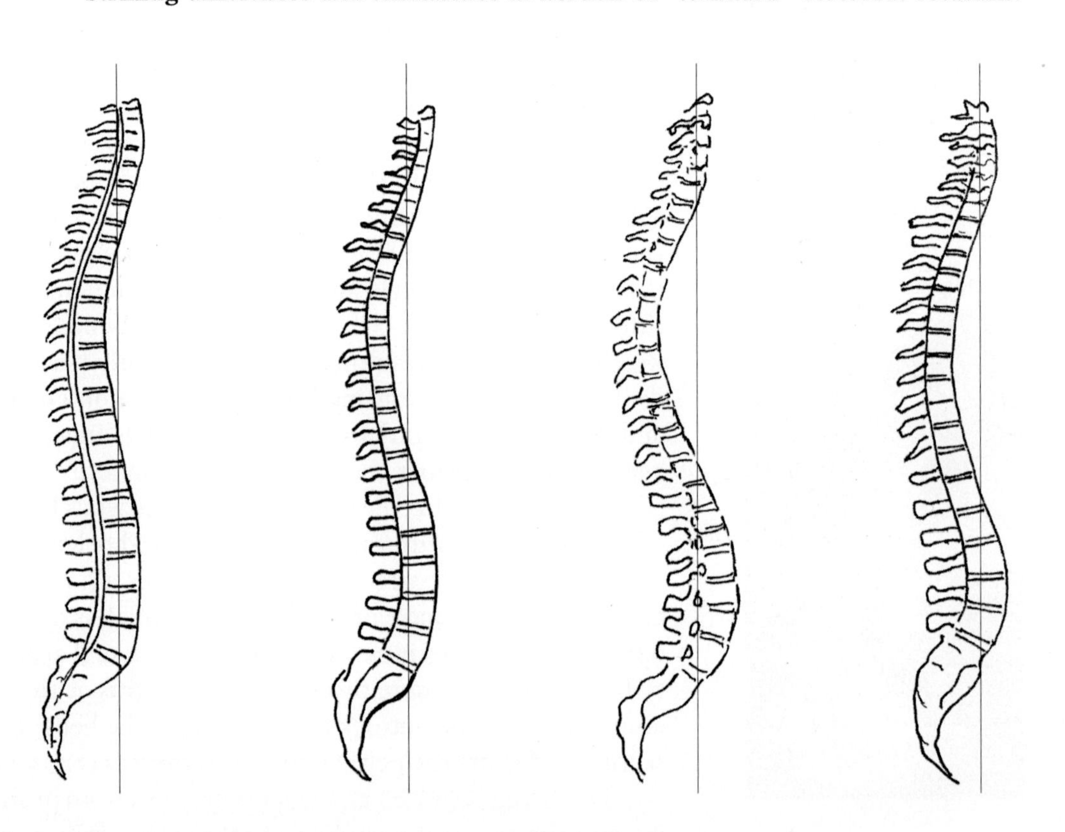

3.13. Well-aligned Spine. A drawing based on the 1938 "standard" spine, CAMP Anatomical Studies for Physicians and Surgeons. *This lengthy spine is free of compensations; it is typical of optimal anterior placement of the pelvis. The plumbline indicates excellent bone support and weight distribution.*

3.14. Well-aligned Spine. A drawing based on a combination of "standard" spines, Frank Netter, M.D., Atlas of Human Anatomy; *and* Textbook of Anatomy *as well as the spinal model I use in my classes. It is thrilling to also see lengthy spines like these, indicating anteriorly slanted pelvic placement. Hopefully, this spinal alignment will renew interest in researching supple spinal shaping and function.*

3.15. Stressed Spine. A drawing based on the 1988 anatomy poster for medical students, Anatomy for Surgeons. *This over-compressed spine (typical of "modern" posture) is full of compensations. The lower (lumbar) spine is over-arched (shortened) and the upper (thoracic) spine is over-curved. This spinal alignment is typical of cumbersome posteriorly angled placement of the pelvis. The plumbline indicates poor bone support and weight distribution. Many contemporary anatomy books in the U.S. and other highly industrialized societies still describe this shortened spine as normal.*

3.16. Stressed Spine. A drawing of a more tucked (flattened) sacral area in the more posterior placement of the pelvis and a shortened back, also described as normal in many recent books on conventionally accepted posture.

Figs. 3.17–3.19

Variations of Stressful "Modern" Posture.

3.17 This drawing shows spinal compensations; pushed back buttocks; locked knees; elevated rib cage; tight, pulled back shoulders; and particularly excessive lumbar arching.

3.18 This drawing shows spinal compensations; held-in abdomen; elevated rib cage; tight, pulled back shoulders; legs too far out front; and particularly tucked buttocks.

3.19. This figure is trying to "relax" out of muscular holding, but her muscles lack elasticity. Her pelvis, legs, spine, rib cage, and shoulders continue to be in poor weight distribution, so her tissues cannot truly relax.

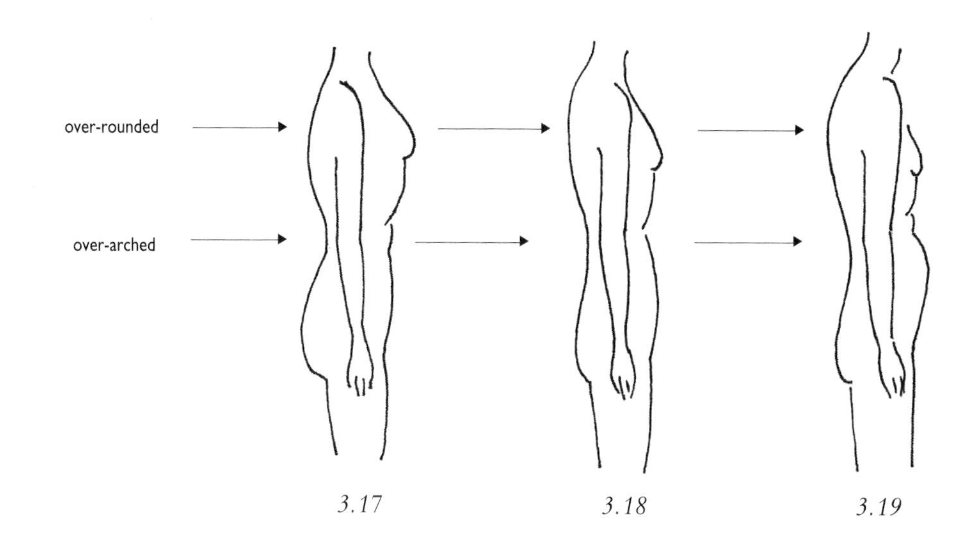

3.17 *3.18* *3.19*

3.20–3.23.

The Shift from Stressful Motion to Supple Motion

The drawings in 3.20 and 3.21 are in the same stressful erect stance as shown in 3.17 and 3.18 (above). Such effort to be erect does not remedy strained motion. The drawing and model in 3.22 and 3.23 are in a centering-balancing erect stance, without effort.

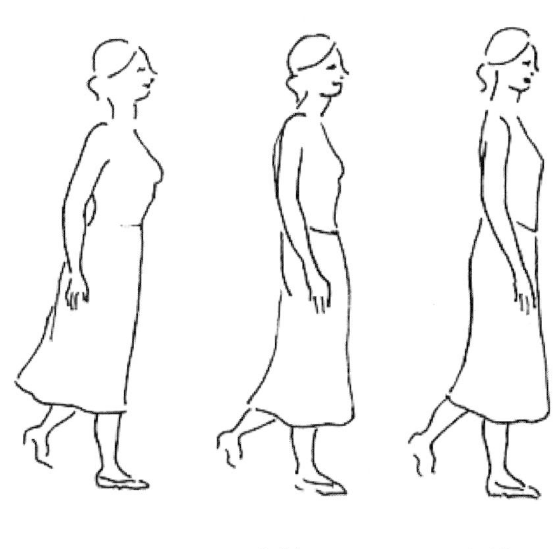

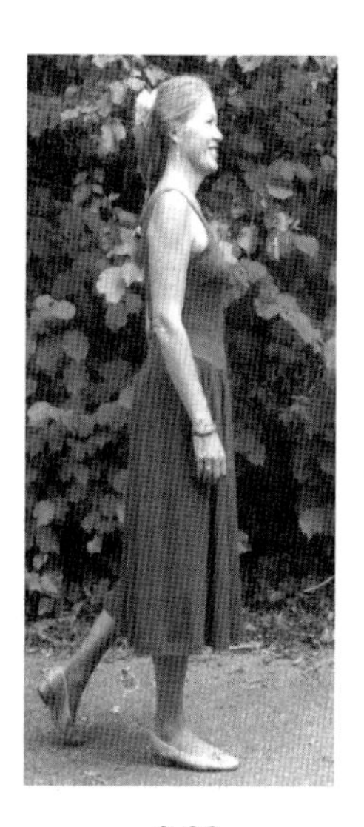

3.20 *3.21* *3.22* *3.23*

we are to our bodies, how we place our bodies, and how we use or misuse our muscles affect the shape of our bodies and our well-being. *Awareness* can enrich *function* when we have an affectionate view of our body and sense the difference between stressful and limber actions. With centering, balancing movements, our soft tissues can reshape without exertion because our principal weight-absorbing tissues, the bones (especially in the pelvic area), become well-aligned to absorb maximum body weight. Our muscles can then recover appropriate tone for increased range of movement [Figs. 3.20–3.23].

Nature shaped us to enjoy great freedom of motion. Our anatomical structure stands the test of time because it is adaptable. We can be comfortable in any activity.

Since our bodies are at least 65 percent water,[9] it is possible to resolve physical distress and regain flexible tissues. As we balance and center our movements, we can imagine a stream flowing through various areas of our body acting as a catalyst for fluid motion. The resulting freedom of movement propels us into improved sensing and a more pliable sense of our being.

Our sensory and motor nerves aid us in sensing both the inside and the outside of our bodies and account for all of our movements. Constrained balance causes long-term tension and compression on nerves and diminishes our ability to sense how to move easily for specific activities or when our bodies need to rest. This disruption of the sensorimotor system may be at the root of many back and joint problems.

The awareness of our movements,—our position in space, and our body weight distribution—originates from our inner (proprioceptive) sensory system. Sensations occur in specialized sensory nerves, the proprioceptors, which, in turn, communicate with our outer senses.

The inner sensory system also regulates the extent of muscular action as well as the production and maintenance of optimal muscle tone, thus preventing the overexertion of muscles. Endurance and resilient posture are dependent on this harmonious muscle tone. Lack of balanced muscle tone results in hypertension or hypotension in the muscles (*hyper* meaning too much, *hypo* too little). When our muscles are hypo or hypertonic, they remain in a state of continuous distress and our sensing capabilities decrease. We rarely notice our body's warnings of potential stress, and it becomes increasingly difficult for our bone structure to absorb our weight comfortably. Thus, many everyday and specialized activities become burdensome.

When we sit at a computer or a piano, we habitually hypertense (i.e., tighten, shorten) our shoulder muscles. This occurs because our upper back muscles (most appropriate for moving our arms) lack elasticity and are permanently over-stretched. Likewise, we tighten and suck in our abdomens in an attempt to counter low back pain. However, such effort results in the flattening and weakening of our pelvis, which is the natural support for the torso. We can learn to tone pelvic and abdominal muscles without muscular clenching (see the *Boat* and *Heart Stretch Lying Down*, pages 90 and 122).

Our posture and gestures are determined to some extent by notions of "correct" posture. Our habitual reactions to messages such as "stand up straight and tall" result in these movements: We raise our ribs, tuck our buttocks, suck in our bellies, force back

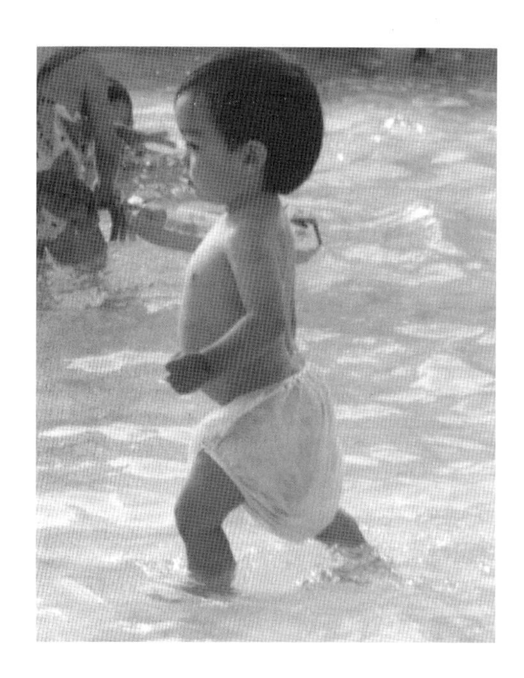

3.24. As very young children, we all moved with resiliency—strong and relaxed.

our shoulders, and raise up our chins—as we try to imitate someone who appears straight. Physiologically, as our anterior pelvic angle decreases, our backs become more curved and shortened, our legs compensate, and we become less flexible. Over time, such overtaxing and "holding" of the body feels normal to us, and we incorporate conventionally accepted posture, as opposed to the postural expression evident in children and resilient adults. Fortunately, we can eliminate these depleting movement patterns. Smooth balance can protect and reduce strain on joints.

Organic images of our bodies can generate insight that assists us with generating relaxed gestures. For example, our pelvis (the center of most bone support) is rich in symbolic and physiological significance. In *The Endorphin Effect*, William Bloom states that "all physical movement in martial arts pivots around the center of power between the hips."[10] He refers to the pelvis as the strongest part of our bodies and recommends that we behold and sense the lower abdomen as "an area of warmth, heat and nurturing fire."[11] *Hara*, the Japanese word for belly, has endless connotations. A hara belly is content, tranquil, fluid, and strong. It is also described as "the physical embodiment of the original Life center,"[12] the inner center of gravity (two inches below the belly-button) where "deep powers have their roots."[13] By regarding our pelvis in this bountiful manner, we will avoid clenching our abdominal muscles, and tucking our sacrum while we remobilize our pelvis.

The *desire to move* is what activates our sensory and motor systems. Our muscles move our bones in a particular direction based on automatic impulses. Certain muscles are referred to as having postural reflexes. They naturally balance weight along the upright spine and appropriately support spinal alignment.

Our bodies have an almost infinite capacity to adjust and readjust [Fig. 3.24]. We can move in accord with this process by letting go of limiting notions and bodily stress. While we firm our bodies with fluid movements, we will be irresistibly drawn to the core of our physicality. The spinal vertebrae and the discs (as well as the joints in their sockets) all articulate equally, regardless of our personality. This *impersonal* functioning is present within us all and offers a common ground upon which to stand. In turn, our muscles are free to move us as we wish, in rhythm with our sensibilities, reshaping us into our *personal* expression.

Firing-up the creative muscle of our mind will spark our first-hand experience of ease. Savoring the poetry of "having a feeling in our bones" will propel us into sensing comfort. We can cherish our superb anatomy; it presents us with tangible proof that we can relax into our bones and appreciate our sinuous flesh.

NOTES

1. Georga-Litsa, *Anatomy Studies* (Athens: Georga-Litsa, 1988): 23; *Gray's Anatomy*, The Classic Collector's Edition (New York: Bounty Books, 1997): 180; and P. H. Abrahams, R. T. Hutchins, S. C. Marks Jr., *McMinns Color Atlas of Human Anatomy* (London: Fourth Edition, Mosby, 1998): 76.
2. *Gray's Anatomy* (1997): 181-182.
3. Frank Netter, M.D. *Atlas of Human Anatomy* (New Jersey: Novatis, 1989); L. F. Edwards, *Surgical Anatomy of the Body* (Philadelphia: The Blackiston Co., 1934): 258; Tom Jones, *Anatomical Studies for Physicians and Surgeons* (Michigan: S.H. Camp and Co., 1938): 43, 89; Carmene Clemente, *Clemente Anatomy, A Regional Atlas of the Human Body,* Fourth Edition (Baltimore: Lippencott, Williams and Wilkins, 1997): 256; and *Surface Anatomy: The Anatomical Basis of Clinical Examination*; First Edition (London: Longman Group UK Limited, 1990): 86.
4. See Martha Plescia in Part IV of this book, "A Physical Therapist's Revelation: The Kentro Approach to Optimal Posture," p. 215.
5. Ibid.
6. Frank Netter, *Atlas of Human Anatomy* (1989) and *Textbook of Anatomy* (United Kingdom: A. W. Rogers: Longman Group, 1992).
7. *Dorman's Illustrated Medical Dictionary* (Philadelphia: BWB Saunders Co., Harcourt Brace, 1988): 902.
8. Deepak Chopra, *Ageless Body, Timeless Mind* (New York: Harmony Books, 1993): 86.
9. Fred Powledge, *Water* (New York: Farrar, Straus, and Giroux, 1982): 14.
10. William Bloom, *The Endorphin Effect* (Piatkus, London, 2001): 137.
11. Ibid: 138.
12. Karlfried Graf von Dürckheim, *Hara* (George Allen Unwin Ltd, London, 1962): 19.
13. Ibid: 43.

CHAPTER 4:

Elegant Exercise, Soothing Stretches

A Love Affair

A rhythm in your muscles
A feeling in your bones.

A melting of boundaries
A blending of tissues.

Form and movement
In love, while

Softly you become
Long, expansive, at ease.

WE KNOW THAT STRETCHING and exercise are important for us. However, the word *exercise* usually incites feelings of frustration and many of us associate the word *stretch* with cajoling our bodies into difficult poses. With the exception of athletes, dancers, and the dedicated few, we seldom follow through with our initial commitment to practice a regular routine—at home or at the gym. After an enthusiastic beginning, we may become discouraged and often shift our priorities elsewhere.

Some people exercise diligently every day because, otherwise, their body starts to feel stiff and tight. Others undertake an ambitious stretching program in the spring after a sedentary winter, only to find that their muscles get overtired or go into spasms due to sudden over-activity.

The KENTRO approach to strengthening and limbering the body fits Webster's definition of exercise: "active use ... a regular series of movements designed to strengthen or develop some part of the body." Practicing balancing-centering guidelines allows us to move from *appropriate* muscles, and to strengthen and render them flexible with

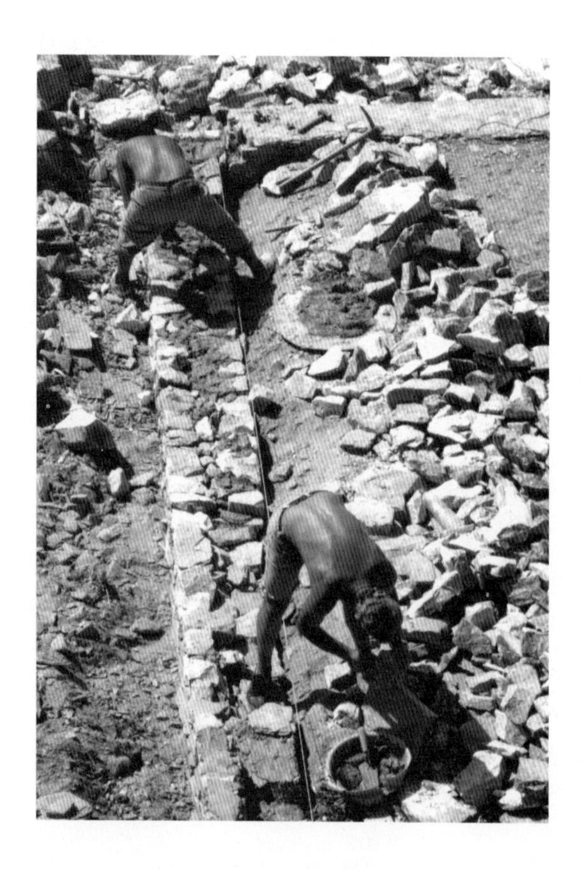

These Greek construction workers have strong pelvic, leg, and back muscles because they bend from the hips, in smooth balance.

an economy of effort. For example, every time we lift from the naturally strong upper back and buttock muscles (rather than from the shoulder and front of the thigh muscle) that very action tones those muscles, as well as pelvic, abdominal, lower back, arm, and leg muscles. Our regular, ordinary actions can dissolve muscular holding and invigorate us.

In the U.S. and other highly industrialized countries, exercise frequently is linked with quick, repetitive, and strenuous workouts. We are often encouraged to build up a specific group of outer muscles independently, with little regard for how we place our bodies while doing so. We are told to count to ten, or some other predetermined number, while we perform a specific strengthening move. But when we count and move quickly, it is extremely difficult to sense a specific area.

To "*sense* a specific area" means to experience clearly the difference between muscles expanding and contracting. Instead of rushing through an exercise to feel the effects in our muscles, we need to sense the muscles to allow them to rest before they work. Wanting only defined, strong surface muscles keeps us from allowing all layers of muscle tissue to function well. Desire for a "body of steel" makes us forget that the body is like everything else in life: the tide going in and out, yin and yang, *expansion* and *contraction*. If we keep our muscles in a constant state of contraction, we constrict the flow of blood to them. They shorten, tighten, and decrease our range of movement.

With decreased mobility, we tend to force our muscles into over-extensions and stretching is not fun. *Webster's Dictionary* has a friendly definition for 'stretch': "to let the body or limbs reach out to full length, as in yawning, relaxing, etc."

KENTRO stretches are akin to a yawn: there is no striving to reach a preconceived goal; there is only letting our body be lengthened and expanded.

We relax and let the stretch start from within, at its own pace. We savor it for a moment (the duration of a yawn or two) and then return to our original stance. We let the stretches be like a *conscious, spirited yawn*.

Giving priority to counting or holding a stretch for a specific period of time distracts us from distinguishing the difference between a relaxed or a strained movement. And we may add new stress to existing stress: we may *push through* difficult poses, without regard to our individual flexibility or strength. It makes sense to avoid goals that unwittingly cause us to extend our torso or a limb beyond their range, resulting in over-stretching of tight tissues.

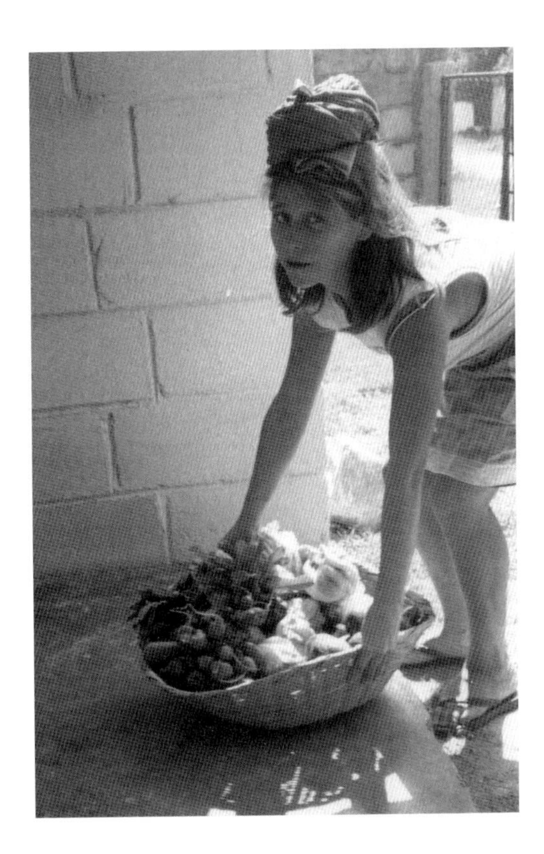

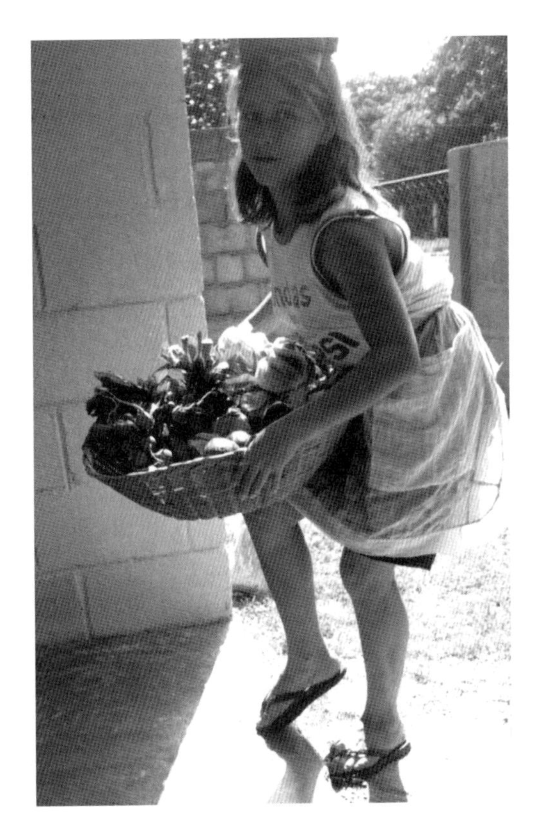

(Left). Maria, a thirteen-year-old Honduran vendor, lets her body relax into a straight back and relaxed shoulders before she picks up the heavy basket. She bends from the hips.

(Right). Her basket is so heavy that she swings it onto her knee before heaving it onto her head. Notice her straight back, relaxed shoulders, and general ease. The weight of the basket is transferred through her pelvis and thighs.

It is worthwhile to find the connections between physical exertion and *how* we move. Ordinary people (and even a significant percentage of athletes and dancers) suffer from back, joint, and neuromuscular problems. For everyone—athlete and non-athlete alike—stressful (out-of-comfortable-balance) movements develop gradually, over years, and are caused by insufficient bone support combined with over-stretched or shortened soft tissues. We easily adapt to these familiar, taxing movement patterns, continuing to miss or not even see the tight shoulder or the twisted pelvis. Typically, we notice small but blunt messages of pain, stiffness, or cramping. As we develop our sensory awareness of muscular functioning, we can learn to sense our body's indication of comfort versus discomfort. This new concept of exercise reinforces productive movement habits, and lets our body reshape us into our optimal expression.

When supple people pick up a heavy object, they unconsciously stretch, and relax their body as they bend—relaxing even while bent—before the action of picking up the object. Such ease and grace is commonly found in people who never frequent gyms, nor practice "warm-ups." We see their bodies get strengthened naturally, through daily activities. Their elastic muscles expand and contract smoothly in proportion to their movements.

This same elasticity is evident in babies. Babies constantly, naturally stretch and "exercise" their legs, pelvis, torso, and neck, whether lying on their backs or being carried on their mother's hip or sacral area.

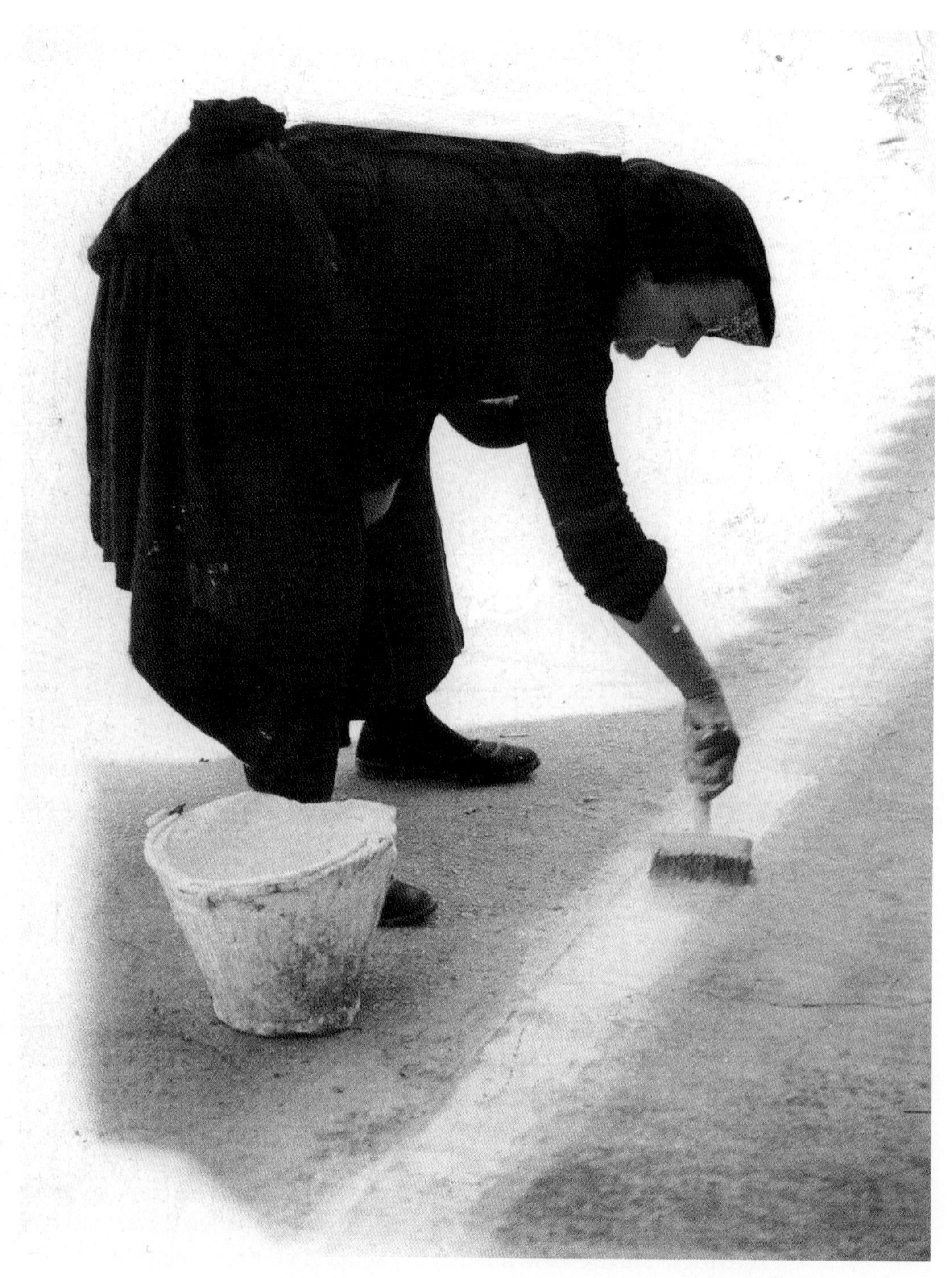

This Greek grandmother is fit and relaxed as she whitewashes the street in front of her house. Notice her bent knees, straight back, and supple shoulder.

These Portuguese men are both sturdy and supple. Their pelvic muscles stretch toward the ground, freeing their back muscles to extend and straighten their torso, without effort.

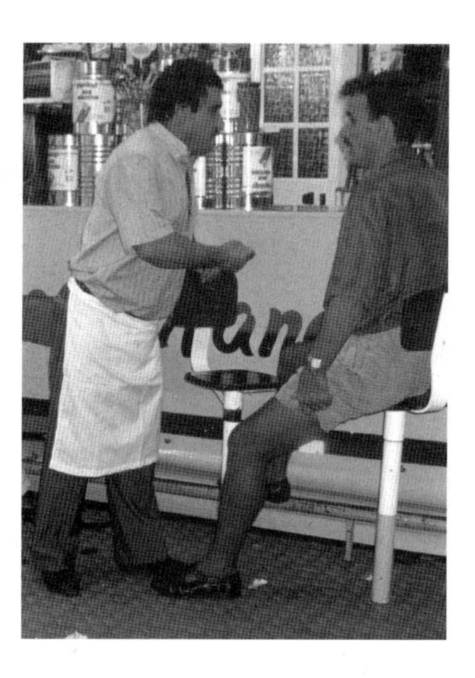

In adulthood, there is value in living the premise of use-or-lose when it comes to our muscular health; yet the use-or-lose idea does not require rigorous workouts. As Deepak Chopra, M.D., wrote in his book *Ageless Body, Timeless Mind,* "As long as you perform regular, minimal activity—the equivalent of walking half an hour a day—you are gaining most of the longevity benefits conferred by exercise."[1] Fitness means adapting well to our environment. We are "fit" when we feel at ease in our ordinary occupations within our personal environment.

Thankfully, we can foster a refreshing and relaxed view of exercise. One half hour a day of walking, or of housework performed in smooth balance, can stretch and tone the whole body thoroughly. For example, by walking with centered balance, stretching (lengthening) and toning (contracting) happen simultaneously in the buttock and leg muscle of the extended leg.

For those who are on an aerobic program, integration of the Kentro guidelines into their routine will help prevent injuries and increase the physical benefits.

KENTRO students report that they feel limbered and get a workout throughout the day.

More than the satisfaction of strengthening a particular muscle, letting our ordinary activities exercise us becomes vitalizing enjoyment of our every gesture.

More than the relaxation of a yawn, letting our body stretch us all day long becomes a continuous pleasure, a quiet delight.

NOTES

1. Deepak Chopra, *Ageless Body, Timeless Mind* (New York: Harmony Books, 1993): 201.

CHAPTER 5:
Balancing with Comfort, Centering with Ease

Each day
my body
moves freely
sensuous
and sweet
to meet
my soul
each day

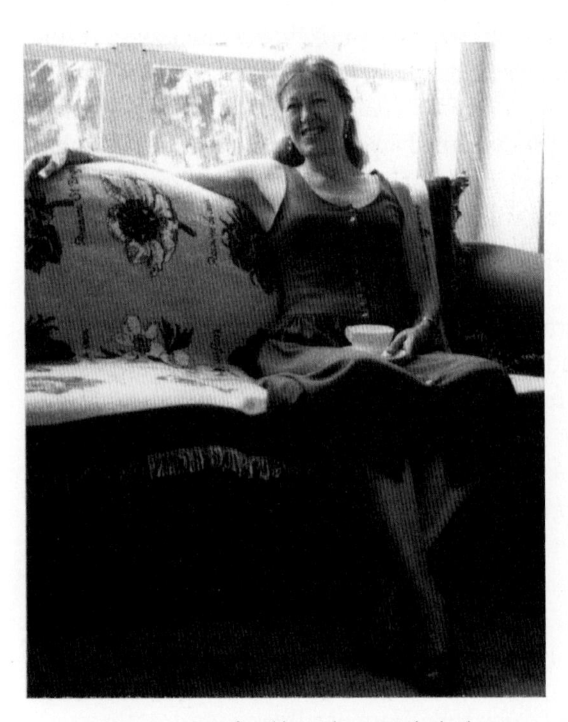

We can sit comfortably with a straight back.

COMFORT AND EASE CAN BE NATURAL to us in our ordinary actions and our rest. We can feel toning in our back, pelvis, arms, and legs while we lift something heavy with comfortable balance. We can sense gentle stretching in our back and pelvis while we sit with centered ease. *Comfort* strengthens our bodies, *ease* lightens our movements.

When we do not balance and center our movements, we tend to feel stiffness and aches after some lifting or being in one position for an hour or more. Our attempts at relaxing our bodies usually result in hunching over. We may feel collapsed, or sluggish instead of strong and open-bodied. Even if we sit in specially constructed "comfort" chairs, put up our feet, or lie down, we still experience distress instead of limberness. We may sit up or sit back at meditation, prayer, or yoga retreats, but find that without specific guidelines , physical suppleness remains elusive. Practicing KENTRO sitting generates true

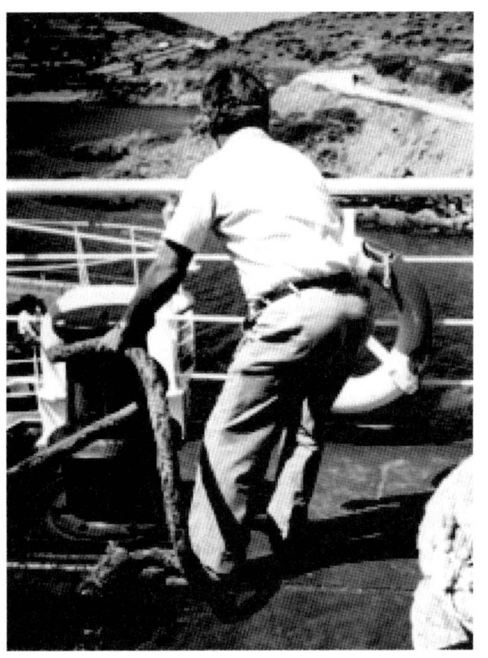

This Greek sailor is in smooth balance while he lifts the heavy ropes. He is pulling the ropes from strong pelvic and back muscles.

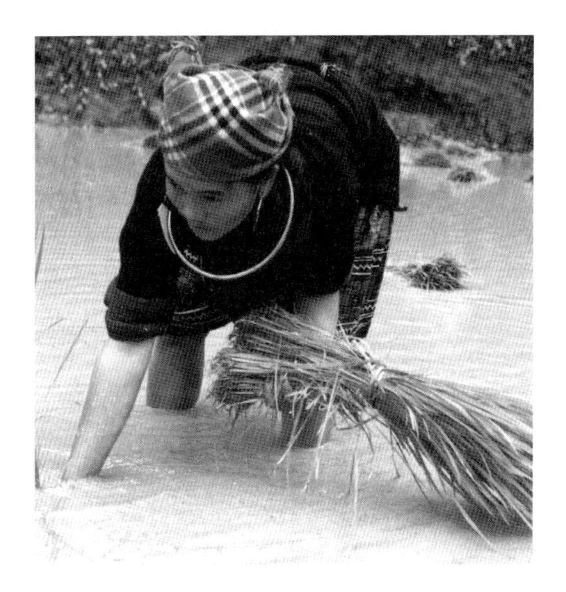

This Vietnamese woman moves with ease all day long as she bends from her hips and relaxes her shoulders, allowing her back to straighten and her upper back muscles to be strong.

comfort. Ordinarily, after sitting at your computer for several hours (and even if you take breaks), your back starts to round and feel weak. Practicing *Elemental Movements* and sitting up on a wedge allows the back to remain erect and limber. Possibly, your neck feels stuck and your shoulders seem burdened. The *Four Directions,* and *Tikanis* keep your neck and shoulders flexible. Vulnerable wrists can regain flexibility with the *Wrist Stretch*. And practicing *Turning* and *Farmer's Rest* keeps your pelvis supple (see Chapter 8-9, and Vignettes 8, 21-23, and 26).

Perhaps when we have not experienced thorough ease, we are confused by and skeptical of the very concept of comfort, associating it with passivity, laziness, complacency, or even selfishness. We may suspect we will "fall apart" from excessive relaxation.

Contrary to this belief, *Webster's Dictionary* tells us *comfort* derives from the Latin, *confortare,* "to make strong." Comfort, then, is inherently vital. Its active meaning is "to soothe in distress; ease." This is complemented by the noun form: "a state of ease and quiet enjoyment; free from worry, pain." This definition of *ease* affirms the interweaving of psychological and physical aspects: "1) freedom from pain, worry, or trouble; comfort; 2) freedom from constraint, or awkwardness; poise; natural, easy manner; 3) freedom from difficulty; readiness; adroitness," and 4) "rest; leisure; relaxation." Let us take to heart the importance of these dynamics.

We can look around the world to see mobility and flow. If we follow guidelines for balanced weight distribution without a caring, centering attitude to our bearing, we

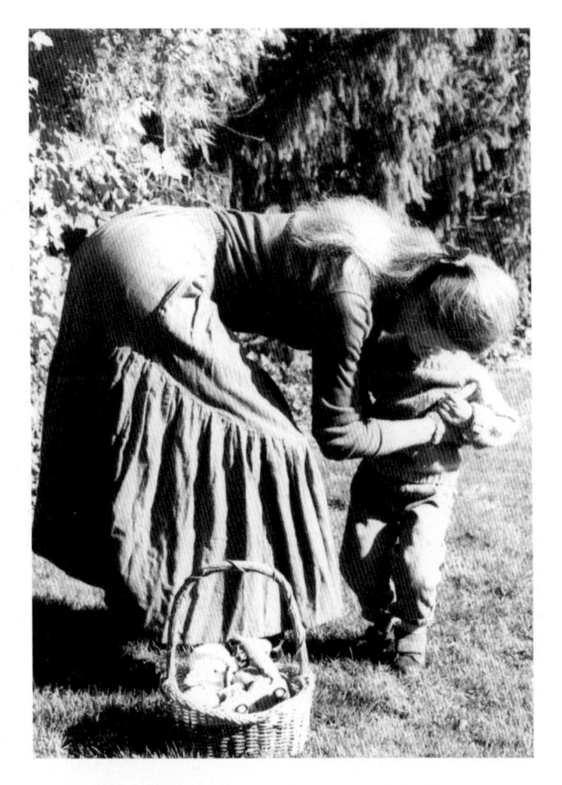

Bending from the hips helps me to lift with ease. Centered-balance grounds me. While I am lifting the child, I feel toning in my upper back, upper arm, pelvic, and abdominal muscles. My back straightens and my shoulders relax.

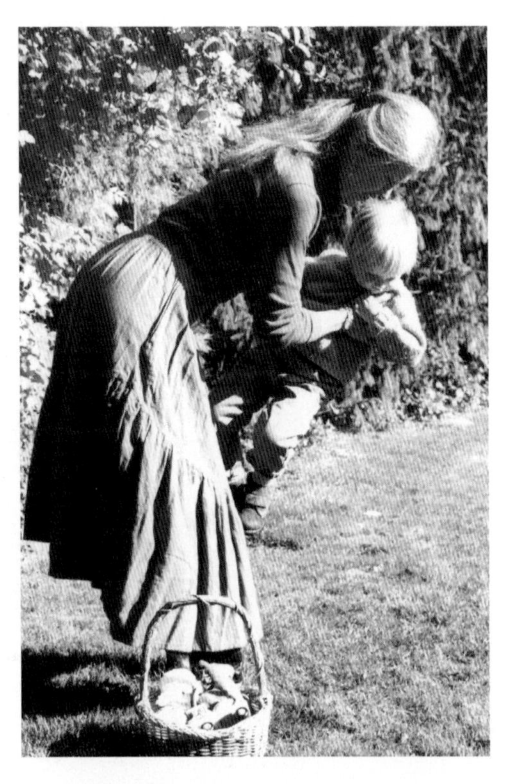

Looking for Elbow Room *is a Kentro movement that releases strain and tones back muscles. Most of my weight and the weight of the child is transferred through my sacral/hip/thigh region.*

may still experience physical and psychic stress due to bodily distress and dislike of our posture. Likewise, if we practice visualizations or similar relaxation techniques apart from effective physical guidelines, we limit the body's potential for growth and renewal. With KENTRO practice, our posture can become a buoyant expression of ourselves in concert with our habitual actions.

At a workshop in California, I invited students to comment on their feelings as a result of applying the KENTRO method. One student said she felt amazing grace in her gestures, which was echoed by other students. Spontaneously, they broke into the song "Amazing Grace." I realized the effectiveness of adding centering to balancing guidelines.

I used to thoroughly dislike washing the dishes. When I bent smoothly from the hips and let my shoulders drop and relax, and my back lengthen, I felt more limberness. However, I did not enjoy this kitchen "task." Over the next few years, I integrated a compassionate attitude toward my body, with gentle stretches (i.e., ***Tikanis, Elbow Room,***

Grounding, Little Moon, and *Four Directions*), into my daily routine. One day, while I was in the middle of washing a casserole dish, I noticed a delightful difference in my kinetic perceptions: My entire body was moving in rhythm with my bending, turning, reaching, and scrubbing. Besides sensing stability in my legs, a continuous straightening in my back, a release in my shoulders and pelvis, and toning in my upper back muscles, I felt grounded and gleeful. My body rocked, exercised, and danced me.

Dishwashing became a sensuous experience.

During a recent KENTRO class, I asked students to focus on a familiar situation that felt burdensome, which we would make more appealing. They chose dishwashing. For contrast, I showed them a stressful approach to washing dishes: Rather than bending forward from the pelvis, I hunched my shoulders over the sink, which automatically rounded my upper back. While demonstrating how to bend forward with flexibility, and move with minimum effort, I played Latin American cumbia music, which helped the students move with more fluidity.

Enjoying our repetitive gestures—including simple kitchen work—is an integral part of our well-being. "Dis-ease" contains physiological as well as psychological connotations. In *Care of the Soul*, Thomas Moore writes: "The word disease means 'not having your elbows in a relaxed position.' 'Ease' comes from the Latin *ansatus,* 'having handles,' or 'elbows akimbo'—relaxed posture, or at least not at work. Disease means no elbows, no elbow room. Ease is a form of pleasure, disease a loss of pleasure."[1] Moore's words amplify the important links between health and release of unnecessary physical strain. *Elbow Room* is one of the essential KENTRO movements that generates spaciousness and broadening in the upper back, promoting mobility in the shoulders and back.

Centering (relaxing of our soft issues) and balance (optimal support of our bone structure) result in feeling "at home" in our activities. While we practice KENTRO movements, such *grounding* helps us to sense our supple tissues; in turn, enlightening feelings of freedom of movement permeate our bodies: The pelvis feels free of the torso, the legs of the pelvis, the arms of the torso, and the neck and head feel free of the torso.

Over time, centered-balance enlivens our native sense of comfort and ease, connecting us vitally with our surroundings.

NOTES

1. *Care of the Soul,* Thomas Moore (New York: Harper Collins, 1992): 164.

Conclusion:
Comfort and Ease Are Natural to Us

Secret Pleasures

if I were to see and enjoy my body
as I see and enjoy
a robin flying, a horse leaping
and a trout swimming.

I would marvel at my body's
graceful bending at the hips,
grounded legs walking the earth,
and limbs embracing babies and lovers.

I would live in the breast of my soul
in a body full of feeling.
I would cherish my body and take care of it.
I would declare my body sacred.

PRACTICING KENTRO MOVEMENTS allows our bodies to recycle strain, and lets us participate with satisfaction in the activities we love: hiking, dancing, playing tennis, meditating, writing, or playing the piano. Simple gestures can increase our youthfulness because the activity itself limbers, invigorates, and uplifts us.

During my first year of teaching, I discovered that we can become more flexible regardless of our age. When I visited my eighty-two-year-old mother in Honduras, I showed her how to sit without effort. In all of my memory, I had only seen my mother sit down briefly. She preferred to stand because sitting caused pain in her lower back. At first she told me she was too old and her postural habits too ingrained to learn to sit differently. Reluctantly, she agreed to try. I showed her how to sit upright on a wedge and taught her the *Boat* stretch to strengthen her back, pelvis, and thighs. After two

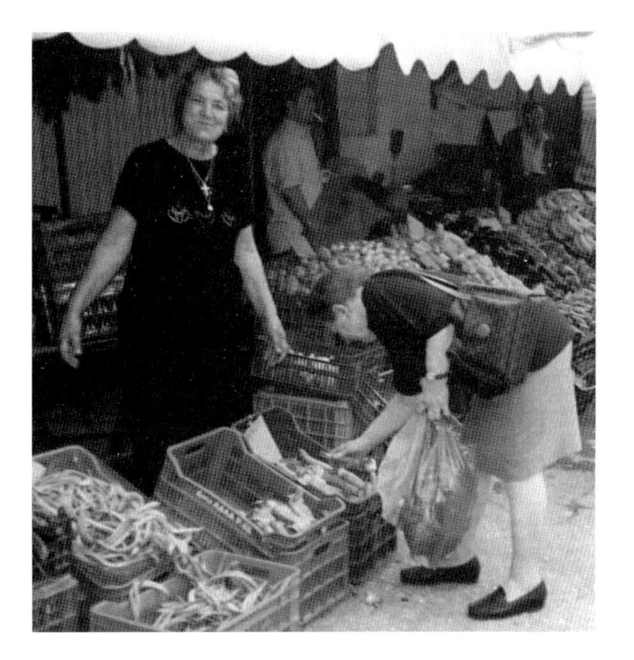

Notice the expansive arms and relaxed, upright stance of the Greek vegetable vendor. The Greek shopper is limber and bends from the hips with a straight back.

weeks of practice, she told me she no longer felt distress in her back while sitting down. Her pain never returned. My mother had fun making wedges for all the dining table chairs, and she continued to practice the basic guidelines that had helped her so much.

My mother was my first elderly student. The significant shifts in her posture inspired my confidence in the inherent malleability of our bodies. Years later, when I had the opportunity to present a series of KENTRO workshops at an assisted living retirement home in Oregon, I knew that having everyone sit in chairs would be the most effective way to teach them. The chairs became both a personalized "gym" and a "place of rest." The students could bend, let go of stress, and exercise gently, all while sitting down. Most importantly, the workshop participants (some in their nineties) learned how to replace agitated, or tiring movement patterns with gentle muscular toning.

In our highly technological society, we are blessed with outstanding conventional and alternative health care. However, even if we follow a healthy lifestyle, and exercise, our bearing reflects the spinal and muscular compensations characteristic of conventional posture. We tend to expect a fairly rapid, progressive deterioration and over-compression of bone structures, lack of agility, joint and muscular distress, and shrinking of our height as we age.

We are encouraged to buy specialized furniture and back supports but are seldom reminded of *using appropriate* muscles for various situations. Many of us are advised to bend, stand, or sit for brief periods of time only. To various degrees, we tend to believe such a restricted view of our posture and motion because we *do* feel vulnerable or resign ourselves to coping with pain.

Much of the inspiration for KENTRO movements has come from pragmatic observations of striking physical plasticity, even in elderly people. We can take a fresh look at aging.

It is not only in developing countries but also in certain industrialized countries, such as Greece, Spain, and Portugal, that we still see an impressive number of women and men of all ages moving with ease, even though they spend long hours typing, weaving, gardening, or carrying merchandise on their heads or bags on their shoulders.

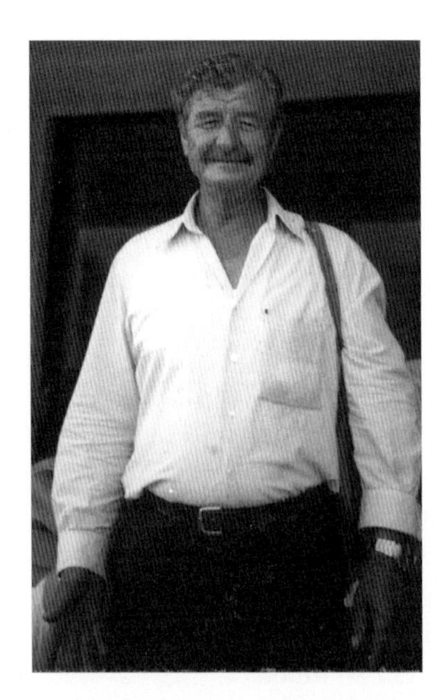

Baba Giorgos is an elderly Greek musician used to carrying a heavy shoulder bag with his instruments. His hips are level and his shoulders stay down, relaxed. He is comfortable.

Centering-balancing movements are like a subtle tonic that grounds us into springiness and prevents premature aging. The loss of physical mobility has more than genetic, chronological, or nutritional components. *How we move* makes an important difference. When we move with strained balance, our tissues over-stretch or tighten as we try to push our bodies "into shape" and "correct" posture, whereas smooth gestures can reform us into pliable posture. Stamina and comfort then become inseparable. Our vertebrae, discs, and joints are able to act as natural shock absorbers. Having to move quickly and unexpectedly or to stay sedentary over a long period of time to meet a work deadline—become far less threatening as we move with more ease.

Our bodies want what we want: harmonious expression. We do not need to *change* our posture; we simply *shift* our body weight into release and relaxation. Our soulful bodies will respond with proportionate reshaping of our malleable tissues. We will be sensing, using, and exercising more naturally strong muscles than before and our back will be healthier. Likewise, limiting beliefs about posture subside. We begin to appreciate the magnificent ways our bodies have adapted to many years of stressful posture, as well as our bodies' renewed resiliency.

Gratitude for our mobile bodies is far more energizing than discouragement about lack of mobility. In your KENTRO practice, "start by being grateful." (My mother's favorite saying.)

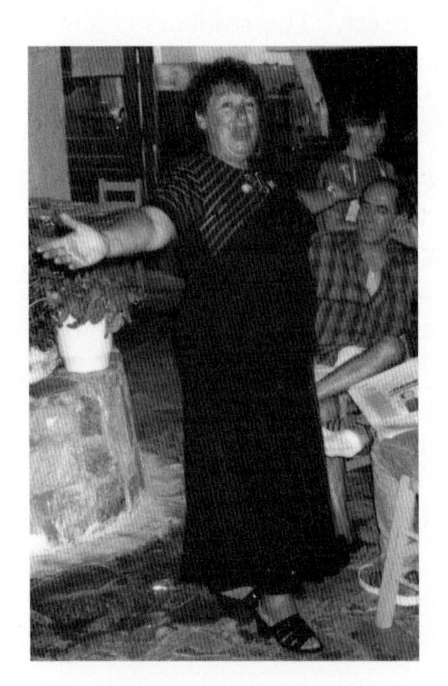

Our bodies are naturally vital, expansive, and expressive.

We can choose to transfigure aging by moving with buoyancy. We can arrive at a place where we began, catching glimpses of the natural, full-bodied expression we experienced as small children. When our sensory memory is aroused, we feel reminders of spontaneous motion. With these sensuous reminders comes the trust that, like children, we will stay in an activity *only* as long as it feels playful, vitalizing, and relaxing.

We can have faith in our personal practice because we can sense the difference between taxing and restful movement. Stiffness and strain can be understood as positive signs: our elastic body is our ally as it signals *dis-comfort* and *dis-ease* in our movements. Once we have a taste of regained suppleness, we can treat ourselves to more of it.

Freedom in our movements can become a close companion to fluidity in other levels of our being. After all, we are no longer trying to tame our posture. Our spirited movements can express us softly, in gentle proportion to our body history.

With each new day, we can craft a joyful physicality.

PART II

The Practice

Feeling looks for a body in form,
form can only find itself in feeling.

RABINDRANATH TAGORE

CHAPTER 6

Keys for Effective Practice

REFER FREQUENTLY to the following list so that you stay in touch with the essential aspects of the KENTRO Body Balance Method.

- Prepare the way for KENTRO movements by first *placing your body into Elemental Placement*: relax your body, let your legs move farther back, sense most weight in your heels, ground your pelvis, level your hips, drop your shoulders (and chin), and lower your ribs to let your back and neck straighten with ease.
- Keep relaxing your body as you practice KENTRO movements *as slowly as possible*, pausing between movements, and *sensing* your movements.
- Keep in mind that a small KENTRO movement can generate deep stretching, toning, and grounding.
- Practice is a process. Your practice is *right* as long as you practice the guidelines caringly and appreciate your body.
- Be sure to integrate KENTRO movements into long periods of sitting down, standing, or reclining.
- Replace limiting notions about your posture with trusting that your practice will generate fluid posture.
- If you are experiencing painful symptoms or are recuperating from an injury, consult your doctor about the KENTRO program. For a while, only focus on restful, gentle, mini-KENTRO movements; consider complementary Cranio Sacral or other mild treatments, massage, acupressure, or whatever suits you.
- As you release strain, expect mild "pulling," aches, or workout sensations, as well as relaxing, expansive feelings engendered by *simple* centering-balancing movements. A brief "dizzy" feeling indicates fuller oxygenation. Whenever you sense strong "pulling" aches, spreading arnica oil or ointment on the area (or placing a hot pad on it) soothes such balancing; taking Dr. Bach flower essences, homeopathic Rescue Drops (available in health food stores) gentles centering yourself to let your body release strain and create tiny readjustments.
- Be practical. Practice KENTRO movements anytime, while you rest or are active.

Elemental Placement Preview

Preparing the Way

- Slow down so you can sense your body; pause in between placements.
- Avoid pushing your body; a playful caring attitude is most effective for postural shifts.
- Elemental Placement is based on Gray's sound anatomical principles; "workout aches" in your muscles will become regained suppleness.

Body Poetics

- Elemental Placement will generate the broadest benefit when you visualize your body as malleable.
- Combine physiological characteristics with the sensuous experience of the elements in nature—water, earth, fire, and air, as you place your pelvis, legs, torso, and head into Elemental Placement.

The Four Key Areas of the Body, and their corresponding KENTRO movements (Movements 1-4, see chapter 8)

- Always practice Elemental Placement before any other KENTRO movement.
- Refer frequently to this section so that you have a clear view of and understand some basic anatomical explanation.
- If you wish to broaden your understanding of anatomy, a recent edition of Henry Gray's original 1857 study of anatomy remains an excellent source. It was not until the 1930s that tucking and tightening the pelvis gained acceptance as a standard posture in highly industrialized countries. This stance, dictated by fashion, distanced us from comfortable balance.

CHAPTER 7

How to Start: Elemental Placement

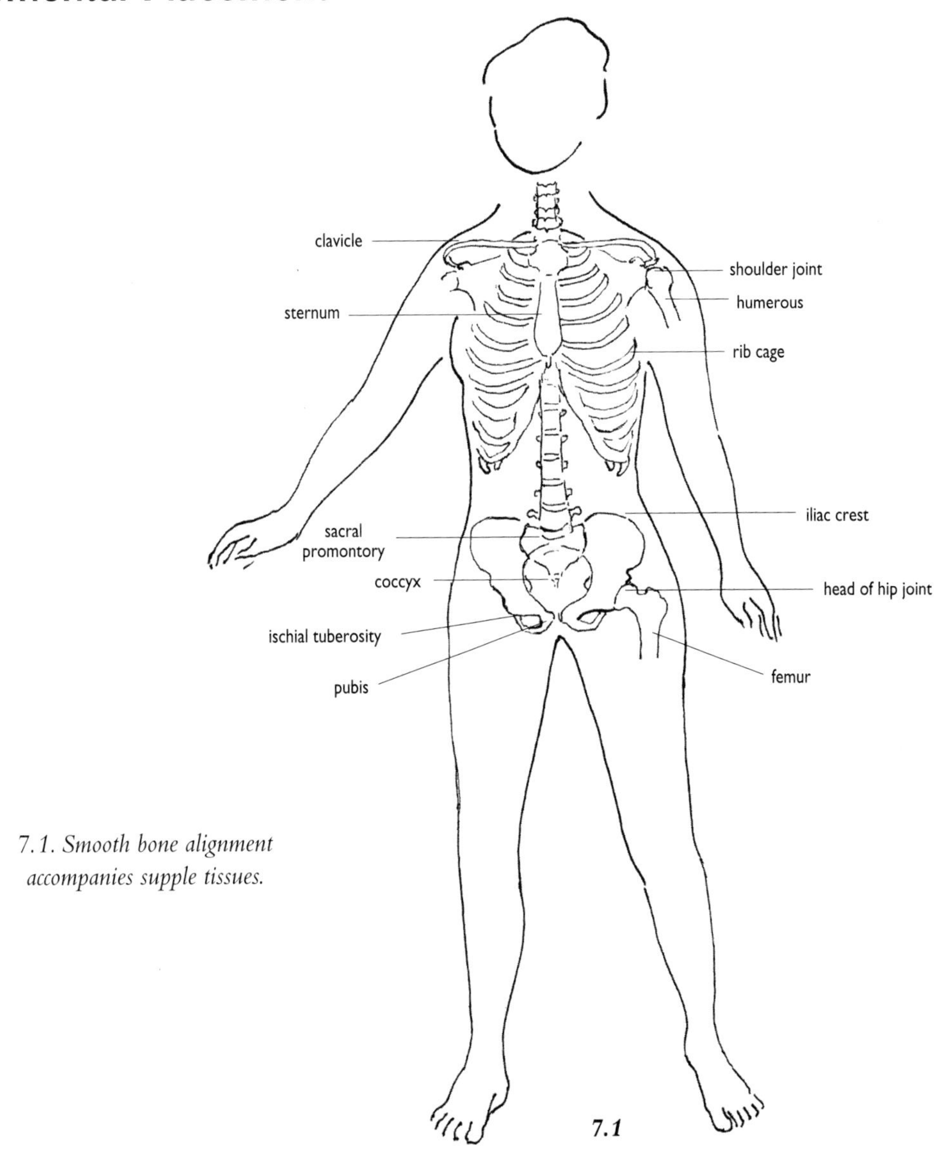

7.1. Smooth bone alignment accompanies supple tissues.

Always practice Elemental Placement before any other KENTRO movement. Center and Balance your pelvis with Grounding, your legs and feet with Little Moon, your torso and arms with Shoulder Roll, and your neck and head with Goose Neck. In time, some centering-balancing of your whole body will happen on its own.

BEFORE ATTEMPTING ANY of the KENTRO movements, start by centering-balancing the four key areas of your body—the pelvis, legs, torso and arms, and the neck and head—with the first four KENTRO movements, which are also the four essential KENTRO movements for Elemental Placement: Grounding, Little Moon, Shoulder Roll, and Goose Neck. The four key areas of your body are always placed the same way. Whether you are standing, bending, sitting, lying down, or walking: ***your legs align with your spine; your pelvis is naturally angled and elastic; your spine and neck lengthen; your rib cage shifts downward as it broadens; your shoulders relax downward, away from your ears; and your chin stays down*** [Figs. 7.1–7.2]. The four essential movements for Elemental Placement precede all other KENTRO movements, whether you are following the Twelve Movements mini-program or the Thirty-three Movements program.[1]

Grounding
Relaxing your body and letting your legs move back, while you shift most weight into the heels. Letting your pelvis shift into a more anterior angle (which happens easily when you bend slightly forward from the hips).

Little Moon
Relaxing your body and letting your lower back straighten (with your diaphragm and abdomen stretching down), while your legs rotate slightly outward.

Shoulder Roll
Relaxing your body and letting your upper back straighten, while your shoulders soften and drop.

Goose Neck
Relaxing your body and letting your neck straighten, while your head moves slightly backward and up.

7.2
These figures illustrate the four key KENTRO movements for Elemental Placement of the four key areas of your body: Grounding for your pelvis, Little Moon for your legs and feet, Shoulder Roll for your torso and arms, and Goose Neck for your head and neck.

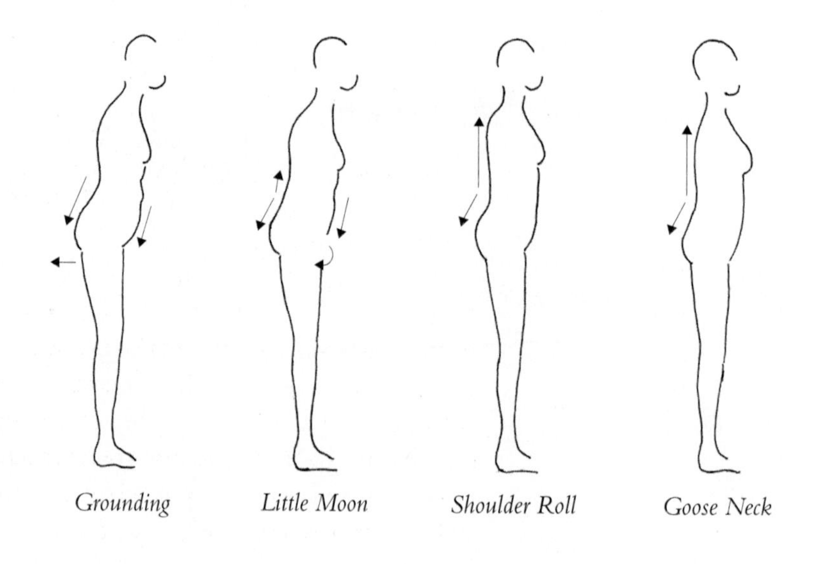

Preparing the Way

- Slow down long enough to sense your body. If your body is stiff and you have been moving out of comfortable balance, rushing into KENTRO movements will simply add more stress. Placing your hands on an area you wish to center-balance will enable you to feel clearly that area.

- Pause *between* KENTRO movements. This will allow your body to make small readjustments. The pause also gives you time to distinguish strain from suppleness and to focus on areas that you wish to relax and strengthen.
- A playful, caring attitude toward your body is most effective for subtle postural shifts.
- Avoid pushing your body into shape. Relax. You do not have to "fix" your posture. By following the Elemental Placement guidelines, your body will reshape you at its own rhythm.
- Elemental Placement is based on *Gray's Anatomy*. By incorporating precise anatomical guidelines with centering relaxation, smooth shifts can occur throughout your body.[2]
- When you bring comfortable Balance to one key area of your body, all other areas benefit. For example, when you balance your pelvis, your back, abdomen and legs can release muscular tightening.
- After a while, the "workout aches" and pulling sensations in your muscles will be replaced by feelings of flexibility. Small shifts in bodily placement cause pulling sensations that you usually experience after exercising or dancing. Yet even slight centering-balance generates some stretching and limbering of strained tissues. The "pulling sensations" last a day or two, until your tissues become more elastic. (See part II, Vignette 10, Blissful Aches).

Body Poetics

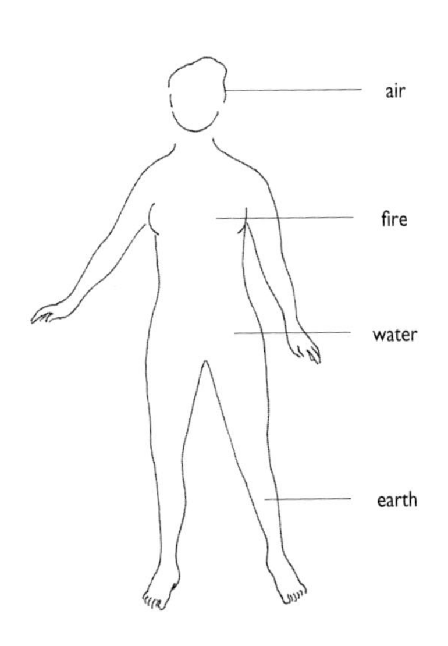

7.3. You can poetically convert the four key areas of your pliable body with the four elements.

- Elemental Placement will yield the broadest benefits when you visualize your body as malleable. This view frees you of notions that equate rounded shoulders with exhaustion, tight tissues with premature aging, and posture with a fixed, "right" form. Not only do we dislike our own posture, but we tend to be influenced by prevalent representations of the body as an instrument to be "maintained." Merging your balancing movements with an appealing and loveable centering image of your body is an effective tool for postural transformation. If it suits your fancy, let clay reflect an organic view of your posture. Sculptors will tell you that once the clay is *centered*, it can take on any shape. You could picture a sculptor within you centering and reshaping "your" clay.
- When you have a pliable, dynamic sense of your body, envision yourself being permeated and reshaped by the continuous movement of natural elements—water, earth, fire, and air. Such images then become part of centering-balancing the four key

areas of your body. Connecting the key areas of Elemental Placement of your body with elemental forces is not essential, but it is energizing and grounding.

❁ Associate your pelvis—the physical center of fluid movement—with water, with flow, with the power of oceans, and with the subtle, lively course of a mountain stream. Your legs and feet are grounded on—earth. Your torso encompasses the expressive, active back, the heart, and the outstretched arms—fire. Your neck and head are the locus of breath, voice, and thought—air [Fig. 7.3].

The Four Key Areas

1. THE PELVIS
Element. Water.

Sensations. Grounding; solidity, fluidity, freedom of movement, a supple "seat," expansion, strength.

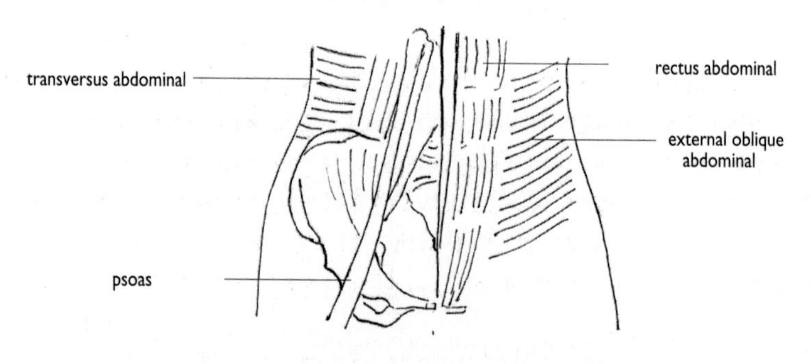

7.4. The front of the pelvis and the abdominal area

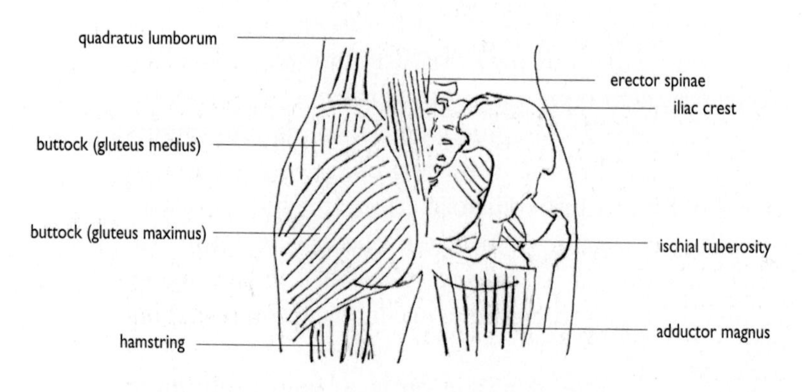

7.5. The back of the pelvis

Structure. The word *pelvis* comes from the Latin for "basin."[3] The pelvis can be the "strongest cavity in our body" when it is in a basin-like, very slanted position [see Fig. 3.3, p. 11, for an illustration of pelvis].[4]

Function. Immediately, we see how important pelvic placement is to spinal health. We bend most easily from the hips because the pelvis is the principal area for an expansive range of movement. The upper part of the sacrum is the base for and articulates with the last lumbar vertebra; this sacral base forms the prominent sacro-vertebral angle, the promontory. Our angled sacrum is the key to comfortably balancing our entire pelvis. Critical pelvic muscles in the abdomen and buttocks can then achieve resilience, expanding and contracting easily, without conscious tightening of these muscles.

Connections. The pelvis is the hub area connecting the torso and legs. Significantly, the pelvis *supports* the spine by *resting* on the legs. The placement and articulation of the strongest, longest bones in our bodies,

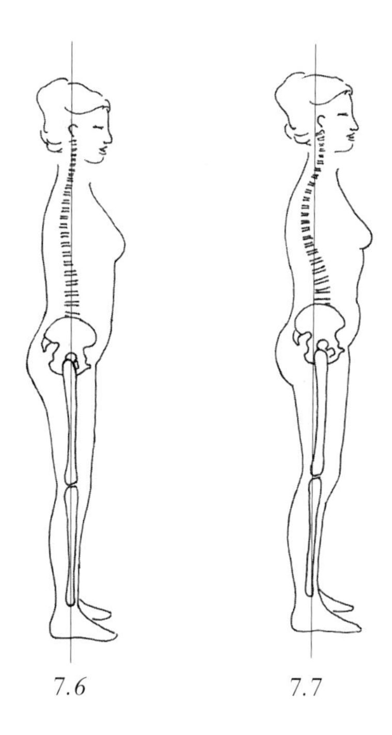

7.6. **Smooth Balance**.
The figure is in Elemental Placement. Her pelvis is anteriorly slanted.

7.7. **Stressful Balance**.
The figure is in uncomfortable alignment. Her pelvis is posteriorly slanted. When the pelvis is less angled, it becomes less supportive of the legs and torso and strains the tissues.

the femurs (thighbones), is noteworthy: when the body is in balanced alignment, femurs function as buttresses for the pelvis. In turn, the strongest muscles, the buttock, and other pelvic muscles are *strong* and *relaxed,* easily supporting the torso. Important back muscles like the quadratus lumborum, psoas, and erector spinae—all of which attach in the pelvic area—can then function well. Like the adductor magnus and hamstring muscles, which have their origin in the pelvic mass, the psoas, buttock, and thigh muscles all function optimally in this position. [Figs. 7.4–7.5]. Since the legs and torso are linked with the pelvis, centering your pelvis into Elemental Placement is accompanied by a slight centering shift in your lower back and legs.

Central Concepts. When we move out of centered balance, the pelvis, legs, and torso become strained, and the pelvis loses its strengthening and relaxing capacity. The basin-like pelvis with its oblique sacral promontory has less of a supportive, balancing angle—it cannot rest easily on the femurs, nor can it gracefully support the spine [Figs. 7.6–7.7]. Consequently, the pelvis, legs, and spine compensate for this discomfort: tissues stress into unnecessary holding patterns as they assume some of the weight-bearing function of bones. Abdominal, buttock, thigh, and lower back muscles are likely to be less elastic. The strong pelvic cavity, now *narrowed*, constricts organs and tissues. In this precarious placement, the legs may lose some strength because when the legs are out of vertical alignment, the ilio-femoral ligaments are chronically straining to absorb the weight of the torso. Likewise, the lower back becomes vulnerable to compensatory arching.

Exercise books tend to isolate certain muscles, such as the psoas and abdominal muscles, blaming them for pelvic and back problems. Concern over these muscles, which tend to lose elasticity through the body's attempts to compensate for pelvic tucking, is understandable. However, the conventional approach to strengthening these muscles is to tighten (shorten) the abdominals and to further tuck (straighten) the pelvic muscles. These exercises, performed in strained balance, tax the pelvic, thigh, and back muscles and increase discomfort [see Figs. 7.13–7.14, p. 47].

By practicing Elemental Placement, you will sense increasing freedom of movement, comfort, and strength in your pelvis, as well as a connectedness with your torso and legs.

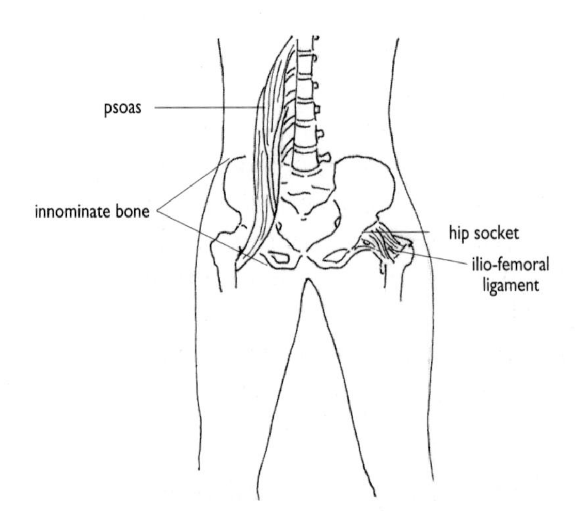

7.8. *Front view of the lower back, pelvis, and thighs.*

2. LEGS AND FEET
Element. Earth.

Sensations. Grounding; standing on your own two feet; upright comfort; stability; sturdiness; mobility.

Structure. Strong femurs (thigh bones) provide the best possible support for the pelvis. The femoral joint is a ball-and-socket joint capable of safely moving in all directions. This movement is assisted by ligaments that prevent inappropriate action and keep the joint snug and protected. The head ("ball") of this joint is fitted closely into the cavity ("socket"). The front of this capsule is embraced by the crucial ilio-femoral ligament, the strongest ligament in your body. This ligament keeps the femur aligned with the trunk and is the "chief agent in maintaining the erect position without muscular fatigue."[5] This powerful ligament plays an important role in allowing balanced placement of the pelvis and legs.]

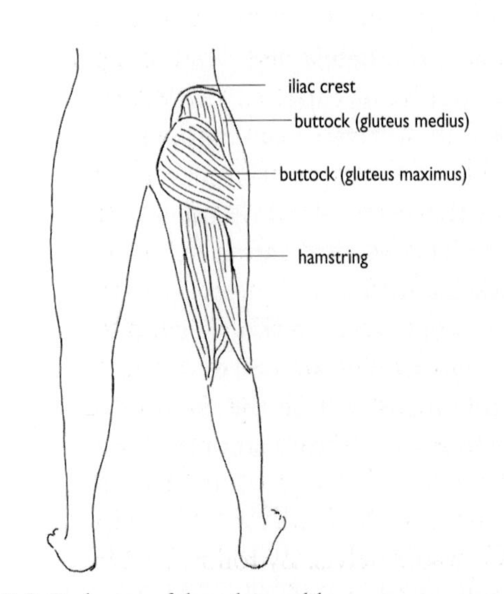

7.9. *Back view of the pelvis and legs*

Function. Elemental Placement of the pelvis with *Grounding* will include the legs shifting slightly back, into more comfortable balance. The trunk can then align vertically with the legs, and this alignment allows the legs optimum mobility, as well as maximum weight-bearing function. The lower extremities (the legs) originate in the pelvic girdle, with the femoral joints fitting into the sockets of the innominate bones [Fig. 7.8]. The leg bones are exquisitely contoured for bearing weight and joint articulation. The principal function of the legs is to provide vertical support for the pelvis. Muscles that attach to the hip joint also promote comfortable balancing of the entire leg. The psoas, which has its origin at the base of the rib cage and along the lumbar vertebra, is one of the prime flexor (bending) muscles in the hip and helps support the pelvis [Fig. 7.8]. The hamstring muscles in the back of the thigh assist the strong gluteus maximus (buttock), which arises from the sacral area and is the main extensor (lengthening) muscle of the thigh and leg [Fig. 7.9]. This powerful, pliable, massive buttock muscle is the principal musculature "for maintaining the trunk in the erect posture."[6] It can be reshaped into resiliency through Elemental Placement.

Connections. The thigh lends muscular and bone support to pelvic musculature and structural alignment. Likewise, the thigh distributes bodily weight over the knees, ankles, and the arches of the feet. When all extremities are in comfortably balanced weight distribution, the knees are relaxed (not bent or locked), and the ankles and feet are flexible yet stable.

The gluteus maximus "steadies the femur on the articular surface of the tibia [leg bone] during standing."[7] When in balance, leg muscles extend or flex the foot and steady the leg on the foot. It then becomes possible for the thickest, strongest tendon—the Achilles (on the back of the calf)—to support the calf and ankle with optimal flexibility for standing, walking, or dancing. The strong heel bone (calcaneus) of the foot plays an important role in weight assimilation because when there is most weight (sensed as pressure) in the area of the heel, the foot can be centered over the main arch in the sole. In flexible feet, heels can bear tremendous weight with the help of the fascia (thin layers of connective tissue that support and anchor soft and hard tissues). The fascia is thickest and strongest where it attaches to the heel. It follows, therefore, that optimal balance of the feet depends on the harmonious balance of the pelvis with the upper extremities; the feet can then play a crucial role in stabilizing ankles, knees, and hip joints.

Central Concepts. A lack of balancing connectedness of the thighs, legs, feet, and pelvis causes the thighs to move forward—out of balance, body weight shifts forward. There is less bone support and lumbar, sacral, and leg tissues endure strain. The important hip and sacroiliac (where the sacrum joins the iliac bones) joints become hyper-mobile instead of a snug fit. Surrounding tissues then are forced to contract continuously to "hold" these joints in place. As the thighs move forward, the buttock muscles and hip ligaments strain to keep on centering body weight over the legs. Too much weight streams through femoral ligaments that were never meant to bear so much pressure. In turn, important muscles like the gluteus maximus and psoas become over-stretched and weakened. Other tissues and organs get less bone support. Abdominal muscles tend to shorten and protrude, pouch-like, which we try to control by tightening these muscles. When we tone abdominal muscles in balanced, vertical alignment, they stretch downward, which lengthens and limbers them. Thigh muscles may also begin to pouch to the outer side of the thighs. Frequently, the outer thigh muscles overstretch and the inner thigh muscles shorten. One or both knees sometimes turn slightly inward or lock (overextend). The feet may compensate by turning too far inward (pronation) or outward (supination), because they are less stable when bodily weight shifts to the front—to the balls of the feet rather than through the main arch of the foot. One hip may be higher than the other—in the absence of a level, stable pelvis. By following Elemental Placement guidelines you can prevent further vulnerability and permit healthy joint articulation.

3. Torso and Arms

Element. Fire.

Sensations. Burden off your shoulders; having a backbone and a broad body; increased breathing capacity; freed arms; upright comfort; a strong, resilient back; heartwarming feelings.

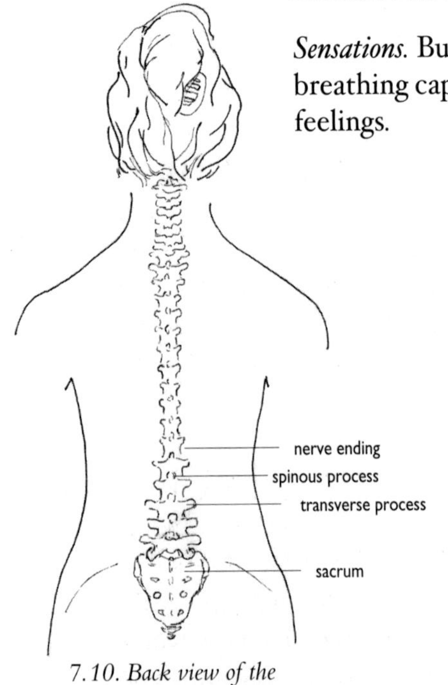

7.10. *Back view of the torso and spine*

Structure. The back has a resilient spine that supports the trunk and head [Fig. 7.10]. Optimally, the spine affords equal space between each vertebra/disc, as well as appropriate space for nerve endings. The structure of the *posterior* (back) side of the spine illustrates clearly that this area of the body is designed for attachment of strong weight-bearing muscles: each vertebra has various processes (small bones that project out of the back and sides of each vertebra) to allow articulation; they also act as levers for muscular/ligamentous attachment. Significantly, there are no such levers on the front of the torso.

The backbone remains in a harmonious, lengthened shape thanks to the erector spinae muscles. These muscles begin as a large, supportive mass in the lumbar area and cover the upper back to "maintain the spine in erect posture."[8] The back is naturally strong because of five layers of weight-bearing muscles.

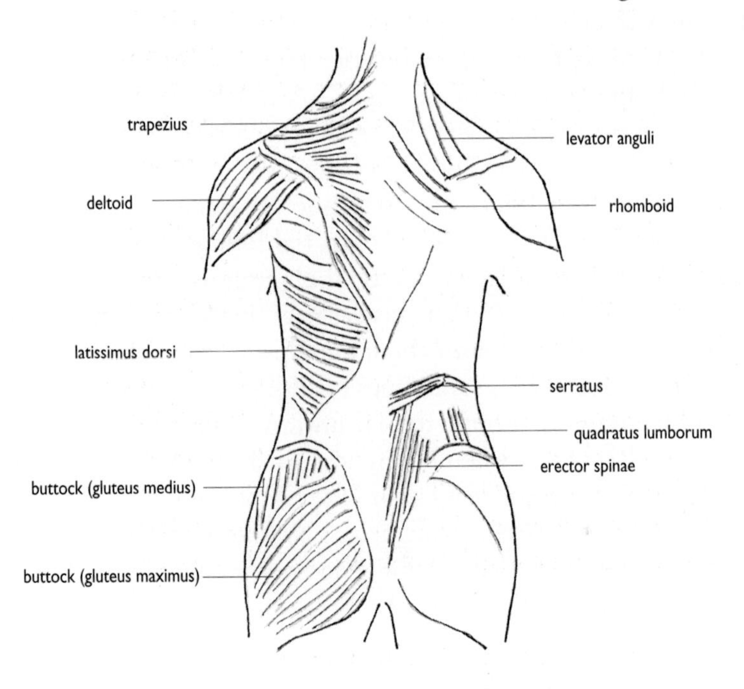

7.11. *Back view of the torso*

Function. Mobility of the torso and arms depends on the intricate balancing-centering connection between the trunk (torso), pelvis, and legs because the pelvis rests on the legs and supports the torso. Include Elemental Placement of the pelvis and legs in all movements of the torso to release tight tissues in the lower back. This link promotes smoother shoulder, arm, and hand articulation. The powerful weight-bearing muscles in the back, such as the internal (fifth muscle layer) erector spinae, counterbalance "the influence of any weight at the front of the body."[9] The levator anguli (second layer) muscle in the scapula (shoulder blade) assists the trapezius muscle, which covers the upper and back portions of the neck and shoulders, in "bearing weights."[10]Likewise, the serratus muscles (on the side of the thorax) assist the trapezius in "supporting weights upon the shoulder."[11] We can also lift weights easily from the naturally strong weight-bearing gluteal muscles in the buttocks-hip region [Fig. 7.11]. These muscles also assist in upper-back muscular action. When the muscles of the back initiate the dynamics of weight-bearing and lifting, the pelvic, abdominal, and thoracic muscles are activated automatically, and thus, are all toned.

In Elemental Placement of the torso, focus on relaxing the entire front of the body and let back and pelvic muscles contract to *avoid* lifting from over-stretched buttock, a tensed abdomen, a rounded back, and strained shoulder (ear-to-shoulder upper trapezius) muscles. Allow the *naturally appropriate* muscles to shape you into comfort and flexibility. The second-layer rhomboid muscles act with the strong middle and interior fibers of the trapezius to draw the shoulder blades directly back toward the spine, preventing over-curving in the upper back. Important postural muscles like the psoas, latissimus dorsi, and quadratus lumborum all connect the lower back to the pelvis.

Connections. Thanks to the angle of the sacrum and its naturally strong gluteal muscles, the pelvis serves as an effective "seat" for the spinal column. As the fifth lumbar vertebra is "much thicker in front than behind,"[12] it forms a small arch with the fourth lumbar vertebra; this tiny natural arch allows the spine to lengthen (straighten) easily, with only slight outward curving in the upper back. The spine is a coordinating center for the structures of the nervous, circulatory, digestive, and respiratory systems, which lie along its vertical axis. The spine can be supple and spacious when it is supported by the pelvis. Respiratory intercostal muscles then can function well, and the diaphragm is assisted by thoracic serratus, abdominal quadratus lumborum, rib cage intercostal, and shoulder pectoral muscles for optimal oxygenation.

The pelvic floor sphincter (eliminatory) and abdominal muscles are naturally elastic [Fig. 7.12]. The rectus abdominalis, the external oblique abdominal, and the lengthy transversalis muscle are connected to the ligaments of the pubic bones and the crest of the pelvic bones. The superficial abdominal muscles assist in breathing out, bending the vertebral column, flexing the pelvis, and allowing rotation of the trunk.[13] The deep muscles of the abdomen pull down the last rib, assist in breathing in, and flex the trunk.[14]

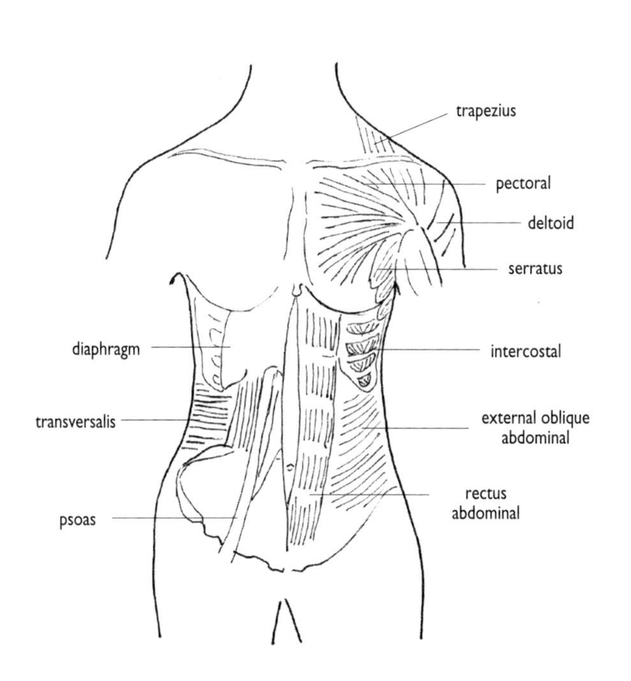

7.12. Front view of the torso

Lower extremity muscles such as the psoas support the alignment of the spine and pelvis upon the femur.[15] Gray does not describe or refer to abdominal muscles as weight-bearing muscles. It appears that these muscles are not intended to be used as *principal*, initiating, weight-bearing muscles. Elemental Placement of the shoulder joints, back, and pelvis allows abdominal muscles to *assist* in weightlifting.

The pectoral (in front of the shoulder), serratus (between the ribs and shoulder blades, in the upper, lateral part of the chest), and the middle and lower trapezius muscles all assist the deltoid arm muscle in raising the arm and in lifting, throwing, or pushing a weight [Fig.7.12]. These muscles are joined by the large subscapular (shoulder blade) muscle, a "powerful defense to the front of the shoulder-joint, preventing displacement of the head of the bone."[16] The deltoid and trapezius muscles, along with teres muscles, all attach to the shoulder blades. Such massive and varied muscular attachments naturally strengthen the upper back. The upper arm muscles, connected to the strong thoracic muscles, are toned whenever arm movements start in the upper back. Smooth function of the upper arm then can extend into comfortable movement of the elbow, wrist, and hand.

Central Concepts. With diminished support from the pelvic area, the spine becomes prone to compensatory curving. Uneven pressure on vertebra and discs causes pronounced inward curving (arching) throughout the entire lower back and outward curving (rounding) in the upper back. In highly industrialized societies, conventional approaches to back health treat such compensations as typical: lower back over-arching is referred to as *lordosis*, upper back over-curving as *kyphosis*. Gray does not mention lordosis or kyphosis. He presents a healthy model of our bodies that is not only refreshing but also essential to our understanding and practice of Elemental Placement.

When the vertebral column, pelvic, and leg bone structures are out of supple balance, the tissues compensate continuously in an effort to support the body's weight. The important paravertebral muscles (which span the length of both sides of the spine and attach to the upper portion of the sacrum) then overstretch and round the spine. The quadratus lumborum lower back muscles (which span from the floating twelfth thoracic rib to the crest of the pelvis) tighten and pull the ribs up and backward, arching the lower back in an effort to counterbalance over-curving in the upper back. Such compensations in the pelvis and torso may be responsible for a disconcerting number of chronic symptoms. When movement is accompanied by stressful balance, not only is the sense of comfort lost, but it seems we lose our sense to use the *appropriate* muscles for weightlifting even in everyday situations. The strong back and pelvic muscles lose elasticity, and the shoulder and abdominal muscles shorten and tighten while we lift, garden, or carry. With balanced lifting, back, pelvic, and abdominal muscles get well-toned.

When the pelvic and torso muscles are weakened, it may seem like nothing more than common sense to set about strengthening them. However, if a weakened muscle

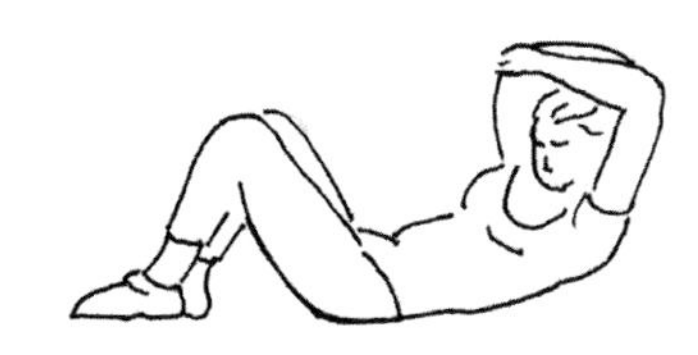

7.13. While we practice the conventional abdominal crunch exercise, the lower back and buttocks over-stretch, the upper back rounds, and the abdomen shortens.

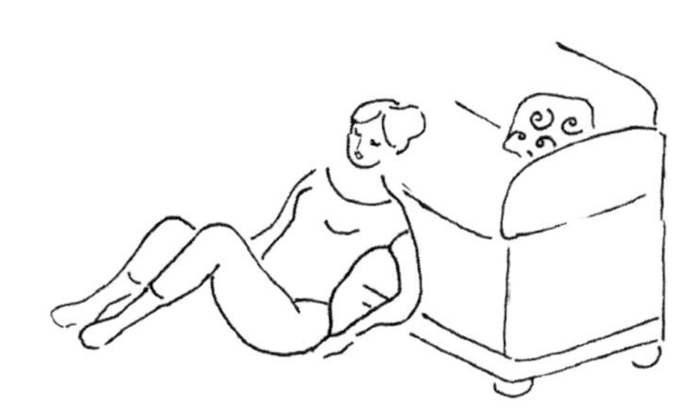

7.14. The KENTRO Boat *movement tones the abdomen, buttocks, and thighs without bodily compensations as long as we keep a straight back, relaxed shoulders, and anterior pelvic placement during the stretch.*

is isolated and then strengthened without *first* experiencing smooth balance, the isolated muscle will be ***strengthened out of balanced relation with other muscle areas*** and is likely to remain overtaxed. For example, toning the abdomen with the oft-recommended abdominal crunch over-stretches the muscles in the lower back and buttock areas, shortens the abdomen, and tends to round the upper back. By contrast, the back straightens, the shoulders relax, and the pelvis stays spacious and *Grounded* with the KENTRO *Boat* toning movement for the abdomen, pelvis, thighs, and back [Figs. 7.13–7.14].

Straining the back, abdominal, and buttock muscles is coupled with a tendency to use tight, upper trapezius muscles for ordinary movements, burdening the body with unnecessary effort. The conventional pelvic tilt exercise tends to increase compensatory arching in the lower back and congestion (strain) in the abdominal, buttock, and other pelvic muscles by pushing the pelvis back and forth. Students who had practiced this conventional pelvic tilt before practicing KENTRO toners reported that they rarely obtained even short-term relief before chronic back and pelvic pain set in again; none of them experienced *Grounding* reshaping of the pelvis or straightening in the lower and upper back. Elemental Placement movements specifically tone but do not stress (shorten) the abdominal muscles while the back straightens and the shoulders relax.

4. HEAD AND NECK

Element. Air.

Sensations. Mobility, a unified body, a head on your shoulders, a strong neck.

Structure. We can sense the neural connection between the head, neck, and torso by becoming familiar with a subtle aspect of the nervous system: the cerebrospinal fluid (CSF). This fluid flows through the ventricles of the brain, the central canal of the spinal cord, and it surrounds the brain's spinal cord as a semi-hydraulic "cushion" in the subarachnoid space. The CSF is considered nourishing for the nerves and protective of the nervous system, and is a vital shock absorber. The back-and-forth flow of the CSF between the brain and the base of the spine is influenced by the alignment of the sacrum, spine, and head. Supple balance in these areas promotes smooth transit of the

CSF fluid. A subtle healing system, CranioSacral Therapy is based on facilitating this flow [Fig. 7.15].

Function. The head rests comfortably on the neck, and the neck can be a supple, strong extension of the spine. Elemental Placement connects all four key areas of the body. The neck and head are the lovely finishing touches to comfortable uprightness. When the legs and back are shifted into alignment, the cervical neck vertebra can follow suit. Young children's bodies express resilient motion: the back and neck are amazingly straight and the head, face, and jaw are at ease. We see similar ease in adults who habitually carry baskets or boxes on their heads. It is unnecessary to learn how to carry weight on the head for increased balance; in fact, it is *not* advisable, unless we have regained thoroughly centered balance and strength. Simply observing as many examples of bodily ease as possible will clarify Elemental Placement. The occipital bone's superior curved line attaches to the broad trapezius, back, shoulder, and neck muscles. The inferior curved line of the occipital bone serves as an outlet for the rectus muscles, which strengthen the back of the neck.

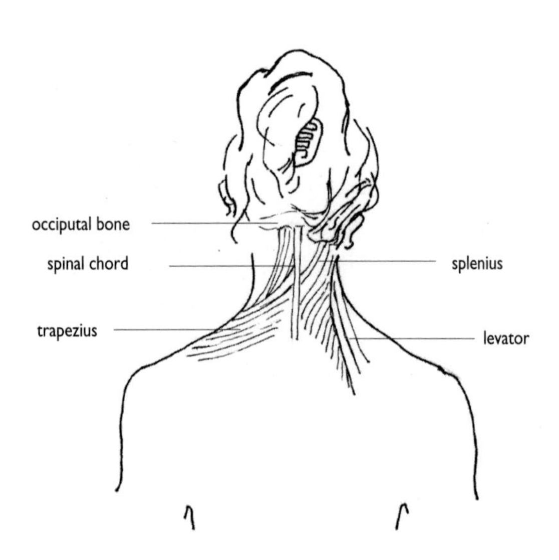

7.15. Back view of the head and neck

Connections. KENTRO students integrate the close connections between the occipital ridges, cervical vertebrae, and thoracic spine when they practice the *Goose Neck* movement, which includes an occipital stretch. These stretches originate in the upper back—which, because it is more structurally fixed than the neck, needs as much gentle stretching as possible—and resolves in a releasing, expansive stretch in the occipital region. Upper back muscles play a major role in the comfortable support of the head and neck. One of the serratus muscles (in the upper back side of the thorax) "draws the lower ribs downward and backward (into balance) and thus elongates the thorax."[17] It also balances and supports the lower ribs. In the same area, the splenius muscles draw the head directly backward, enabling the trapezius to keep the head erect. Farther down, the erector spinal muscles in the lumbar region and their prolongations exist in harmonious relationship with the trapezius muscle.

Central Concepts. When the upper back curves, the neck compensates by over-arching. As a result, the back of the neck becomes over-compressed and the front of the neck over-stretched. By holding the shoulders and chin up, head and neck movements become restricted. Spinal CSF may not function smoothly in this contracted position. The occipital region feels jammed and the jaw becomes tight; the head may tilt forward and, by habit, everyday movements start from strained shoulders. By practicing

Elemental Placement for the fourth key area of the body, compensations in the head and neck resolve slowly, especially as the body regains a supple neck and the relaxed angle for the head: chin down, eyes level with the world [See Fig. 7.6, p. 41].

Over time, Elemental Placement will bring you relaxation and strength while it unites the four key areas of your body and helps pulsate them with life.

NOTES

1. The Twelve Movements mini-program includes the Elemental Placement movements 1–4, as well as movements 5–12: *Bending, Sitting Up, Sitting Back, Tikanis, Leg Rotation, Boat, Lifting,* and *Prayer.*
2. If you wish to broaden your understanding of anatomy, a recent edition of Henry Gray's original 1857 study of anatomy remains an excellent source. Keep in mind that *Gray's Anatomy* was written before the "modern, flattened, lean, and tight" look emerged in highly industrialized countries at the beginning of the twentieth century. It was not until the 1930s that tucking and tightening the pelvis gained acceptance as standard posture. This stance, dictated by fashion, distanced us from comfortable balance.
3. *Webster's Dictionary.*
4. Henry Gray, *Gray's Anatomy*: 179.
5. *Ibid,* 272.
6. *Ibid*, 426.
7. *Ibid*, 431.
8. *Idib*, 343.
9. *Ibid.*
10. *Ibid*, 341.
11. *Ibid,* 382.
12. *Ibid,* 43.
13. *Ibid,* 365.
14. *Ibid,* 367.
15. *Ibid,* 417.
16. *Ibid,* 384.
17. *Ibid,* 342.

CHAPTER 8:

Elemental Movements

(KENTRO Movements 1-4)

FIRST KEY AREA: THE PELVIS (Grounding Movement)	Element: Water
Function	**Sensations**
• Is naturally slanted, due to the angled sacrum	*Fluidity*
• Supports the torso for comfortable balance	*Elasticity*
• Is the center of most bone support	*Strength*
• Is the *center area* for moving freely	*Grounding*
• Is supported by the legs	
• Possesses naturally strong buttock muscles	

1. Grounding

PREPARATION: Stand in profile to a long mirror, to check your alignment.

A. Place the inside of your left hand on your lower back (with your fingers on the arch in your spine and the palm of your hand on the muscles). Place the palm of your right hand on the top of your right buttock muscles, letting your fingers fan out.

B. Contrast discomfort with comfort. Start with discomfort: briefly move your pelvis and legs about one inch farther out in front of you. Note increased arching in your lower back; most of your weight (pressure) is on the balls of your feet. Immediately shift your body back into an upright stance.

C. Comfort: your body and let your torso bend slightly forward, and let your pelvis and legs shift out back one or two inches (without tucking or sticking out your buttocks), while you press your *right* hand slightly downward on the buttocks (so they stretch away from your torso). Let your abdomen stretch downward. Your left hand will stretch your lower back slightly upward to release and straighten it. *Let weight shift to your heels until there's about 95 percent pressure in the heels and 5 percent pressure in the big toes. Sense straightening in your lower back, expansion in your pelvis, and increased stability in your legs.* You may think that your buttocks are sticking way out and that your torso is hunched. Your mirror verifies that this is an illusion. FORGET about being upright. So far, you have only focused on the first movement—Grounding—the foundation for more resiliency above and below the pelvis. It may take some weeks of frequent Grounding (and of muscular release of strain) for you to *feel* the Grounding happening. *You will feel more limber and more "weight" in your pelvis, as well as more strength in your legs. Smooth, balancing placement of your legs supports the legs and is essential for pelvic* Grounding.

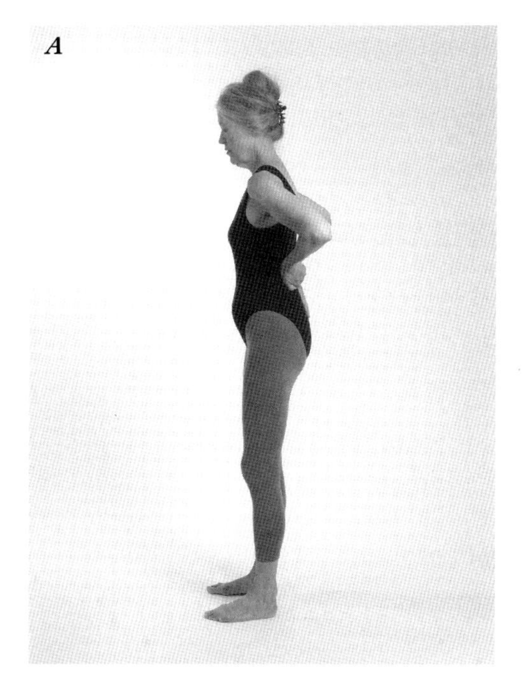

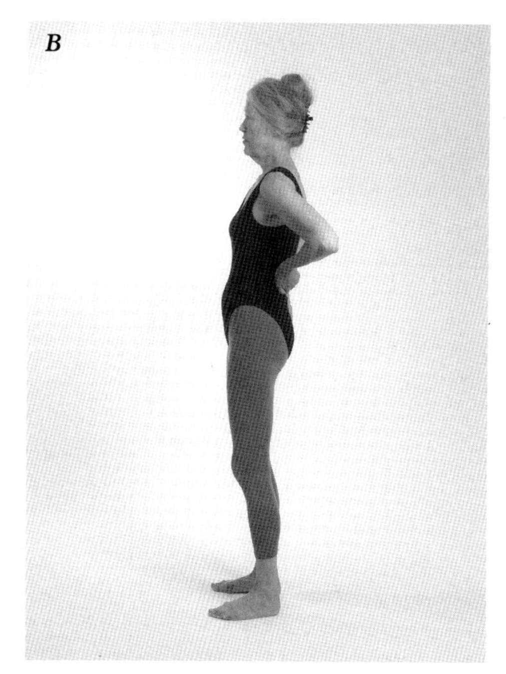

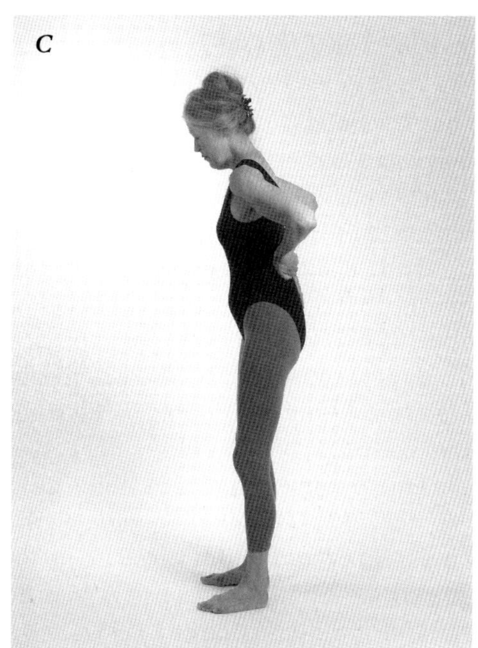

GROUNDING

BENEFITS: *Grounding* your pelvis relaxes and harmoniously realigns your pelvis, legs, and lower back; it limbers and strengthens your core pelvic muscles. Only when your pelvis is grounded can your legs optimally support your body weight and can your back straighten.

HELPFUL HINTS: Sticking your buttocks out, arching your lower back, raising up your rib cage, tightening your belly and tucking your buttocks are counter-productive to Grounding. Practice it anywhere. Practice Lying Down and Prayer before Grounding is helpful.

VARIATIONS:
There are additional approaches to fostering fuller experience of Grounding. Practice A, B, and C by keeping your left hand on the lower back, but moving your right hand onto your diaphragm and relax that muscle with gentle downward pressure. Try A, B, and C by placing the palms of both of your hands onto your pelvic (innominate) bones with downward pressure; your pelvis will *feel* heavier but also like a relaxed "seat."

Your Clay-Like Body

Grounding is an enhancing attitude toward ourselves, permeated by profound physicality: it has its genesis in our creative core, where our sensuous artist mixes form and flow, balance and centering, water and earth. The word *ground* means: "the base, the bottom of anything," and "foundation."The ground is the bottom of the sea, as well as the surface of the earth. Fundamentally mysterious, water and earth together suggest our basic nature: malleable clay. Shifts in our fluid bodies invite shifts in other levels of our being.

Our clay-like bodies are like a path that leads us to nature, to our personal place in nature. To ground ourselves is to return to our senses, to feel our pliable bodies in all our daily gestures. Our pleasurable sensing guides us to say "yes" to life. The stuff we are made of connects us to ourselves.

This intimate connection is our home ground; it is the process of being at home—at ease—in our bodies. Grounding movements allow us to feel like welcome guests in our activities and everyday life. We sense an inner belonging, and we move in harmony with everything around us, deepening our humanness. Ordinary, down-to-earth gestures—carrying a child, sitting at a desk, mopping, or repairing a fence—then become our grounding resource. When we sense and feel our movements, simple activities can vitalize us.

It is our nature to be shaped by our inner sculptor, who first molds a base—the legs on which the pelvis rests, and who then molds the torso, arms, and head on top of the supporting pelvis. We do not need to have our feet on the earth to ground our whole body. Our grounding movements emanate from the solid yet mobile pelvis: this

Grounding: Your Clay-Like Body

This Greek sailor is grounded: His pelvic muscles stretch out behind him (for counterweight) as he bends from the hips. His back straightens, and his shoulders drop. Notice his sturdy stance: His shoulders stay down as he pulls the rope with upper back muscles; his pelvis stretches and "sits" on his hips. Most of the weight distribution goes through the pelvis and the hips.

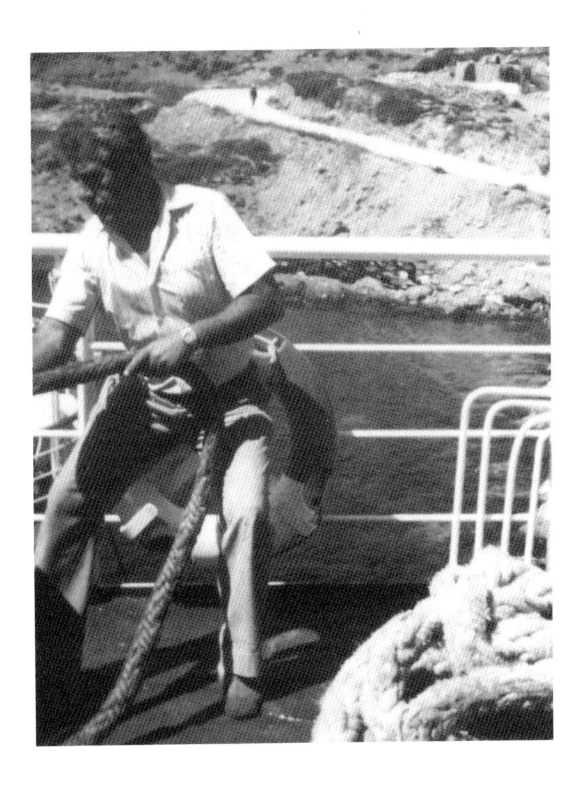

main area for weight assimilation feels like a supportive "seat" we can settle into, as well as being the appropriate area for initiating our movements in a flowing manner. Grounded movements then ripple throughout our bodies, releasing stress. When our pelvic muscles are tight and overstretched due to strained motion, our torso muscles likewise tighten and overstretch. Our pelvic muscles are designed to be naturally toned and limber by lengthening and expanding away from our torso. This suppleness is a prerequisite for our torso muscles to also lengthen, expand, and remain elastic.

The verb *to ground* means "to found on a firm basis" and "to instruct [a person] in the elements of first principles." The KENTRO guidelines encompass Gray's sound anatomical principles. Yet only when comfortable balance merges with a relaxed, affectionate approach to our body—the principle for centered ease—can grounding happen.

By centering and balancing our actions, we feel shapeable yet stable, "on firm ground." We give in to grounding—and feel uplifted.

SECOND KEY AREA: THE LEGS AND FEET
(Little Moon Movement)

Function

- Support the pelvis for comfortable balance
- Align vertically with the spine
- Include the strong thigh muscles
- Are bolstered by the femurs, the strongest bones in the body

Element: Earth

Sensations

Stability
Standing on your own two feet
Sturdiness

2. Little Moon

PREPARATION. Stand next to a chair or table with one-foot space between your feet and your left hand on the chair. Shift into Elementary Placement—Grounding.

A. Align your legs by bending slightly forward and verifying that the center of your knees is in line with the center of your foot (the space between the second and third toe). Slowly shift your body-weight from one leg to the other, to *sense balanced weight distribution, with level hips.*

B. Spread the fingers of your right hand over the top of the right pelvic (innominate) bone with the palm of your hand reaching toward the right sacroiliac joint. Keeping your hips level, shift your weight to your left leg, then relax your buttocks and let your right hand slowly pivot your right leg outward—from the hip area, allowing only slight pressure (weight) on your right heel. *Sense a slight outward stretch in the right front crest of your pelvic bone and thigh, and a slight stretch in the sacral area of your right buttock.* After a brief moment, shift equal weight to both legs and Ground yourself again.

C. Align and center your left leg by placing your left hand onto your left front pelvic crest, shifting your weight to your right leg. Repeat "A" and "B" for the left leg. After a brief moment, shift equal weight to both legs. You may *sense* a *slight "pulling" sensation (release of strain) in the inner thigh, hip, and sacral areas.* Now you are ready to shift from this broad stance into smooth alignment of your feet as described in "D."

D. With most of your weight in your heels, and a slight amount of weight *only* in your big toes, slowly slide your feet about an inch toward each other, while your hands apply a slight outward pressure on your crests (to keep your pelvis and legs centered). You will see that your arches are uplifted (more pronounced) than before the Little Moon. *Sense a pleasant stretching throughout the inside of your thighs as these shortened muscles extend, increased toning in your buttocks and spaciousness and stability in your feet.* Stay in this stance for the duration of a few yawns.

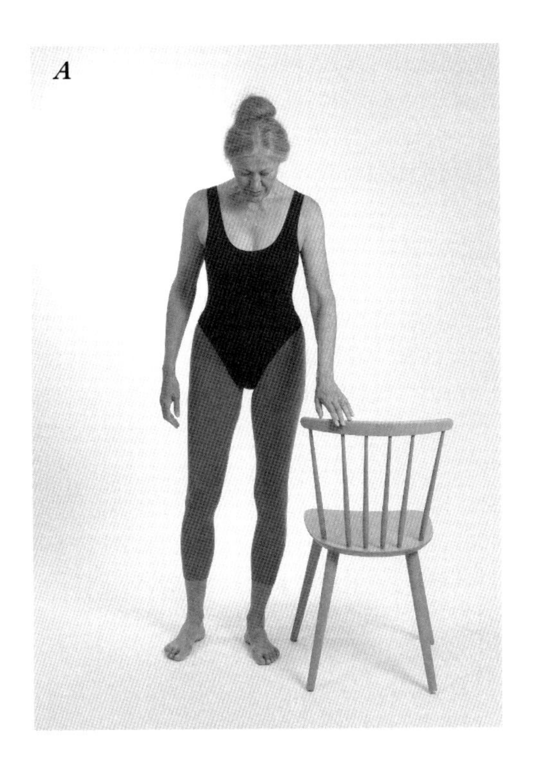

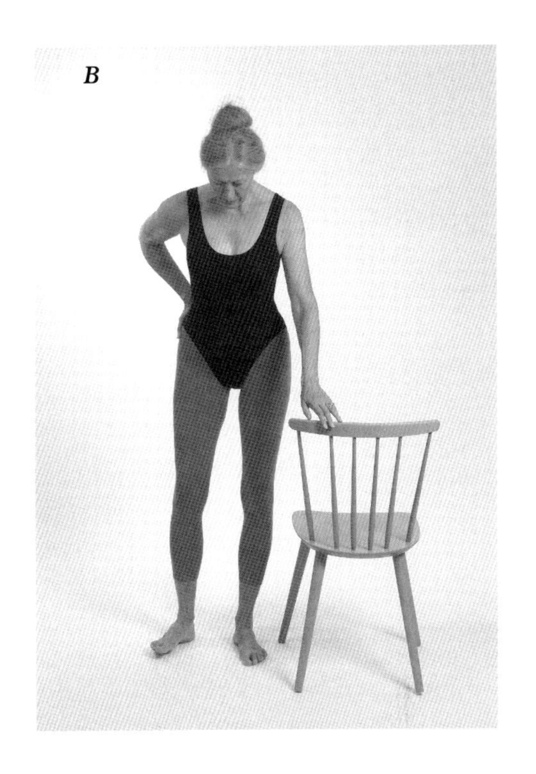

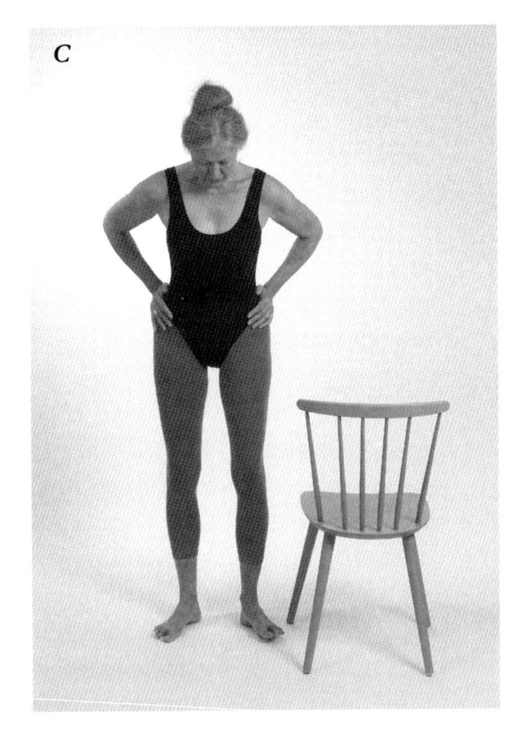

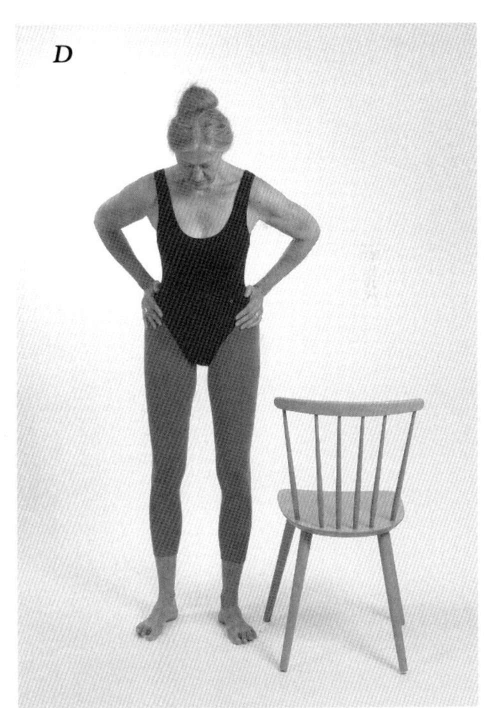

Little Moon

BENEFITS: *Little Moon* is the most effective KENTRO movement for realigning your legs and feet into centered balance. It relieves pronation (too much weight on the inside of the foot) and supination (too much weight on the outside of the foot). The Little Moon movement allows the strong hipbones to support the pelvis and limbers and tones your pelvis as well as your legs.

HELPFUL HINTS

Prevent tucking or twisting your pelvis. Notice whether your foot leads when you rotate your leg outward, which moves your foot out of centered alignment with your leg. After a few months, you will *feel* more supple in the hip and sacroiliac areas. Practice Little Moon in bed and waiting in line. Practicing the Pelvic Rock, Turning, and Belly Dance before Little Moon is helpful.

VARIATIONS

Practice the Little Moon while you are lying down on your back with your knees bent and your hands on the crests; slowly extend one leg at a time.

Body Ecology

Ecology is the branch of biology that deals with relations between living organisms and their environment.Our bodies can move in supple relationship with our activities. Ecology is a composite of the Greek *oikos,* house; and *logos,* understanding. *Our bodies are our constantly reshaping houses.* Our senses and feelings reside in this fluid house. *We move into our house—into well being,* by letting spaciousness and limberness permeate us.

We start to feel at home when we perceive the blending of muscle, bone, breath, sensing, and feeling. Throughout the day, our bodies realign us into smooth support of our bodily weight, so we can move as we wish.

We do not have to match our bearing with idealized posture. Our body has the innate capacity to heal and reshape itself at its own rhythm, in concert with the rhythms of nature, which is constantly reshaping herself.

With centered balance, every sensuous reshaping of a specific area creates a release throughout our entire body. *We are at home* when our movements arise freely: our resilient nature becomes unhampered and uncultivated, simple and gracious. Over time, our body can reveal itself exuberantly:

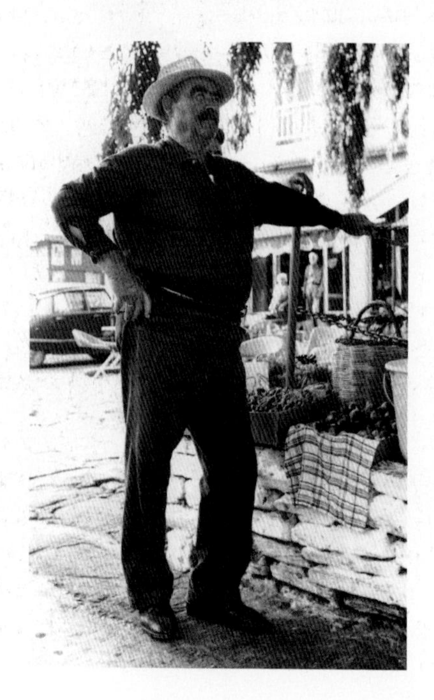

This Greek vendor connotes fitness—vital comfort in a relaxed stance. His right leg placement is similar to the Little Moon *movement.*

we will experience a letting go and a centering, which seems like tiny explosions of ease.

I recall admiring some "volunteer" sunflowers that cheered my garden, their broad faces thick with edible seeds. I exclaimed to my friend, Kevin, "How do they do it? They are so tall and sturdy!" Kevin replied, "They follow their nature." Of course! It's as simple as that. And so it is with us.

We are embodied in a nomad—our bodies take us places, and we are guests in this familiar form; it houses our deep selves. When we feel stiff or limited by our body, we may wish to disassociate from our body, in an effort to "manage" it. We may try out mind-over-matter visualizations. Paradoxically, this is the opportune time to *associate* with our body—which continually adapts and balances our motion as best as it can, so we can go on playing the piano and playing tennis.

Free is at the base of the word friend. Centering and balancing our actions connect us with our body, our ally, and our movements suit our daily living. Simple activities then sustain and season this intimacy. *Fit* refers to adapting well to our environment. This is our ecology: feeling fit, effusive, and relaxed in our gestures, linked with the rich, ancient clay of our surroundings.

I regularly refer my patients with chronic pain and postural dysfunction to Angie. I know the results will be transformative for them because I have experienced the changes myself. Angie's understanding of the dynamic relationship between gravity, our neuro-musculoskeletal systems, and the expression of Self in the world is unparalleled. KENTRO relieves pain and prevents injuries and gently works to resculpt our bodies and our experience. Body armoring slowly melts away as we find ourselves solidly and safely balanced in our world. I use the KENTRO principles everyday in my practice as a massage therapist and CranioSacral therapist. They are easy and fun.

—Judith Sanford, Massage Therapist, CranioSacral Therapist, Ashland Institute of Massage (Oregon)

THIRD KEY AREA: THE LEGS AND FEET
(Shoulder Roll Movement)

Element: Fire

Function

- Support the neck and head
- Include strong back muscles for comfortable weight-bearing
- Allow relaxed shoulders
- Include the elastic abdomen

Sensations

Broad front, relaxed shoulders
Strong backbone
Full breath
Upright comfort

3. Shoulder Roll

PREPARATION. Stand facing a long mirror and practice Elemental Placement—Grounding and Little Moon. Have a hand mirror nearby.

A. Place the inside of your right hand on your diaphragm (tummy area) and the palm of your left hand on your lower back, with the fingers touching the groove in your lower spine. Let your torso shift slightly forward by bending from the hips, letting your diaphragm soften. This allows your entire rib cage to shift into more comfortable alignment and relaxes the tight muscles in your diaphragm. You may think that your lower back is more rounded; however, under your left hand, you will have a *sense of a longer, more even groove in the spine and lengthened muscles in your lower back.* Slowly return to an upright position with your right hand putting a slight downward pressure on your diaphragm. *Sense a release in your lower back and diaphragm*, which prepares the way for realigning your upper back and shoulders.

B. Return your left arm to the side of your body and place the fingers of your right hand onto the front of your left shoulder joint, *to sense your left shoulder's movements.* Slowly roll your left shoulder forward, out in front of your body, an inch or so (which will push your right fingertips slightly away from your shoulder joint), and continue with C.

C. Let your right fingertips put slight pressure onto the left shoulder, guiding it into a slightly diagonal downward and outward direction (away from your ears). Relax your shoulder. *Sense a release in your shoulder and expansion in the shoulder blade area.* Let your left elbow move slightly back (about one inch), relaxing your arm. *Sense your left shoulder moving slightly farther back* on its own; your shoulder blade area broadens and flattens. You may *sense a slight "pulling" in your shoulder/shoulder blade muscles.* This is not new stress. It is a sure indication that tight muscles are beginning to release strain. In the mirror, you will see broadening in the front, top part of your torso, where the pectoral muscles expand when your upper back expands. Drop your right arm and stay in this stretch for the duration of several yawns. Keeping your left arm by the side of your body, apply the A and B guidelines to your right shoulder.

D. Pick up the hand mirror with your right hand and turn your back to the wall mirror. Repeat A, B, and C for your left shoulder. You will notice broadening in the left shoulder blade muscles as well as flattening, and straightening in your upper back.

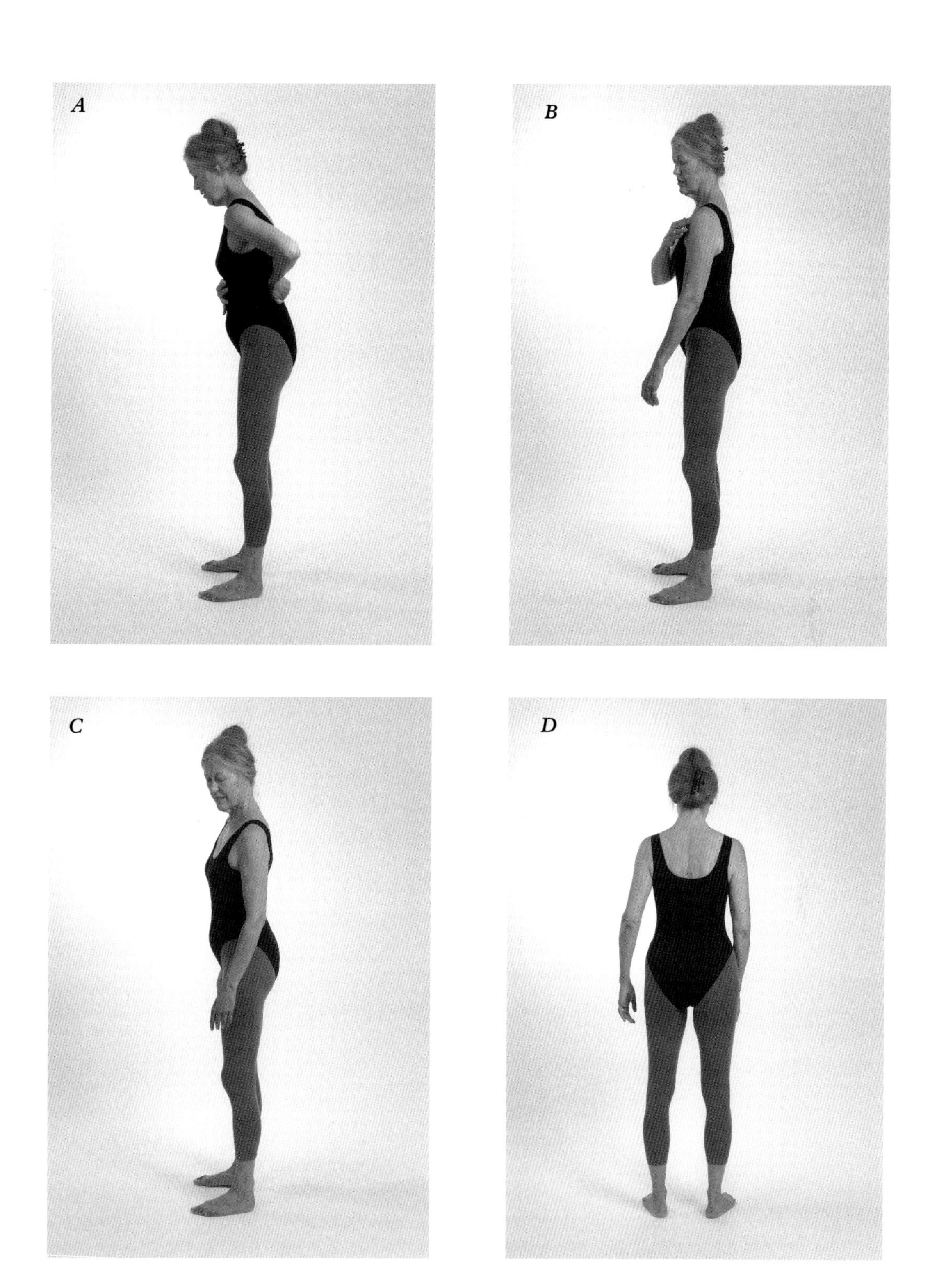

SHOULDER ROLL

BENEFITS: The profoundly relaxing *Shoulder Roll* is essential for regaining elasticity in your shoulders and back. Likewise, it slowly increases straightening in your upper back and assists your rib cage into comfortable spaciousness.

HELPFUL HINTS: *Pushing* your shoulders back or raising up your shoulders or rib cage is counterproductive. For contrast, push your shoulders back. You will *feel a disagreeable strain in the shoulder blade area.* You will see bunched-up, tightened upper back muscles and arching in your mid/lower back. Relax out of this effort. *Always* start the Shoulder Roll with lengthening your lower back and relaxing your diaphragm for comfortable balance. Practice Shoulder Roll anywhere, after Grounding and the Little Moon.

VARIATIONS: Broaden the Shoulder Roll by accompanying motion in your shoulder with a sweeping movement of your entire arm.

Sense and Sensibility

Centering and balancing our movements expands our sense of restful and energizing motion. Ordinary actions become vitalizing threads in the fabric of our identities, as long as we exercise our senses and take the time to feel our movements. Our life is filled with an abundance of color, sounds, aromas, forms, and movement. Our gestures are part of the sensuousness that defines the quality of our day-to-day experience.

'Sense' and 'sensibility' are companions. These two words blend into and resonate with one another. 'Sense,' (from the Latin, *sentir,* "to feel, perceive,") is "the ability of the nerves and brain to receive and react to stimuli through ... sight, touch, taste, smell and hearing." This description focuses on our physical experience of the world through our five senses. 'Sensibility' transcends 'sense' to encompass our emotional and mental faculties as well; it is our ability to feel, our capacity to be affected emotionally or intellectually, our delicate, sensitive awareness or responsiveness. In many situations, we are discouraged from trusting our perception. Even the phrase, "be sensible," suggests rational thinking, devoid of personal feeling. Yet it makes sense to use as many of our faculties as possible for personal expression.

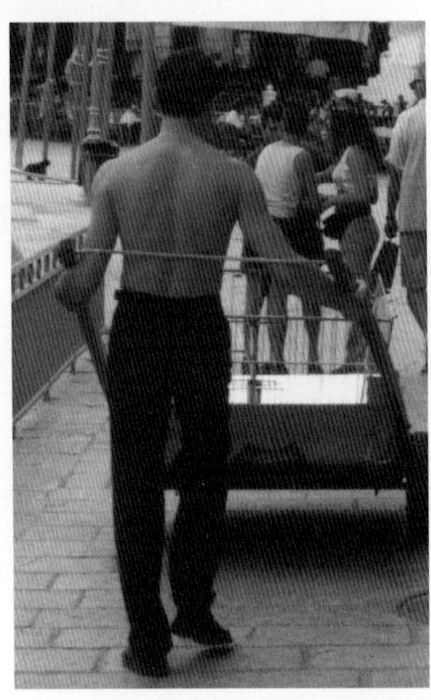

This Greek man is pushing a cart using his upper back muscles. Notice the even groove in his limber, strong back. His back remains straight and his hips remain level. By practicing Shoulder Roll, *we can regain the relaxation in our shoulders as is evident in this man.*

When we focus on posture, we have a tendency to separate the realms of thought, sensing, feeling, and bodily expression. At times, we only observe the sensations of tingling or warmth caused by stretching, without noticing how we actually *feel*, which may range from tense and overtaxed to rested and dynamic. We may believe that our bearing, at least for the moment, is "correct," yet we may feel stiff and uncomfortable. We tend to get lost in external appearances, in "perfecting" the shape of our bodies.

Before I began practicing KENTRO movements, my upper back would round whenever I tried to relax while standing or sitting down. I tried to "think tall," lifting my torso from an imaginary string at the top of my head. However, my ribs lifted up, my lower back arched, causing my back muscles to become even more strained than before; then when I relaxed, my back would round again. Later, when I experienced comfortable balance and ease, my muscles regained limberness. My back straightened—I "grew" one and a half inches taller—without straining to stand tall.

Combining sense with sensibility results in enjoying our appearance, hand in hand with the pleasure of sitting, bending, or walking with suppleness.

Such delight is supported by a neurological network that connects our beliefs with subtle perceptions. In her book, *Molecules of Emotion,* Candace Pert, a research professor in the Department of Biophysics and Physiology at Georgetown University School of Medicine, addresses this biochemical process. Pert presents us with an exciting new bridge between physiology and the psyche. Specialized cells, called neuropeptides, act as both messengers and mood-enhancing endorphins. These neuropeptides are composed of strings of amino acids that branch directly off of our DNA.

Pert and her colleagues discovered that a neuropeptide in the nervous, endocrine, or immune system attaches to a corresponding receptor mechanism for emotional information exchanges in the body whenever rebalancing is needed. Approximately sixty of the neuropeptides Pert has traced "account for the physiological manifestations of emotions—for enlivening emotions ... for flowing energy."[1] A dialogue takes place between the neuropeptide and its receptor, and the receptor can be altered. "This means that even when we are 'stuck' emotionally, fixated on a version of reality that does not serve us well, there is always a biochemical potential for change and growth."[2]

This innovative, neuroscientific research demonstrates that physical structures (e.g., joints, muscles, nerves, and protein chains) are influenced by life-enhancing feelings that are biochemically identifiable.

There are key areas in our body, where sensuous information is concentrated. Almost every peptide receptor that concerned Pert's team could be found in the *back* segment of the spinal cord, which is the "principal site for sorting (receiving/processing) the entire range of our bodily sensations and feelings."[3] By practicing smooth balancing movements, we actively lengthen and limber our backs. The KENTRO emphasis on integrating balance with centering is supported by Pert's premise that there are "almost infinite pathways for the conscious mind to access—and modify—the unconscious mind and the body."[4] She goes on to explain: "Your mind, your feelings are in your body, and it's there, in your somatic [physical] experience, that feeling is healed."[5]

The practice of KENTRO guidelines fuses *Gray's Anatomy* and a caring view of our body with Pert's neuroscientific findings on emotion; by attaining flexibility in our back and in our entire body, we can awaken and amplify fulfilling feelings. Students remark that when their back untwists, they experience a gentle unfolding of their sensibilities, in proportion with a new sense of inner and outer strength.

Fourth Key Area: The Neck and Head (Goose Neck Movement)

Element: Air

Function

- Are supported by the torso
- Include resilient neck motion
- Provide strong neck muscles

Sensations

Mobility
A head on your shoulders
Looking straight ahead

4. Goose Neck

PREPARATION. Stand in front of the mirror. Balance and center your pelvis, legs and feet, and torso with Elemental Placement. Relax your entire body.

A. Place your fingertips on the small occipital grooves behind your ears (just under the base of your head). You may just *detect* subtle indentations.

B. While applying slight pressure from your fingertips onto the occipital grooves—slowly let your neck move forward, and let your fingertips put upward pressure onto the grooves. Keep your head in the same position (chin slightly down) throughout the stretching. Keep your head level, your shoulders down, and your torso relaxed and upright. This stretch begins in your upper back. *Sense your shoulder blades flattening and your back lengthening. Feel your head lift up and a stretch throughout your neck and upper back.* Remain in this position for the duration of several yawns. Keep your fingertips in the occipital grooves. Step B is *essential* because you must first create elasticity in your upper back before your neck can stretch back *without* effort.

C. Slowly bring your neck and head upward and *slightly* backward. Your head will appear much more aligned: you *feel* like you "have a head on your shoulders." Let your fingertips put continual upward pressure on the occipital grooves as your head moves into more alignment. Your neck will *feel longer*.
Take your fingers off the occipital grooves. *Relax* and forget about the Goose Neck (until you practice it again) to avoid stiffening your neck into the "right" posture. Repeat the stretch as often as possible.

BENEFITS: The *Goose Neck* movement relaxes and tones your neck muscles and aligns your head more vertically with your spine and legs. It helps your face to relax.

HELPFUL HINTS: Prevent pushing up your chin or rib cage to force your head back into alignment. Remember that your legs, pelvis, and torso are reshaping; eventually your head will shift farther back, and shortened muscles at the back of your neck will be toned. Practice the Goose Neck anywhere.

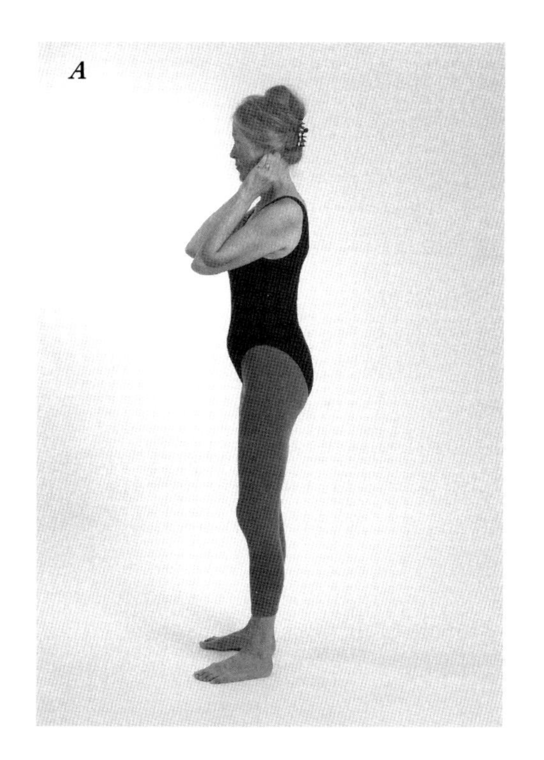

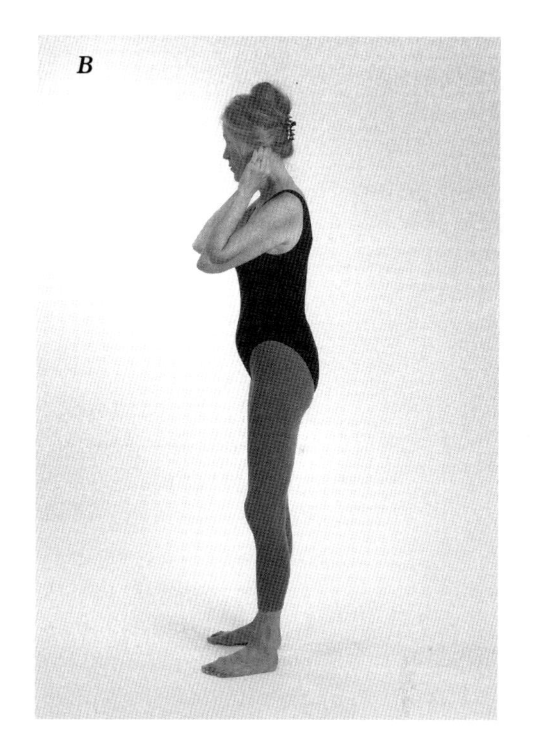

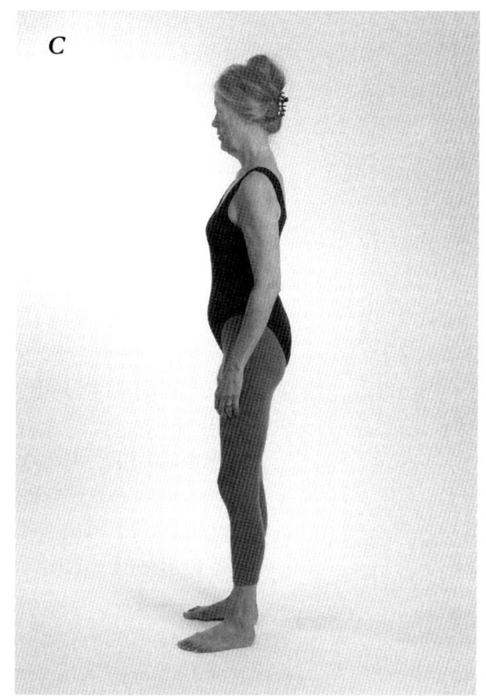

GOOSE NECK

VARIATIONS: Practice the Goose Neck to the *left* and to the *right* so neck tissues get stretched in various directions. Try lying down on your back, raise your head off the pillow about two inches only for an *instant* because the muscles at the back of your neck get deep toning. With your fingertips in the grooves, roll your head from side to side. Try out a horizontally inclined "figure-eight." Let your fingertips (in both grooves) "draw" a tiny circle toward the ear lobes, followed by a tiny circle toward the center of your neck.

Body Aesthetics

In *Anam Cara*, John O'Donohue writes that "there is nothing in the universe as sensuous as God. The wildness of God is the sensuousness of God. Nature is the direct expression of the divine imagination. It is the most intimate reflection of God's sense of beauty."[6]

We embody nature. It is the nature of our movements to reflect divinely inspired beauty and sensuousness. Our thoughts, feelings, and movements all emanate from creation. Visualizing our bodies as malleable allows them to be continuous, spirited expressions of creative energy. The wellspring of this energy is at our core, where an inner artist restores us.

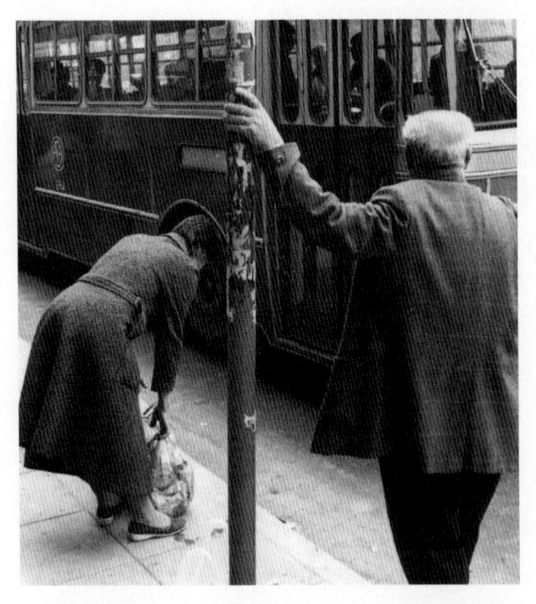

The Greek man on the right is raising his left arm from the shoulder, which uses muscles that tighten them. Yet the woman's shoulders are relaxed because she is grounded: Her pelvis stretches away from her torso, and her back is straight as she lifts the groceries using her upper back muscles.

The word "aesthetic" derives from the Greek, *aisthetikos*, for "sensitive," and *aisthanestha,* "to perceive." Simply stated, we can choose to respond aesthetically to our bodies, sensing and feeling our movements so we can regain zestful mobility.

The KENTRO method aims to enliven our sensibilities so we may sense dynamic comfort in all of our gestures. We can shed mechanistic imagery and rigid ideas about posture that make us feel stuck in our bodies. KENTRO practice fosters a playful acceptance of our current physical state. This compassionate centering attitude, combined with balancing guidelines, brings us into the present moment, invigorating our capacity for free movement.

Focusing on body aesthetics has yielded life-enhancing expression in my everyday activities. Over time, I've sensed my creative energy moving beyond the realm of art and into everyday life. During my years of painting and showing my art in galleries, I was often discouraged by my body's chronic stiffness and tightness. I believed my body was naturally weak and assumed strained posture was normal. While recuperating from a debilitating back injury, I became more flexible by integrating balance into my movements. When I included centering relaxation with balance, my everyday occupations overflowed with refreshing experiences. My body spread out luxuriously when I stretched out to rest. Whenever I would sit down to paint for several hours, I moved in rhythm with the brushstrokes. I sensed more tranquility during meditation. Stirring a casserole or vacuuming felt like a dance. When I took long walks, my body felt grounded. Repetitive movements became creative acts, generating resilient gestures.

Gleefully, I began to trust I could live my life with more spontaneity. When I remembered to listen to my body, I felt encouraged to follow *what I felt moved to do,* and I did my best to avoid *should*s. My interests and inner discernment guided my movements. I did fanciful things that I hoped would expand my understanding of supple motion. I went to Greece for three successive summers to learn traditional Greek dance and to paint, meditate, and soak in nature. As a result, my projects became more diverse and innovative.

My own experiences are echoed by hundreds of KENTRO students who have gradually become more poised, comfortable, and grounded. Above all, I have seen these students—representing a wide variety of occupations, cultural values, diets, and lifestyles—become more fluid in their lives.

Sensing the quality of our actions is essential to enjoying our everyday life. Rigid intellectual constructs about "proper" posture take us outside our bodies and ourselves. We can come home to our senses. We can stop *fixing* our postures when we can *feel* our posture reshaping us into flowing motion.

John O'Donohue offers this observation about the sensory system: "To be sensual or sensuous is to be in the presence of your own soul."[7] Exercising our ensouled senses can reconnect our bodies with subtle areas, bringing delight into our activities. When we place ourselves in the vibrancy of the moment, our senses respond to our need for rest or action. Our bodies love this affectionate attention. When our pliable bodies shift us into ease, we experience our true nature. We are not born merely to survive; we are born to thrive.

NOTES

1. Candace Pert, "The Wisdom of the Receptors: Neuropeptides, the Emotions, and the Bodymind," *Advances,* (vol. 3:3 Summer 1986): 15.
2. Pert, *Molecules of Emotion* (New York: Scribner, 1997): 146.
3. *Ibid,* 141.
4. *Ibid.*
5. *Ibid,* 293.
6. John O'Donohue, *Anam Cara: A Book of Celtic Wisdom* (New York: Harper Collins, 1997): 50.
7 *Ibid,* 59.

CHAPTER 9:

The Remaining Movements

(KENTRO Movements 5-33 and their Vignettes)

5. Bending Forward

PREPARATION. Stand in profile to a long mirror with at least a foot of space between your heels. Practice Elemental Placement.

A. Place the inside of your left hand on the top of your buttock muscles and the inside of your right hand onto the base of your rib cage (to sense a relaxation in the diaphragm). Begin by bending from your level hips. Let your torso slowly come forward while you slightly bend your knees, letting your buttocks muscles relax and stretch; *sense Grounding.* Keep most of your weight in your heels. *Sense your buttocks extending and expanding out behind you, away from your torso.*

B. As you bend your torso farther forward, continue to Ground your pelvis, drop your shoulders, and bend your knees. Keep opening your thighs to center your legs (the center of the knees in line with the center of the feet). Place the inside of your right hand on your lower/mid back (with your fingers touching your spine) to feel your spine straighten. Your left hand will help you *sense keeping your ribs down*. Keep your neck in line with your spine.

C. Bring your arms forward and place your hands on the pelvic crests. Keep most of your weight in your heels and relax your ankles (folds in the skin indicate release). *Sense stability in your legs and muscular toning throughout your thigh muscles, with extensive stretching in the back of your thighs—the hamstring muscles.* As you bend even farther, it is essential that you continue with A and B so that your body weight can be assimilated in the sacral and hip region. Let your pelvis "sit" on your hips. *Sense additional letting go, comfort, and stability as you let the legs support your grounded pelvi.s*

D. Return to an upright stance with both hands onto the top of your pelvic bones. Combine slight pressure of your hands on your pelvis (to help pelvic muscles to keep on expanding, relaxing—away from the torso) while slowly straightening your legs, and bringing your torso up; keep your back as straight as possible and your ribs and shoulders down. *Sense that your pelvis feels more elastic, and like a "seat," your legs feel strengthened, and your torso feels longer.*

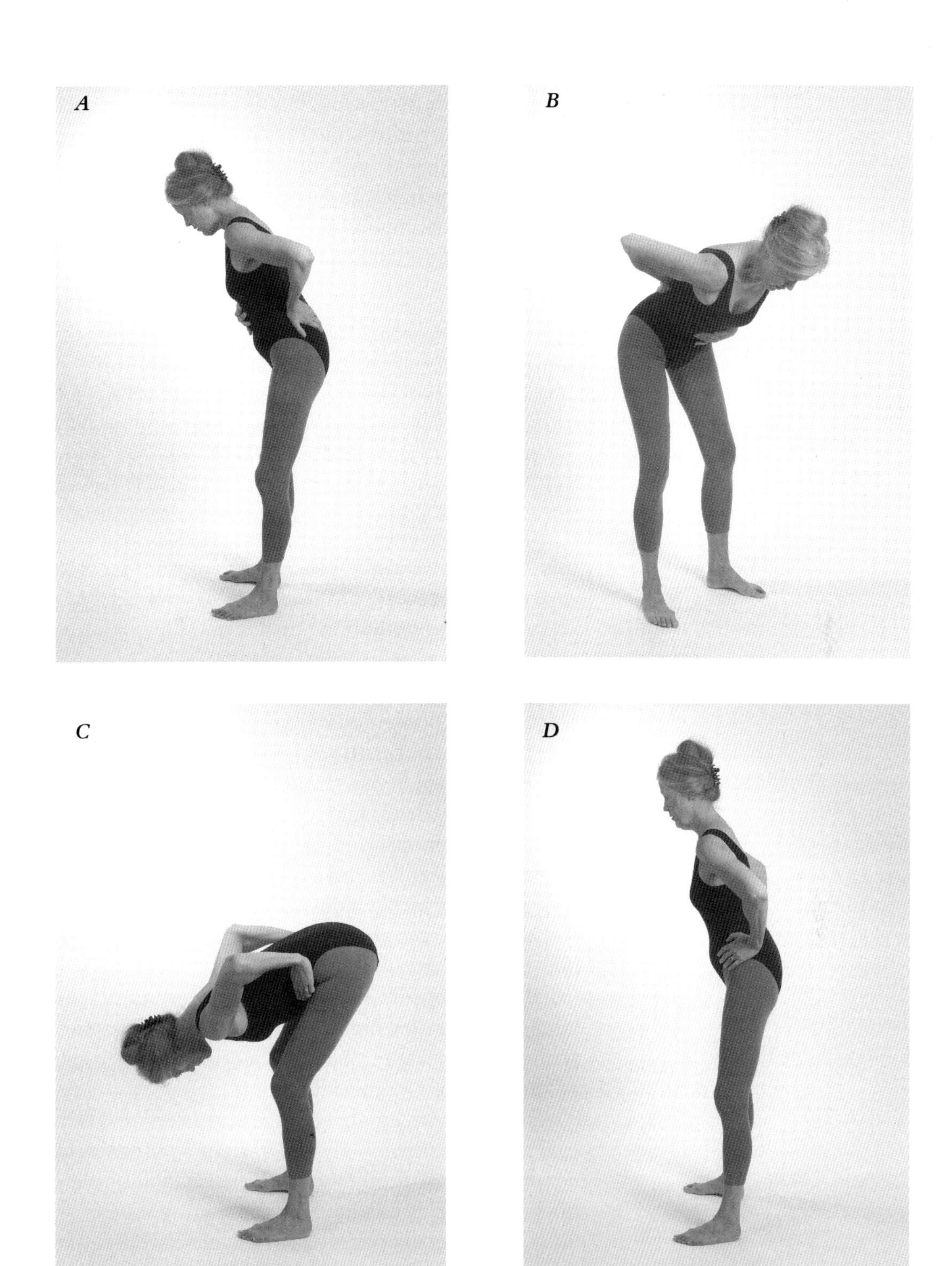

Bending Forward

BENEFITS: *Bending Forward* in centered balance is the easiest placement for *sensing* and fostering grounding in your pelvis and stretching in your back. This movement stretches and tones your hamstring muscles most gently and efficiently, and it stretches all leg muscles harmoniously. Bending Forward is both energizing, relaxing, and improves circulation. Every time you bend forward, you remobilize your pelvis and release strain from both your pelvic and back tissues.

HELPFUL HINTS: Prevent weight (pressure) on the balls of your feet, lack of symmetry in your pelvis or legs, sticking out or tucking your buttocks, twisting or tightening your pelvis, twisting, arching, or curving your back or neck, and pushing up your rib cage, shoulders, or chin. Always let your inner thighs open outward for pelvic mobility. Give yourself enough practice time for your buttock and hamstring muscles to stretch and become supple before you attempt to bend forward with your head close to the ground. Practice Bending anywhere. Prayer, Pelvic Rock, and Pelvis Up the Wall are helpful before Bending.

VARIATIONS: Try Bending Forward and place both hands on top of a table. Follow the usual guidelines for Bending Forward, and slowly "walk away" from the table, a few inches at a time. Ground yourself with each small step. When your pelvis starts tucking, immediately move your feet closer to the table.

Activities in Balance

In some contemporary theater, dance, and sports, we see examples of the straight back, angled pelvis, dropped shoulders, and open, broad front emphasized in KENTRO guidelines. Certain activities are still practiced in smooth balance. The beauty of these gestures, once typical in highly industrialized countries such as France and the United States, can inspire us to shift our movements into resilient body expression.

Photographs of American actors and musicians from the early twentieth century illustrate the powerful presence and liveliness resulting from such expansive kinetics. These images convey restful posture free of muscular stress.

Today, actors, acrobats, singers, dancers, and musicians are often told to have an open body and upright bearing. Instructors who lack comfortably balanced motion, however, will find it difficult to offer optimal physical guidelines for these professionals. Comfortable balancing movements can broaden the effectiveness of the visualization or relaxation techniques taught in these settings.

We are used to hearing *posture* defined as correct or incorrect, as a thing unto itself, independent of activity. With physical centering, we can experience posture as fluid movement in action.

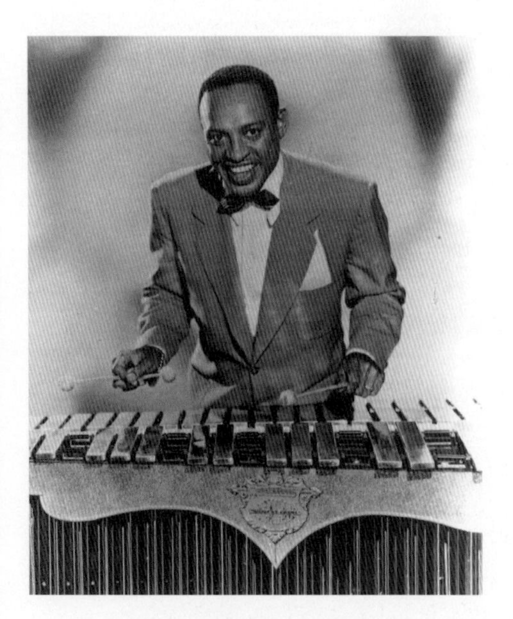

Lionel Hampton (c. 1940).
He bends comfortably from his hips, his back straightens, and his shoulders drop and relax.

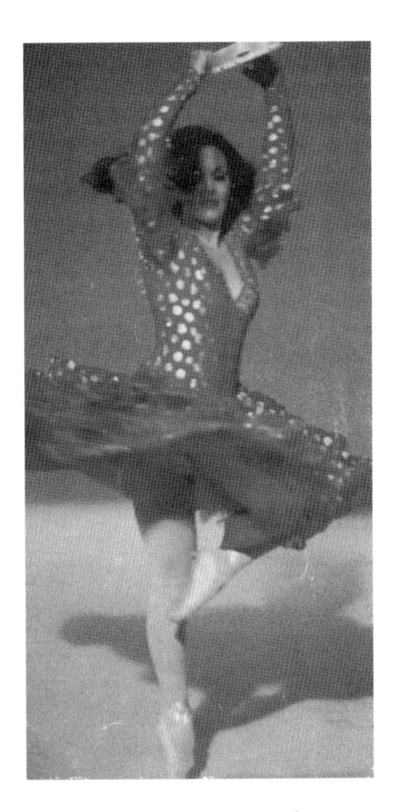

Cecile is dancing in smooth balance: Her leg is in line with her spine, her arms lift from her upper back muscles, the front of her body is broad and long, and her head and neck are relaxed. She illustrates that we can ground ourselves even when we wear heels or dance on our toes.

Marcel Marceau, the renowned French mime who has been performing his art for over fifty years, still moves with limberness. He continuously bends from the hips, gliding and walking with big strides. He does not push up his rib cage or force his shoulders back, yet his body appears youthful. Marceau communicates his ideas and feelings effectively through his slow, dance-like balancing movements.

While teaching Cecile, an American ballet choreographer and dancer who lives in Paris, I gained insight into the shift away from comfortable posture that occurred in highly industrialized countries during the 1930s. Cecile habitually pushed up her rib cage and forced back her shoulders. After she practiced KENTRO centering and balancing movements for remobilizing her body, Cecile's back straightened, her shoulders dropped without effort, her knees regained flexibility and her legs and spine showed a more vertical alignment. Cecile commented that practicing the KENTRO method reminded her of when she had studied ballet with two older Russian ballet masters many years ago in New York. They would exclaim, "No bones!" when Cecile lifted her chest in an effort to become upright, and "Legs under!" to indicate that the dancer's legs were not in stable placement.

Cecile understood "No bones" to mean the teachers did not want her lifting her rib cage, which made her ribs protrude and shortened her lower back. Nor did they want her tucking her pelvis and placing her legs (and weight balance) in front of her torso. By "legs under," they meant aligning her legs with the spine (placing the legs under the pelvis instead of out front). The ballet masters were trying to warn her against unnecessary effort and stiffness. With this in mind, Cecile especially appreciated KENTRO's specific, comprehensive movements and tools for equilibrating her whole body into smoother balance, which was typical of early twentieth century Russian ballet.

Contemporary acrobatic dancers, such as the U.S. Pilobolus dance group and the performers of the Canadian Eloize circus, have amazingly flexible pelvises and backs with an even groove along their spines, from the base of the neck to the small of the back. Likewise, some award-winning athletes (e.g., Carl Lewis, who for many years was

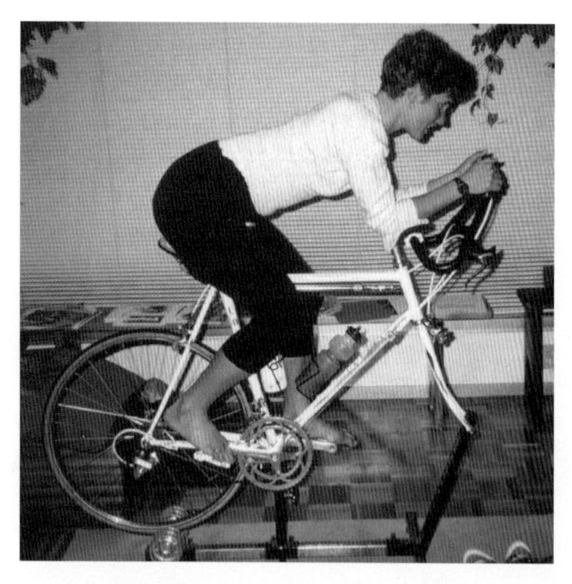

Triathlon medal winner Krista Whelan is demonstrating how to sit on a bicycle in smooth balance. Notice her grounded pelvis, straight back, and relaxed shoulders as she achieves toning in the upper back muscles. For ordinary bike riding she could slightly raise her torso so that her neck would be more in line with her spine.

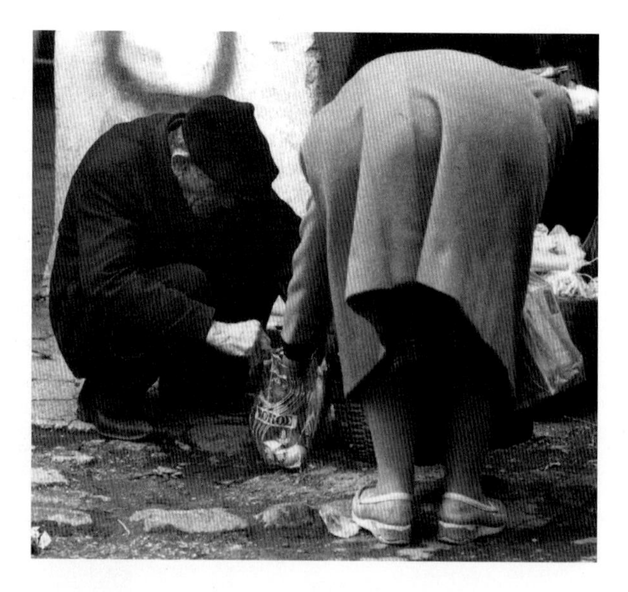

The Greek woman on the right is bending from her hips in smooth balance. The man on the left, who is squatting, only remained in that position for a few moments. Squatting (with more flexibility than this man) is a typical way of sitting for people in many ground-dwelling societies around the world. Since such people have squatted from childhood into adulthood, their pelvic and leg musculature is significantly more supple than the musculature of people who move with strained posture and are used to chairs. When our muscles lack elasticity, squatting tucks our pelvis, rounds our back, and places too much weight on the shoulders and delicate knees. We can avoid severe strain by practicing KENTRO *Bending to regain flexibility and strengthen the upper back, pelvis, and legs.*

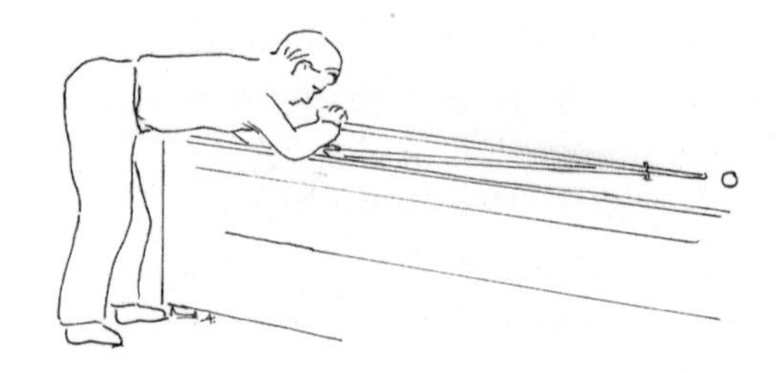

Notice the flexible pelvis and straight back of the billiards player. In this steady stance, his shoulders drop because he plays from his upper back muscles.

among the fastest runners in the world) embody grace, well-proportioned strength, and the resilient anterior pelvic slant in their movements.

I was delighted to watch an American dolphin trainer move with flowing, balancing gestures as he bent over to feed the dolphins. I also find top ice-skaters fascinating because of the fluid balance (slanted pelvis and straight back) and suppleness exhibited in their movements. At a Louisiana restaurant and dance hall, I noticed the relaxed uprightness and sensuous movements of certain couples dancing to traditional Cajun music. Their backs were long and straight, their shoulders down, and their pelvises mobile. Prizewinning pocket billiards players demonstrate similar ease when they bend from their hips, letting their back lengthen and straighten as their shoulders relax. They play from their upper back muscles and turn from the hips and feet to avoid twisting their backs. Strong martial arts Aikido instructors move with the grounding anterior placement of the pelvis.

No matter what we are engaged in—work, performance, or relaxation—we can prevent unnecessary injury, exhaustion, or strain by practicing KENTRO guidelines. Instead of pushing our bodies into peak performance of a sport or art we love, we may decrease effort and increase our muscular elasticity. Rather than getting frustrated when an enjoyable activity results in aches or pains from stressful movements, we can be energized by it. We can welcome harmonious movements into our dancing or playing of an instrument or sport.

After ten years of trying endless treatments and therapies for back pain, KENTRO Body Balancing worked like a 'miracle'. I had severe, chronic back pain, and sciatica, and no other form of therapy — chiropractic or stretches — had relieved me. My back pain and sciatica are now gone and my muscles and joints have become more flexible. This is the first time I am enjoying the journey.

—Krista Whelan (California), Second in 1993 World Triathlon Competitions

6. Sitting Up

PREPARATION. Place a wedge toward the front edge of a chair (see "The Art of Wedge-Making," p. *78*). Stand in front of the chair and practice Elemental Placement.

A. Place your hands on the top of your pelvic bones and bend forward with level hips. Ground your pelvis, let your back straighten, and center your legs. Allow at least a one-foot space between your knees.

B. Sit down on the edge of the wedge and bring up your torso slowly while your hands put downward pressure on your pelvis, to help you *sense your pelvis stretching away from your torso*. Your chin, rib cage, and shoulders stay down. Let your left thigh slant slightly diagonally downward. Have at least one of your thighs at a diagonal slant to place your pelvis and torso into comfortable weight distribution. You will be sitting farther forward on a chair than you are used to.
   Center your right leg as you extend it slightly out front. Your right leg will act as a counterweight so you can bend forward or turn your pelvis easily from your hips.

C. Repeat Elemental Placement. Place the palm of your left hand on the base of your rib cage and the palm of your right hand on your lower back, with your fingers on your spine. Bring your rib cage an inch or so forward, into the palm of your left hand. *Sense a softening in the diaphragm (base of the ribs) and a lengthening and straightening in your lower back muscles.* Relax your abdomen so it can stretch downward, toward your feet. Shift your torso and head with the Shoulder Roll and Goose Neck movements. *Sense broadening in your upper back; your shoulders will be down and your head farther back.*

D. Practice a Goose Neck. *Sense that your head is farther back.* Drop your hands onto your lap and stay in this gentle stretching for the duration of several yawns. Repeat A, B, and C as often as you like. In time, you will be comfortable sitting for several hours, as long as you integrate Elemental Placement stretches and vary Sitting Up with Sitting Back or some other KENTRO movements.

BENFITS: *Sitting Up* on a *wedge* realigns your body and relieves you of muscular strain because your torso and pelvis can be smoothly balanced and centered. Practicing guidelines for Sitting Up generates surprising upright comfort and mobility.

HELPFUL HINTS: Prevent sitting too far back on the wedge (which flattens it), tucking your pelvis, tightening your abdomen, arching your lower back, or curving your upper back (which pushes your shoulders and head forward). After following the A, B, and C guidelines, prevent "holding" yourself up; just relax. When you *feel* "pulling" aches in your back—from balancing releases of strained tissues, take a break by leaning forward (forearms crossed and onto your desk), or Sitting Back, or place yourself into the soothing Prayer (on the floor). Practice Sitting Up anywhere. The Prayer and Farmer's Rest are helpful before Sitting Up.

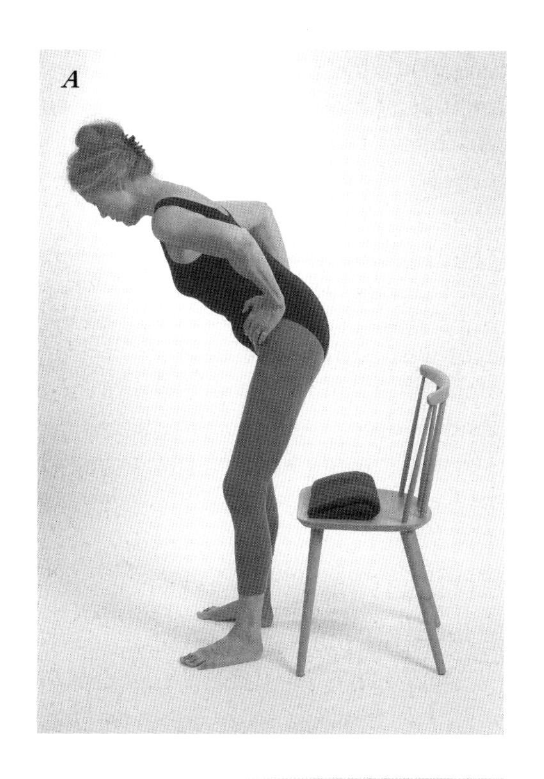

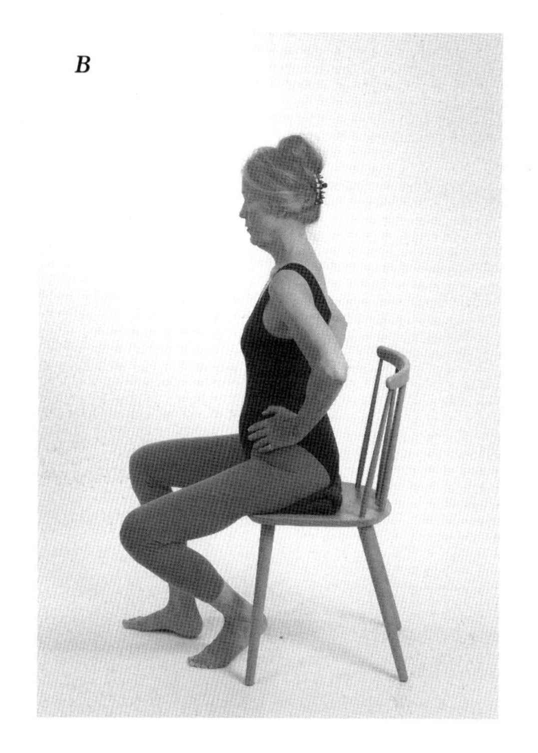

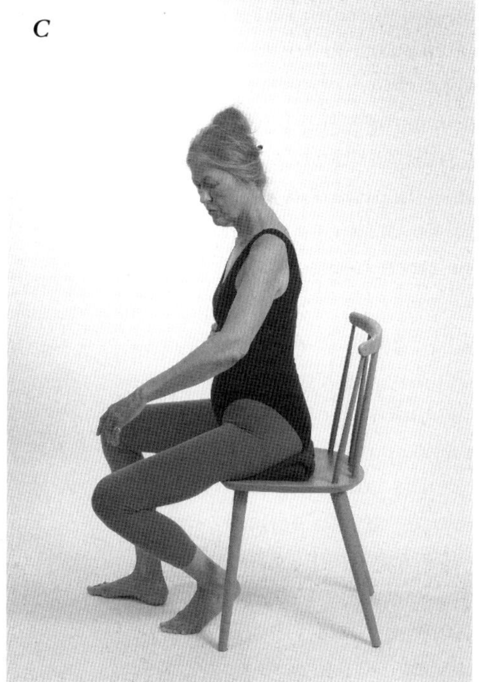

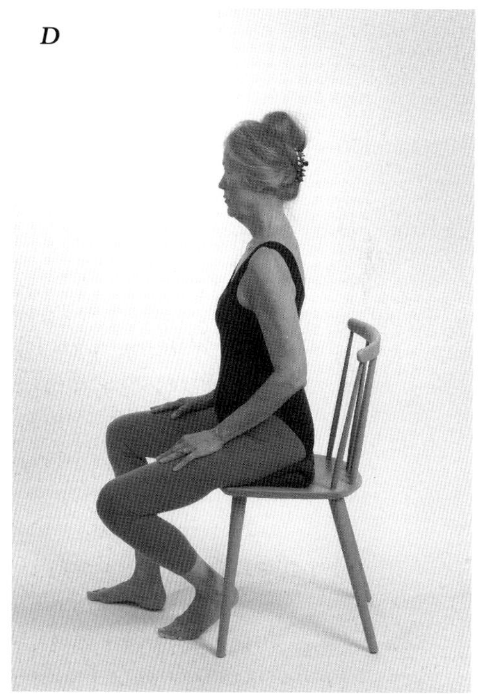

Sitting Up

VARIATIONS: Experience more comfortable Sitting Up when you sit on the downward sloping edge of a sofa or when you sit on a wedge placed on a stool. Try sitting on a table, as you do not need your feet on the ground for Grounding yourself because grounding happens in your pelvic area.

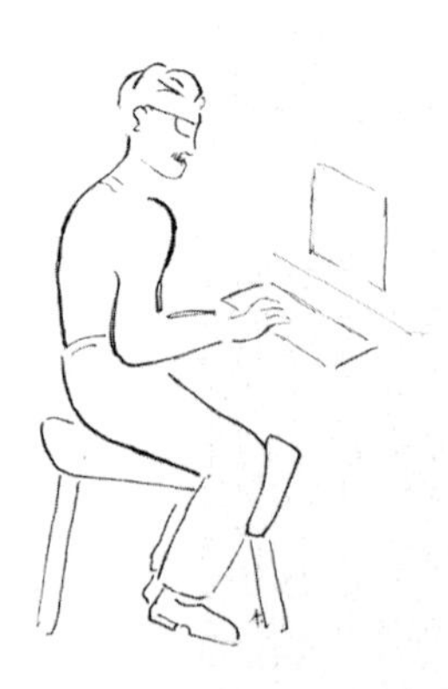

When we sit on this specialized chair with a tucked pelvis, there will be too much pressure (weight) on the knees.

Keep Your Furniture

Often, when we attend a meeting or visit a friend, we sit in a chair or recline on a sofa to *rest.* But if we move out of comfortable balance after sitting, instead of feeling rested, we will feel stiff after a short period of time. We experience aches and distress in our back, pelvis, neck, or shoulders. We might begin to think that it must be unhealthy for us to bend or sit for more than half an hour at a time, since these actions feel taxing, and even reclining can tire our back.

We are frequently told our furniture is to blame for our discomfort. Some of us buy costly orthopedic furniture or opt for plush easy chairs, surrounding ourselves with the "right" kind of furniture in hopes of soothing our aching bodies.

For many of us, sitting on specialized chairs with bent knees on a knee rest places too much pressure on the knees. We may actually sense strain on that delicate part of our bodies as well as on our backs. Nor do we find our ergonomic chairs all that helpful; we invariably have to get up and walk around, stretch, or lie down after a short period of sitting. The cushioned armchair causes us to tense and round our backs.

Fortunately, by simply *creating a shift* in how we bend, sit, or recline, we can move past such disappointment into increasingly fluid postural expression. As a result, we can find satisfaction in the everyday utility of both our new *and* old furniture. Such ease of movement allows us to experience furniture as *supportive:* our flexibility increases as we sit at our desk, bend over the kitchen counter, or stretch out in our favorite chair.

Practicing KENTRO Balancing guidelines enables us to sense how to sit or recline comfortably on any chair or sofa, as long as we allow Centering relaxation to happen.[1] We can type, paint, or play the piano without tiring. The key is to bend, sit, and recline while sensing expansion in the pelvis, lengthening (straightening) in the back, and harmonious weight distribution and release of stress throughout our body. We can keep our backs from stressful over-arching or over-curving by using soft, pliable fabric wedges or pillows to *fill in* concave areas on couches and chairs. We can feel vitalized, even while resting on a sofa.

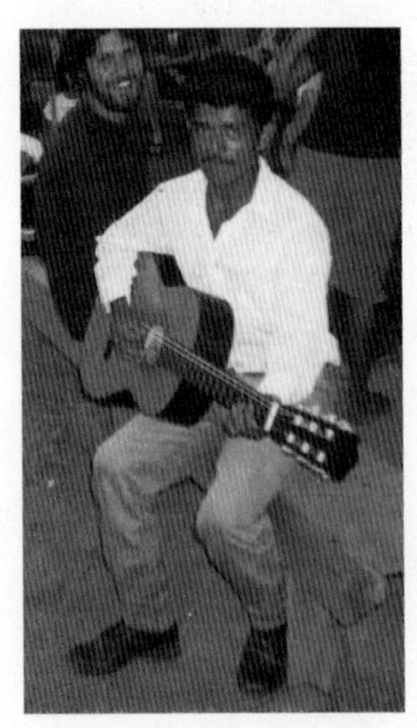

This Honduran musician sits comfortably on a bench, his shoulders down, his back straight, and his left thigh at a downward slant to ground his pelvis.

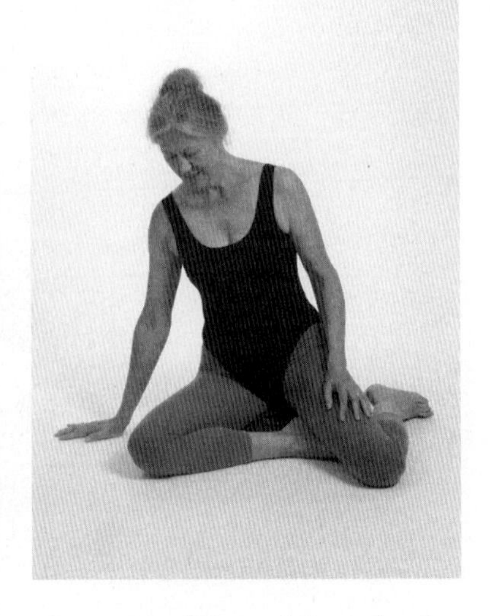

A variation of Sitting Up *on the edge of a wedge—on the floor.*

This photo shows Thomas Edison (c. 1893), sitting upright without effort; his pelvis and thighs slant, his back is straight, and his shoulders are relaxed.

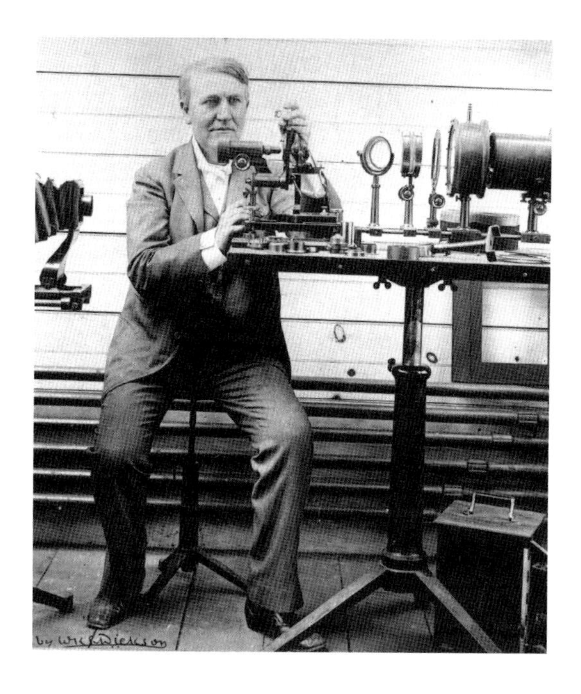

These balancing and centering feelings enable us to experience dramatic shifts in how we view ordinary furniture. All furniture becomes practical, offering convenient opportunities to tone and limber our bodies. A humble metal chair can serve as an at-home meditation center, a prop for stretching, or a dance school barre. Sensing resiliency as we bend, sit, and recline can dissolve the belief that we are being controlled by our furniture, thus generating an agreeable relationship with these familiar objects.

We see our old home or office chair—formerly "wrong" for us—with fresh, affectionate eyes. We are more than at ease in it; we can take pleasure in its shape, history, and craftsmanship. Instead of being discarded, the old chair becomes a most special chair because it has also become a helpful chair. Seats at the cinema or restaurant, and even our car seat, can become quiet allies in extending our leisure and relaxation.

I have had lordosis (swayback) and hip dysplasia since childhood. I studied Iyengar yoga for ten years and I was contemplating quitting my job because my body ached so much at the end of the day from sitting at a computer. After studying KENTRO for the past six months, I can sit comfortably with ease for as long as necessary. The simple KENTRO guidelines give immediate results. My body changed right away, and my activities are more efficient, relaxed, and fun.
—Jeanne Benioff, Software Consultant and Singer (California)

7. Sitting Back

PREPARATION. Stand in front of a chair and place a thin rectangular pillow or soft fabric even wedge (around 6–8 inches high, 1 inch thick, and 10 inches long) on the floor nearby. Practice Elemental Placement.

A. With your hands on your pelvic bones for level hips, relax your pelvis and bend forward. Sit down, bend forward, pick up the wedge, and place it on your lap.

B. Place the inside of your left hand onto your diaphragm; let this muscle soften to realign your ribcage into relaxed placement. You may think that you have rounded your lower back, but by placing your right hand on your lower back, you will *sense a straighter, more even groove*.

C. You are now ready to recline back from your hips. Keep your left hand on your diaphragm (to help you focus on keeping the rib cage down), and your right hand on your lower back (to focus on straightening it). Bend back very slowly so you can *sense your torso lengthening.* Pick up the wedge with your right hand and place it so that, as you recline, it will be at the base of the shoulder blades (always place the wedge above your sacrum). As you place your upper back onto the wedge, your shoulders will be momentarily out front.

D. Drop as much bodily weight as possible from your upper back onto the wedge, a little like "gluing" your heart area onto the wedge. This allows you to be as "weightless" and relaxed as possible, with your ribs down. *Sense your upper back straighten and your shoulders relax*. Notice that your upper torso *feels more open and broad*. Let your neck be in line with your spine. Momentarily, place the inside of a hand onto your lower back to reassure you that there is no arching. Also, place both your hands on your shoulder blade muscles and gently "lift" up your upper back to extend it even more and "glue" it on the wedge. Your upper back will straighten with the Shoulder Roll. Stay in this placement as long as you *feel comfortable*.

BENEFITS: *Sitting Back* in centered balance will allow you to be comfortable enough to take a nap or meditate over a long period of time. Placing the wedge in your upper back fosters a beginning of easy, gentle, well-supported bending backward. There is no reason to only sit upright; Sitting Back, along with leaning forward into the Farmer's Rest results in a variety of releasing stretches for your back. With a wedge, you can sit back in relaxation on any seating that has a back. An even wedge can "straighten" the indented back of a seat or sofa, allowing your back to straighten without effort and for you to be in Elemental Placement.

HELPFUL HINTS: You do not need a wedge for your pelvis because weight is mostly assimilated by your upper back. How far back you place your pelvis on a seat for *Sitting Back* depends on the angle of the back of the chair. If it slants back, you can place your pelvis toward the back; if the chair is straight-backed, scoot your pelvis farther up front so that your weight is distributed through your upper back. When the wedge for your upper back is too thick, it will round your back and bring your shoulders out front.

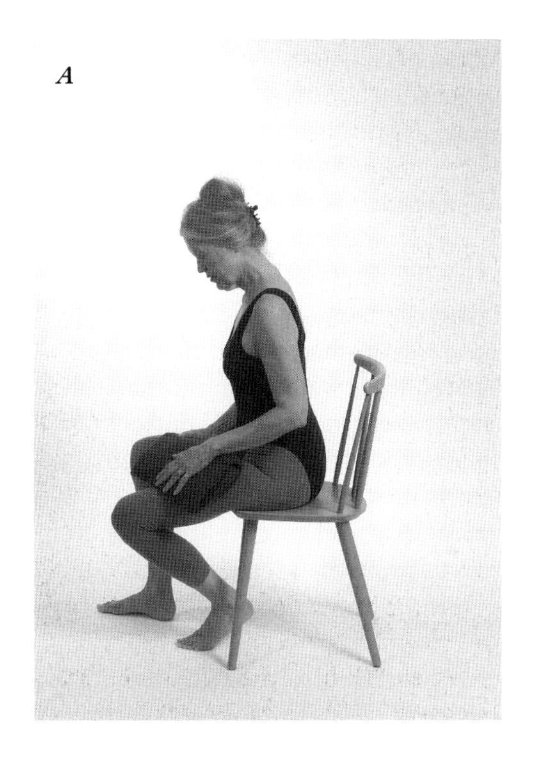

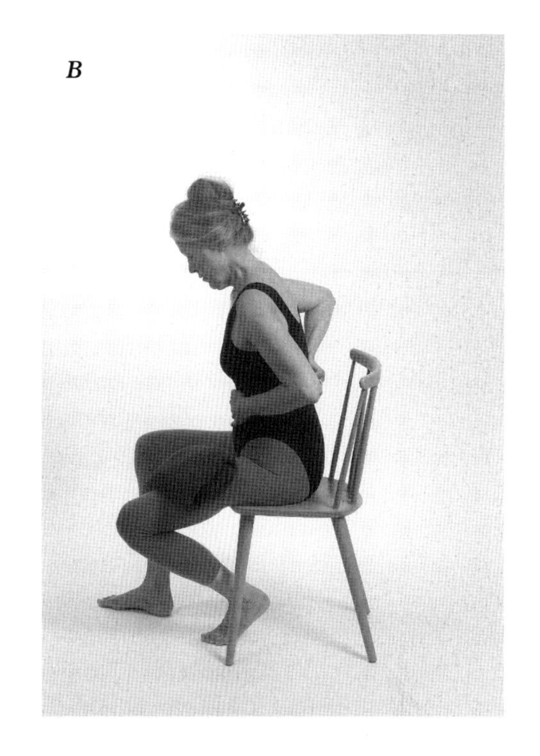

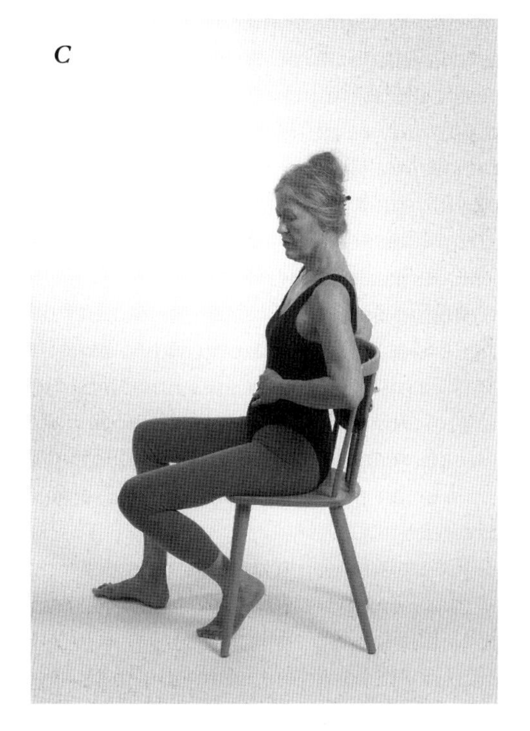

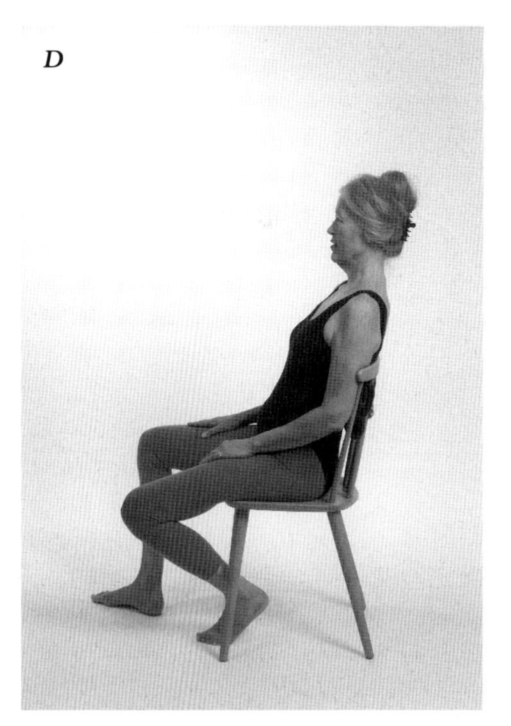

SITTING BACK

Placing the wedge too far down your back will cause arching in your lower back. Prevent tucking your pelvis, arching your back, or pushing back your shoulders. Practice Bending Forward and Farmer's Rest before and after Sitting Back.

VARIATIONS: Try out *Sitting Back* in the car, on the sofa, in an armchair, and in bed.

The Art of Wedge-Making

Conventional, manufactured foam wedges are designed to support "weak" areas, such as the neck, back, and pelvis. However, foam wedges have a fixed form, which generally accommodates a rounded back, arched neck, and tucked buttocks (with hopes that sitting will be more "bearable"). Thus, these wedges act as a crutch and may fix the body into further compensations. Some foam models are fabricated with specific arching, which puts pressure on the lower back or neck, augmenting the arching already present in that area; other models extend over the sacral area, increasing pelvic tucking. Because these wedges "maintain" uncomfortable posture, tissues cannot lengthen and expand into soothing balance.

In contrast, homemade wedges for Kentro practice are adaptable and can be molded to the height and bodily shape of the user, in concert with the size and shape of the furniture. Every time we sit or recline is an occasion for us to sense afresh the difference between constrained postural placement and flowing Elementary Placement. The more we experience physical flexibility, the more we can perceive how to place our flexible wedges so that they enhance our mobility.

Sitting or reclining can generate powerful shifts into fluid posture, as long as we employ a piece of soft fabric or a sweater, folded into a "wedge" for Elemental Placement of our bodies . Use of such informal wedges allows us to relax in saggy sofas or uncomfortable seats—as long as we know how to shape and place these wedges for our own comfort. They make the simple act of sitting up at a desk, piano, or dining table, or reclining on a sofa or deck chair, an enjoyable experience. The back straightens easily, shoulders and neck release strain, the upper back muscles are exercised, the front broadens, and the pelvis is freed, regardless of our placement or the shape of the furniture. We can place ourselves into lasting comfort, free of muscular effort.

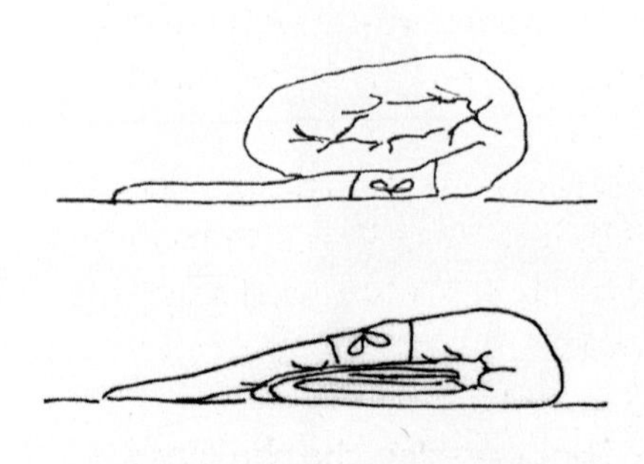

(Top) Loosely fold your wedge fabric, leaving about six inches of the fabric flattened out.

(Bottom) Turn over your half-made wedge, and smooth down only the thin edge that you will sit on.

Without an adaptable wedge, muscles in our pelvis, back, and shoulders easily tighten or weaken into compensatory function. When we try to relax, our buttocks tuck, our backs round, our shoulders droop, and we tire, even while sitting on specially cushioned, ergonomic seats.

Malleable wedges connote an aesthetic approach to postural expression: we develop our sensibilities to hand-shape

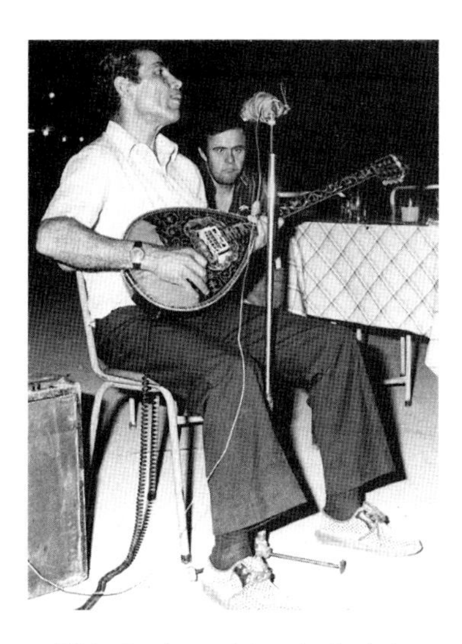

This Greek musician sits back in comfortable balance: His back is straight and his arm is positioned so his fingers play from the heart area-upper back muscles.

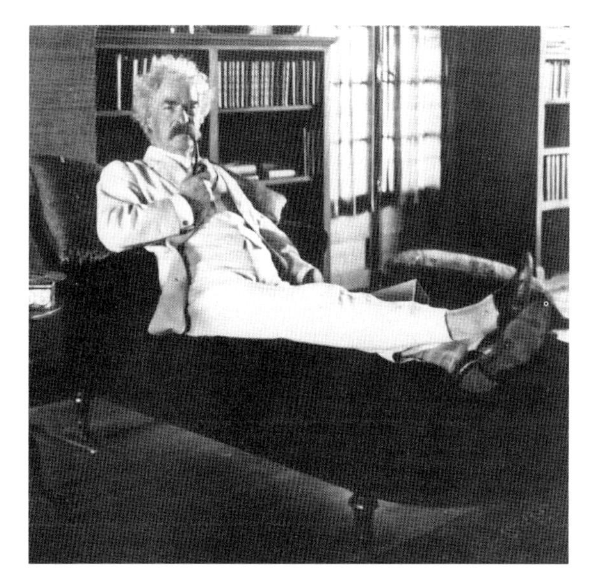

In this photo of Mark Twain, notice how he bends comfortably from the hips to sit back. His back is long and his shoulders are dropped.

them as we wish and in accord with the situation. The root of the word "art" is "to join, fit together," and its principal meaning is "the ability to make things; creativeness."

A personally shaped wedge harmoniously joins the sitter to the seat.

Practical, hand-made wedges of our own creation broaden our sense of smooth balance and amplify our feelings of centered relaxation, while we luxuriate in bending, turning, or resting on seats, sofas, and floors with sinuous, supple gestures.

Reshapeable wedges can be made out of a small bed or sofa pillow, sweater, jacket, cut-up blanket, sweatshirt, or soft fabric (like fleece). When we carry extra clothing with us, such as a jacket or shawl, they can instantly be converted into an efficient wedge. Over time, we will become familiar with the appropriate texture, thickness, and softness of fabric to create appropriate wedges for various areas of our body.

For sitting upright, form the front part of the wedge thinner than the back part and place the wedge close to the front edge of the seat (especially if the seat slants down in the back as shown in Sitting Up, page 72). This situates the pelvis at a balanced angle. Most of the weight is absorbed by this main center, allowing the trunk to be easily supported by the pelvis. The pelvic muscles then relax and spread away from the torso, which prevents over-compression or over-stretching of the back muscles; the chest and whole front broaden, and the shoulders go down.

If the hips are uneven due to injury or tight tissues, the wedge can be slightly thicker (in the back) under the lower hip to allow equal pressure and stretching in both hip and sacral muscles. When the lower back feels severely compressed, lessening the

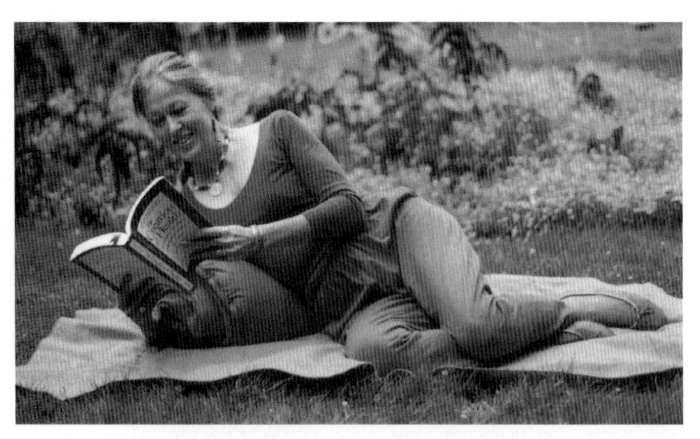

The fleece wedge under my arm and torso allows comfortable placement: The weight is off my shoulders, my back straightens, and my pelvis is relaxed.

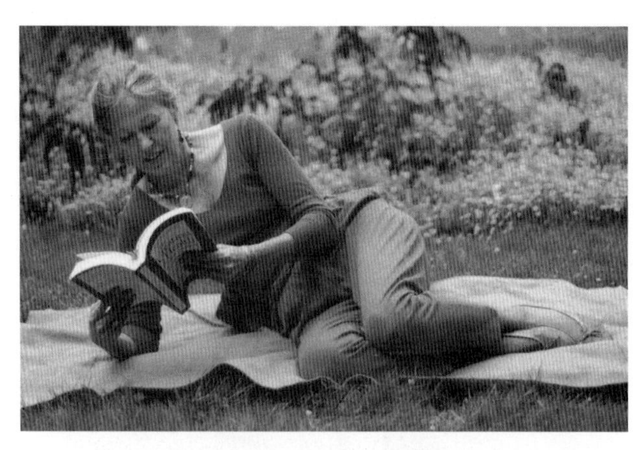

In this uncomfortable placement, my shoulders strain, my back rounds, and my pelvis tightens.

(Left) We can sit back comfortably in any folding chair or airplane by placing a thin, flat wedge in our upper back. A thin wedge placed at the base of the shoulder blades allows my shoulders to relax and my back to straighten.

(Right) Without a wedge, my shoulders are out in front because my back is rounded and the entire front of my body is congested, shortened. The result is overall uncomfortable placement.

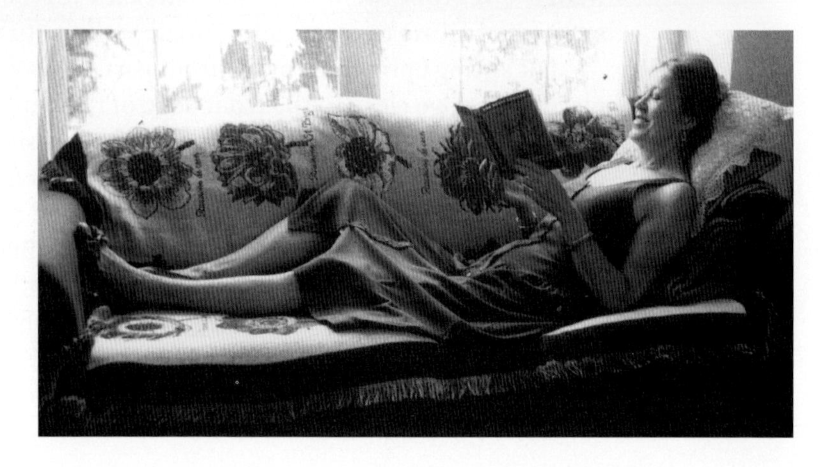

The pyramid-shaped wedge made with two pillows and a small blanket allows comfortable placement: My back is straight, my neck and shoulders are relaxed, and there is no muscular strain in my abdomen or pelvis. My upper back and upper arm muscles will benefit with slight toning while I hold up the book.

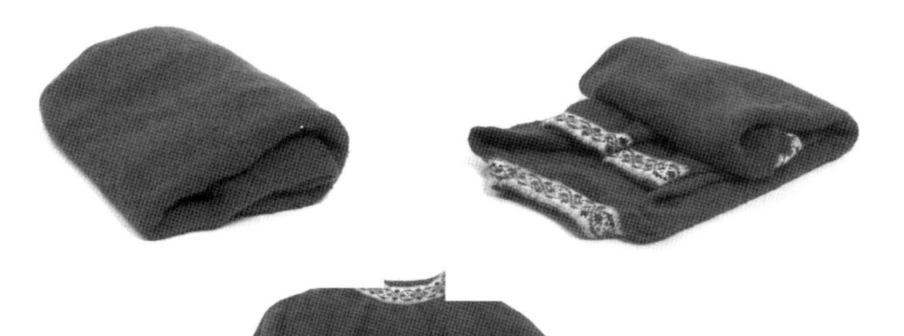

(Top left). This is the wedge used throughout the main thirty-three KENTRO movements.
(Top right). Unfolding the wedge.
(Bottom). And voila, a soft Peruvian sweater.

thickness of the wedge allows a smoother straightening in the lower back. If the pelvis is especially tucked and the sacral area flattened, thickening the wedge will gently reshape the natural arch between the first sacral and fourth and fifth lumbar vertebrae.

When we desire to lean back in a seat, the fabric is removed, flattened, shaped into a narrow rectangular wedge, and placed on the upper backside of the chair as shown in Sitting Back, page . It should be thick enough to fill in the concave indenture of the chair, but wide enough to span the base of the shoulder blades and the upper portion of the lower back. This allows the spine to lengthen evenly along the back of the chair, leaving space for the shoulders to relax. Naturally, a taller person needs a slightly broader wedge than a shorter person. Likewise, the wedge is adjusted according to the curvature of the sitter's upper back. Then there is space for the shoulders to go down and for the upper and lower back to straighten.

When reclining on a couch, bed, floor, or the ground, several pillows or a blanket create a wedge substantial and long enough to easily straighten the back. Reclining on one side of the body is comfortable when the wedge is placed under the shoulder and upper arm to allow the back to lengthen. As long as the wedge is soft, yet thick and firm, it will take as much weight as possible off the shoulders, neck, and back.

Our lives improve when we live and travel with these simple fabric wedges. An all-day car trip no longer tires our back if we place a wedge under our shoulder blades; this fills in the curvature of the car seat, enabling our back to straighten and our shoulders to relax. It is easier to relax in the dentist's chair when we place a very thin, flat wedge under our shoulder blades, so our back, neck, head, and shoulder muscles are at ease. We can avoid a stiff neck and aching in our back from a long airplane trip by stacking two airplane pillows (doubled) behind the shoulder blades. Reading a book in bed or on a sofa for hours at a time can be relaxing when our back stretches out onto a thick pyramid-wedge of pillows or blankets. Using pliable wedges promotes resiliency.

By using a pliable wedge in all sitting and reclining situations, we can center and balance ourselves into pleasurable comfort while we are active or at rest.

8. Tikanis

PREPARATION. *Sit up*, placing yourself on the edge of a pliable wedge. Practice Elemental Placement.

A. Place your elbows close to the side of your body. Relax your abdomen and pelvis. Keep your shoulders down and your elbows close to your body. Slowly open your forearms outward combined with the Goose Neck. Let your upper back (shoulder blade area) muscles contract slightly, until there is two to three feet of space between your hands.

B. *You have opened your arms wide enough* as soon as you have an odd *sensation of your shoulder blades "colliding." You are in the full stretch.* Your shoulder blades do not "collide"; small inter-shoulder blade muscles simply are functioning again. Stay in the stretch long enough to say to yourself "Tikanis?" (Greek for "how are you"). *Sense significant expansiveness—flattening and broadening in your upper back.* Stay in this stretch for the duration of a yawn.

C. Come out of the stretch slowly. Let your neck and head move upward and *slightly* backward. Let your forearms rest on your lap, slightly farther back than before. You will continue to *sense lengthening and straightening in your upper back and neck, your shoulders will be more relaxed, and your head will feel more comfortably aligned.* Your body may seem more peaceful. Repeat the *Tikanis* several times, with short rests in between.

BENEFITS: The *Tikanis* generates unique multi-directional stretching in your upper back; it realigns, relaxes, and tones your upper back and shoulders. This gentle movement effectively prevents and alleviates stress and strain in your upper back, shoulders, and neck.

HELPFUL HINTS: Prevent raising your ribs, arching your lower back, or pushing your shoulders back (tightening shoulder and shoulder blade area muscles). Practice Tikanis before typing, drawing, and lifting. Practice Looking for Elbow Room, and Four Directions before Tikanis.

VARIATIONS: Try Tikanis while you are lying on your back. In this placement, the Goose Neck movement is a strong toning stretch for the muscles on the back of your neck, so only raise your head about an inch off your pillow, and only momentarily (to be gentle to your neck muscles).

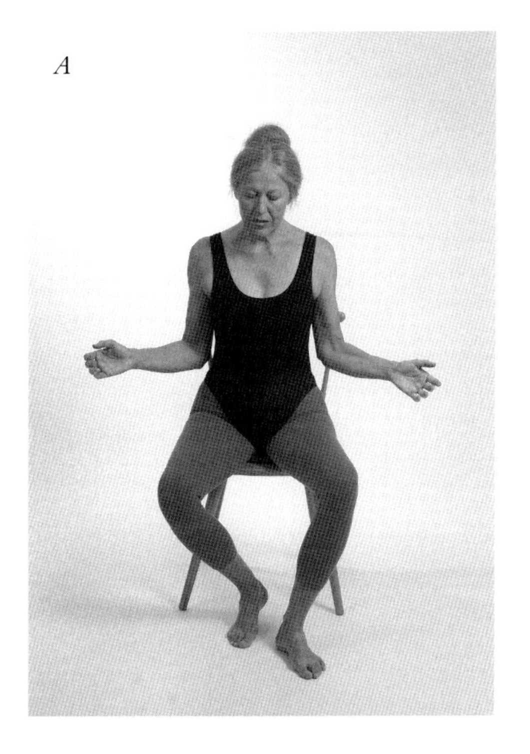
A

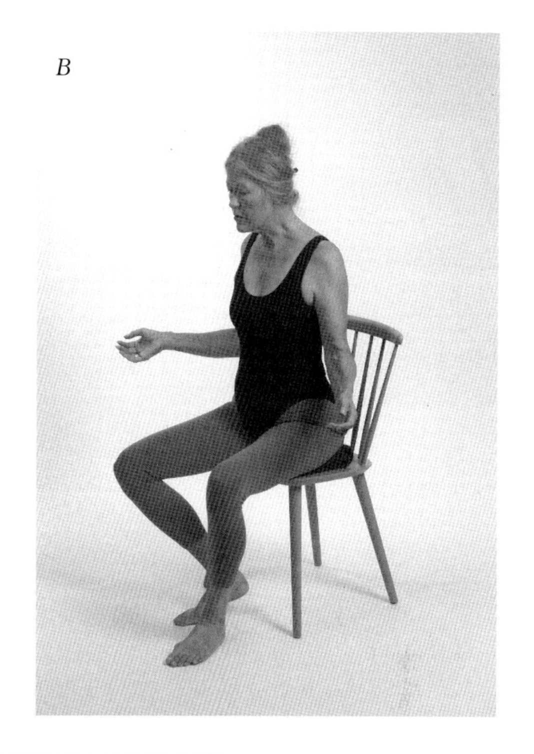
B

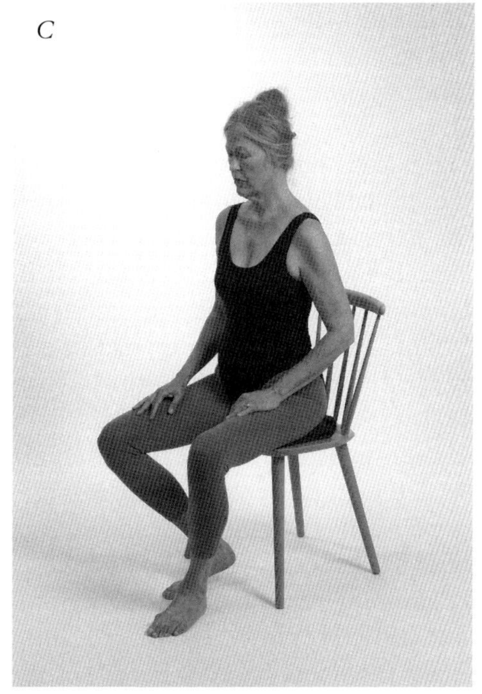
C

Tikanis

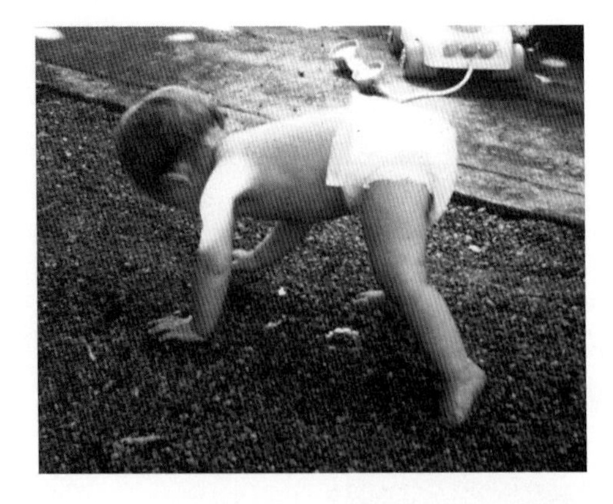

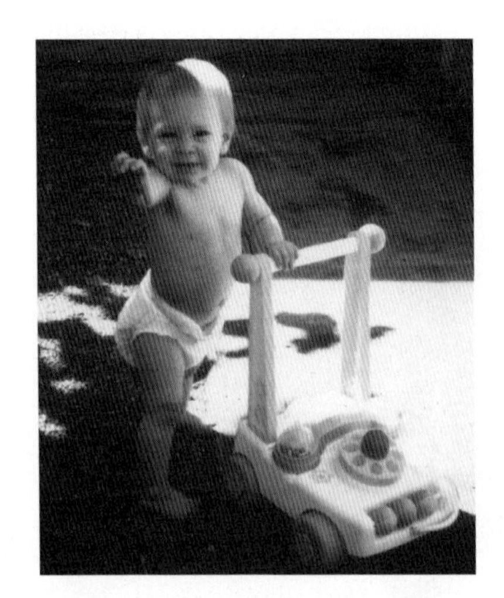

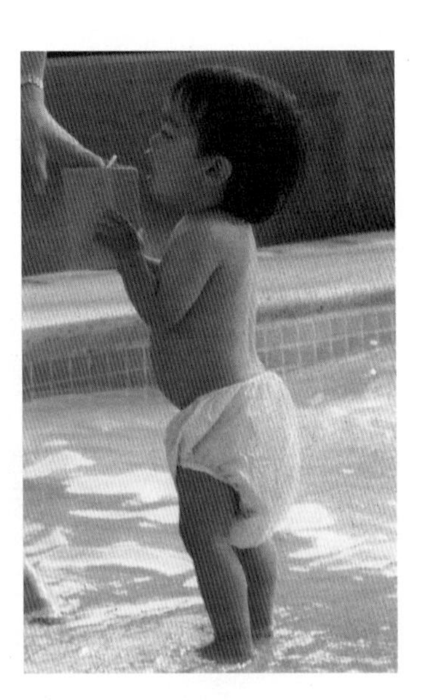

(Above left).
This American infant senses that most of her bodily weight is easily assimilated in her sacral/ hip area. She relaxes her shoulders, moves her arms from her upper back muscles, and keeps her back straight.

(Above center).
She stays in comfortable placement while she raises her arm, without raising her rib cage or arching her back.

(Above right). This American toddler senses smooth balance. His back is straight, his legs align with his spine, and his pelvis is at its natural angle.

KENTRO and Children

The posture of small children provides a wellspring of inspiration for KENTRO practice. Their pliable little bodies reflect the innate resiliency common to all of us when we were young.

As babies we were in constant motion, stretching and exercising our arms, legs, back, and neck. When we see infants expanding their whole body, accompanied by gleeful sounds and smiles, we are moved by their physical joy, and momentarily connected to their dance we respond pleasurably to the rippling life force in their movements. The artist at our core loves fluidity.

The mobility found in infants is amplified in small children. Children live in their bodies. They feel their way into the experience of each activity. They trust their sense of equilibrium as they explore a myriad of gestures. Children have a natural desire to move, and they love full-bodied motion. They shape their reality through fine sensing and keen self-expression.

Utterly sensuous and supple, children are energy in motion. Their kinetics are vital because they fully perceive their world. They find natural stability and poise by trying out physical attitudes again and again, playfully and without effort, until they feel secure and grounded in their bodies. We see them bending naturally from the hips and lifting or doing actions from their upper back muscles. They have not yet heard about "correct" bodily placement and carriage; they do not tuck or tighten their pelvis or force their shoulders back. Whenever they briefly round their shoulders, they do not loose the *even groove* throughout their back because they are so resilient. Although their heads are quite heavy in relation to their bodies (similar to an adult carrying a heavy basket on his or her head), they unconsciously master centered ease.

The expansive gesture of this Greek boy with a straight back, relaxed shoulders, and grounded pelvis is similar to the KENTRO *Tikanis movement.*

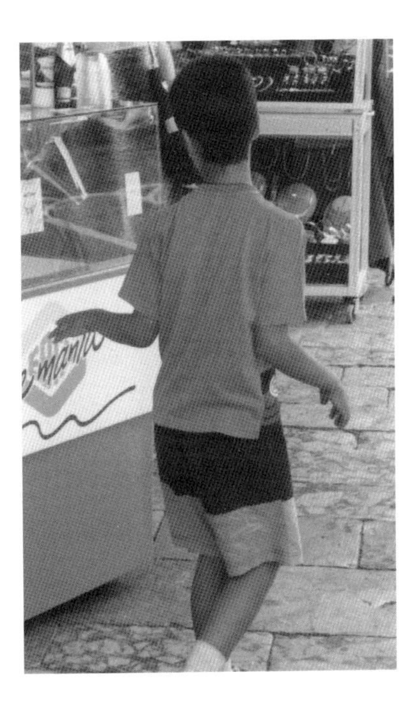

Practicing KENTRO guidelines encourages a fresh approach to our actions, an approach rooted in sensing our way into energizing, agreeable bearing. The guidelines allow us to discern relaxation and toning in our muscles. As we center and balance ourselves, we begin to regain the malleability of our early years.

It is likely that children are influenced by the postural habits of the adults around them. We can often see three- and four-year-olds begin to tuck their pelvises and curve their backs if they see adults doing so to "relax." They tense their muscles when a parent or teacher warns them, "hold in your belly," "lift your chest," or "your buttocks stick out too much." In time, the child's free movement is affected.

As adults, tightening our musculature to conform to intellectual notions of an attractive body shape curtails our flexibility. Our dynamic motion and our sensory discernment may decrease. Perhaps we only are in touch with our bodies when we are active: running, dancing, or exercising. We may believe we have to control our movements, so we continue to push ourselves into uncomfortable postures.

Supple balance can renew the liveliness we experienced as toddlers. We are designed so that our bodies can move us into delightful ease all day long. This, surely, is grace.

9. Leg Rotation

PREPARATION. Place a mat or blanket on the floor and lie down on your back, keeping your knees bent. Shift your body into Elemental Placement.

A. Allow around a foot of space between your knees so that your hips and entire pelvis can be in balanced comfort. Place the palms of your hands on the crests of the pelvis. Level your hips by *sensing* even pelvic crests and equal amounts of pressure (weight) under both buttocks muscles.
B. Relax your abdominal muscles but contract your left buttock just slightly to raise your left bent leg—one foot straight up off the floor toward your left shoulder as preparation for the rotation itself.
C. With your right hand putting pressure on the right side of the pelvis (so it stays in symmetry), let your left thigh rotate slowly outward (less than a foot) before it goes downward (in guideline D). *Sense toning in your right buttocks and abdomen (without any tightening of these muscles on your part).* In fact, you will *sense abdominal, buttocks, and thigh muscles being toned.*
D. When your left leg rotates downward, you complete a half-circle movement. Set your foot down, keeping one foot-space between the knees. Stay in the Leg Rotation original position the duration of a yawn. After one rotation, rest a moment before you rotate your leg again, so that your body can make fine readjustments. Alternate sides. Start with two rotations on each leg. In time, you can build up to six rotations for each leg in one session.

BENEFITS: The *Leg Rotation* is a highly effective, basic *relaxing* and *toning* KENTRO movement. This rotational movement creates releases throughout your pelvis and thighs. Likewise, important pelvic and thigh muscles are stretched and can regain efficient functioning.

HELPFUL HINTS: Prevent tightening your abdomen, which over-stretches your buttock muscles, and raising your leg from tightened abdominal muscles or arched (shortened) lower back muscles. Initiate the Leg Rotation from your buttock muscles, without any goal of rotating your inner thighs as far outward as possible (which might tighten your lower back). Practice Little Moon and Pelvic Rock after the Leg Rotation.

VARIATIONS: If you are recuperating from a hip/sacral injury, practice an effective, "passive" leg rotation by simply giving your left heel the "message" to lift off the ground without *actually* raising it (making the outward half-circle rotational movement with your foot staying on the ground). Increase toning of your abdominal, pelvic, and thigh muscles, with more extension (straightening) in your leg. Let your ankle "draw" a horizontally inclined "figure eight" configuration.

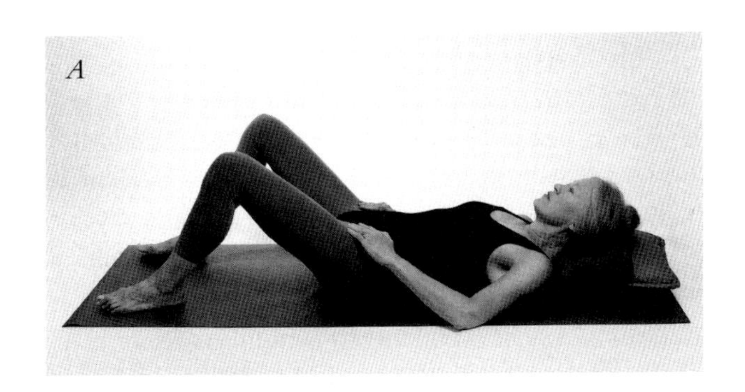

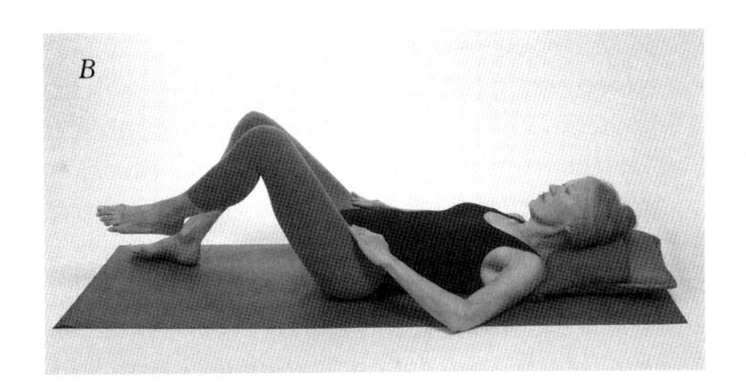

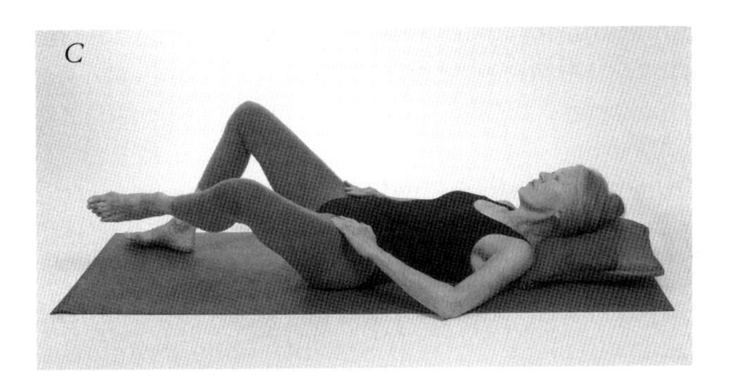

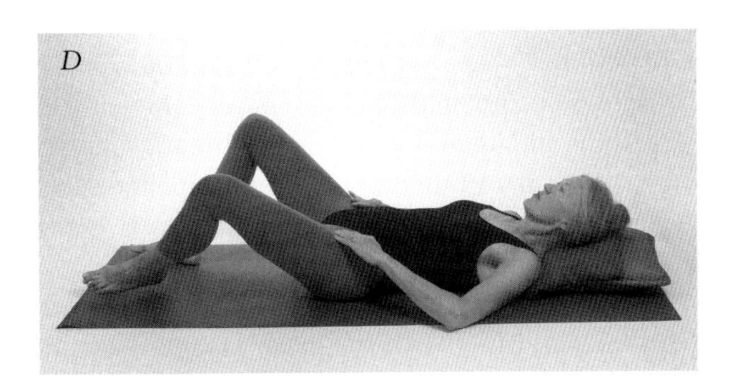

Leg Rotation

KENTRO and Meditation

Centering movements provide the basis for a physically fluid meditative experience; they reflect a restful approach to our body, allowing it to stretch, both metaphorically and physically, between earth and sky (see Vignette 28, Living Between Heaven and Earth, p. 182). In this process, there is no need for commands—no "chest out," "belly in," "shoulders back"—because there is no notion of idealized posture.

Comfortable balance involves minimal effort; practicing small postural shifts generates physical suppleness. When our body is at ease, we can meditate anywhere, anytime, during ordinary actions and rest. However, people who are unfamiliar with sensing *comfort* tend to associate this word with passivity and a lack of drive or stamina. As a result, we accept discomfort and stiffness as normal. Even sitting down quietly is a tiring experience when we do not have clear guidelines for sensing relaxation.

Some books on meditation indicate that comfort will come in time; that the pains we feel in the back, ankles, or shoulders are from a resistance to letting go of stress, or that the meditation itself will help us transcend the pain if we detach ourselves from our bodily sensations. But, these suggestions are difficult to follow where we have strained bearing.

There are a variety of wonderful mindful practices that focus on awareness and inner tranquility. We can choose meditations based on sounds, images, or breath to help connect with our inner life. Yet when we experience pain or feel ill-at-ease during a meditation, our focus strays easily and often. Most practices encourage us to sit upright and seek a firm yet agreeable seat, but rarely are we given clear recommendations for such sitting.

I learned about supple sitting a few years before I started teaching KENTRO Body Balance. My husband had encouraged me to learn Transcendental Meditation (TM). Although I enjoyed the instruction and felt motivated to practice, I felt a lot of physical distress during my sitting, which I found distracting. By using a soft fabric wedge, I learned how to sit without any muscular "holding," without struggle. Taking time to seat myself as cozily as possible made an enormous difference in the quality of my practice. I found myself spending less time formally meditating and more time mildly shifting my body so it could continuously let go of strain during the sittings.

After a few years, placing myself into enjoyable balance became such a satisfying approach to becoming calmer and more energized, *sitting itself became my full meditation.* In a natural, unplanned way, I added breath, images, and prayer to my daily habit of sitting; physical and mental releases happened gently. And some of my most special meditation experiences occurred while I was sitting with my eyes closed in a Paris subway or while dancing in Greece.

When I was invited to teach a workshop on Sitting at Jikoji, a Zen center in Northern California, I met with the guest Japanese Zen master, Kobin. I was heartened by similarities between Zen philosophy and KENTRO guidelines: a quiet, inner focus; restfulness on all levels; and the quality of being in the present moment. Kobin's emphasis on a soft, strong *hara*—Japanese for the belly, physical center, and essence

This sitting position can be comfortable for a long period of time, as long as we alternate sides by raising the left knee off the ground (and dropping the right knee onto the ground). The wedge allows me to ground my pelvis, keep my back straight, and relax my shoulders. The placement of the right leg is similar to a passive Leg Rotation *movement. Japanese Zen Master Kobin encouraged me to teach this approach to relaxed sitting meditation.*

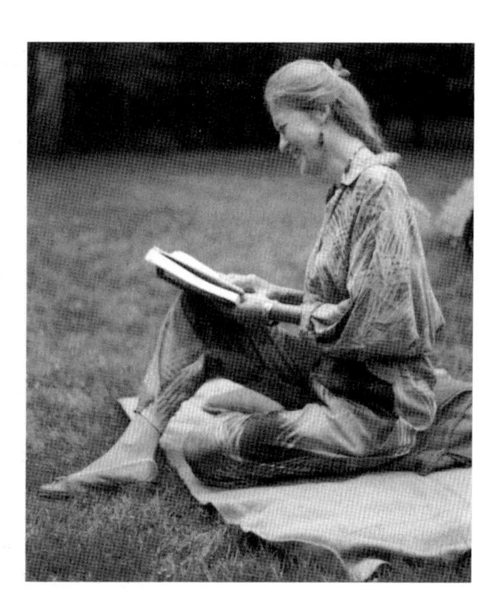

of our mysterious being—resonates with the KENTRO focus on allowing our belly and pelvis to relax (and stretch downward) during centered sitting.

I showed Kobin a limbering approach to sitting on a low stool or pillow, with one knee bent on the floor and the other knee bent out in front. With the deftness of a master, Kobin immediately tried out this manner of sitting and felt the relief it allowed. He asked me to teach this unconventional way of sitting to the participants, as he had noticed much unrest in their customary placement. Kobin himself sat upright, light as a feather, perhaps similar to the way his ancestors sat in balance many generations ago.

I was grateful I could offer guidelines to help the meditators integrate flexibility in their shoulders, back, and hips with the flow of their meditation. I showed each person how to clearly feel the difference between a taut belly and a toned belly, and how to sit upright by snugly resting within themselves while their torso rested on their pelvis. Once the students felt more at ease in their sitting, with relaxed back, shoulders, neck, and legs, they were on their way to alert calmness.

The word *meditation* has at its base *med*, which means "to measure, consider, reflect."We can infuse this definition with perceptive sensing and feeling, bringing physicality into meditation. We caringly *sense, consider,* compare, choose, and practice specific movements for more ease; we *reflect* centeredness in every balanced action. In this way, mindfulness expands into "bodyfulness." Activities like archery, cooking, and typing all can feel equal in flow, beauty, and fullness: we hold the bow and arrow, chop the leeks, and write our essay with a straight, strong back, relaxed shoulders, and resilient pelvis.

Practicing KENTRO movements with such affectionate attention allows us to relax physically and psychologically into a soothing visit with our creative core. Our thoughts, gestures, and activities can be imbued with peaceful, sensuous experience.

10. Boat

PREPARATION. Place a mat on the floor (or use a thick, soft carpet). Lie down on your back with your knees bent and practice Elemental Placement.

A. Raise your torso, bend your elbows, and extend your arms out behind you; keep at least one foot-space between your knees. Relax your belly and shoulders.
   Keep your shoulders down, allow around two feet of space between your hands, and spread your fingers out behind you or toward the side of your body. *Ground* your pelvis by relaxing your abdomen and buttocks—focus on *those muscles stretching away from your torso.* Notice pressure (weight) on the base of the buttocks, *the ischial tuberosities.* Let your abdomen stretch downward, toward the ground.

B. While relaxing your abdomen, slowly bend farther back from the small of your back, let your hands move slightly farther back until you sense expansion in your pelvis and lengthening in your back. *Sense a slight "pulling" toning sensation in the muscles at the back of your neck. Feel extension and expansion in your back and pelvis and relaxation in your shoulders and abdomen.*
   Keeping your hips level and your abdomen relaxed, contract your left buttocks for the duration of a few yawns. "Tell" your left heel to lift off the floor *without actually doing so.* You will sense *various pelvic and abdominal muscles being activated—toned, even though you did not start out by tightening the abdominal muscles! Also detect toning in the thighs.* Rest a moment. As with all KENTRO toning stretches, the restful interval between stretches should be longer than the duration of the actual stretch itself so your body can do small releasing readjustments. Alternate sides.
   You can also "lift" both heels off the floor (*without actually lifting them*) while you keep on relaxing your abdomen and lengthening your back.

C. Relax your entire body. Unless you have a hip injury, actually lift your left foot about half an inch to an inch off the ground.
   Alternate sides. You can start out with a few stretches on each leg and, after a few months, stretch seven times at one sitting.

BENEFITS: The *Boat* is an amazing strengthener for all pelvic core, thigh, lower back, and neck muscles. This movement is helpful for realigning your pelvis/thighs into comfortable articulation, and it also energizes your entire body.

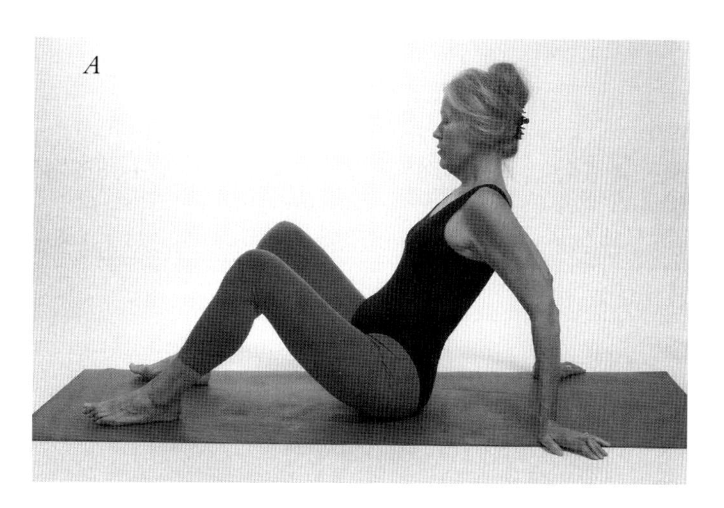

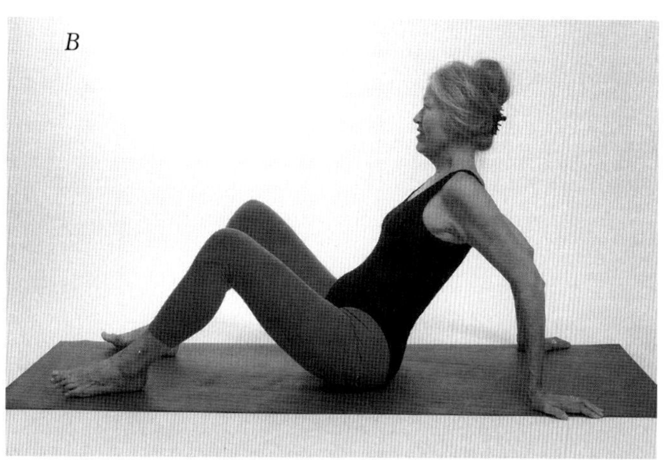

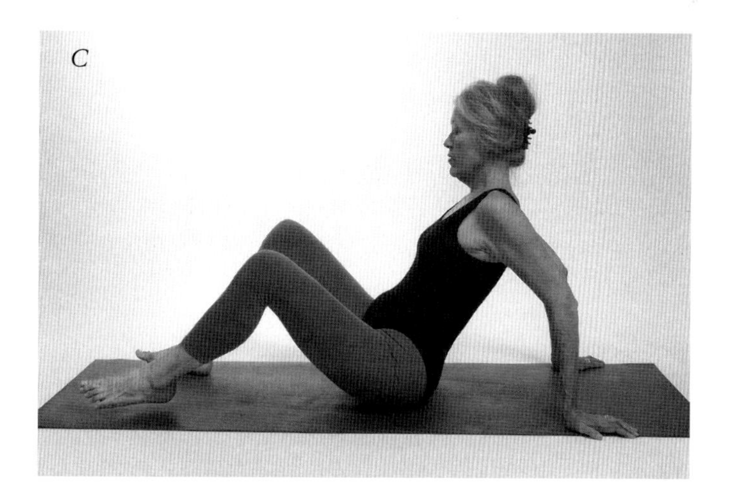

BOAT

HELPFUL HINTS: Prevent tucking your pelvis, tightening your abdomen, raising up your rib cage, rounding your upper back, or stressing your shoulders. If you have a vulnerable or injured hip or sacral area, *only* practice a few passive Boat movements, *without lifting your heel off the ground. You will still sense toning in your pelvis, thighs, and back.* If your abdominals are weak, you will benefit with the Boat. Practice Leg Rotation, Tikanis, and Pelvic Rock before the Boat.

VARIATIONS: Experience the most comfortable placement for the Boat by sitting on the floor with your back to the base of a sofa. After several months of practicing the Boat, try *barely* lifting both heels simultaneously off the ground, for the duration of a yawn and with long rests in between stretches.

Blissful Aches

Practicing KENTRO movements generates relaxation and toning that is often accompanied by pulling or slight aching sensations—the harbingers of ease. During this process, our joints are actually realigning into more comfortable balance while our soft tissues extend, flex, expand, and contract more harmoniously. The "pulling" that arises while we center and balance ourselves signals increased muscular elasticity.

We can relish these feelings. They are reliable indicators of healing shifts in our bodies.

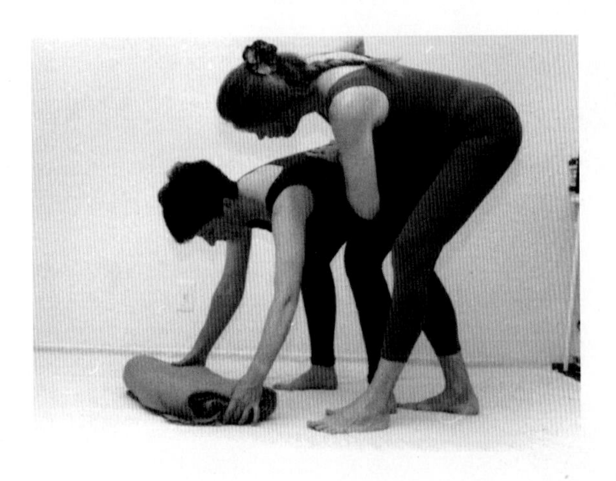

While Cindy bends forward in comfortable balance, she experiences "pulling" in her pelvis, back, and thighs, indicating releases, toning, and extension in these areas of her body.

Most of us have negative associations with any type of aching. In the past, our aches were probably followed by pain resulting from an injury, or we may have experienced joint or muscular aches from moving in a stressful manner. It is common to interpret a new situation based on similar experiences in the past. So we may automatically assume that centering aches are bad, even if we feel more supple. Physiologically, these KENTRO positive pulling sensations—similar to the muscular "workout" feelings from playing a sport or dancing—confirm that our back is straightening and broadening.

A KENTRO movement for a specific area, such as the Boat for the pelvis, can produce workout feelings throughout our bodies, including our thighs, diaphragm, and upper and lower back. These sensations herald releases dependent on each person's body history, practice, and sensuous awareness. Instead of following the stressful notion, "no pain, no gain," these mild aches relax and renew us.

Such unique aches are never overwhelming, and they vanish within a few hours or days, once our bodies have increased flexibility. When we stay in a balanced position for long periods of time, such as bending to wax a floor, we may feel a strong, uncomfortable pulling in the backs of our legs. We can stretch gently by taking many short breaks. Rubbing arnica massage oil (or ointment) on a stretched area is also helpful.

Shortly after I first started teaching the KENTRO program, my vacuum cleaner broke down. I decided to practice bending forward by sweeping the living room carpet with a small Chinese broom that had a one-foot-long handle. Over the next two weeks, my back stretched and straightened with ease, but I felt terrific pulling in the hamstring muscles on the back of my thighs. From this, I learned that bending forward in balance is an effective means of strengthening the legs.

Since then, I continue to feel releases in regions of my body where tissues were tight due to injuries from my youth. I feel as if my body is shouting, "Hurray! I am finally getting limber!" Practicing simple movements like Grounding, Prayer, Looking for Elbow Room, and Little Moon eventually transforms aches into freed postural expression. In time, as our bodies become more supple, our mind welcomes these precursors of resiliency.

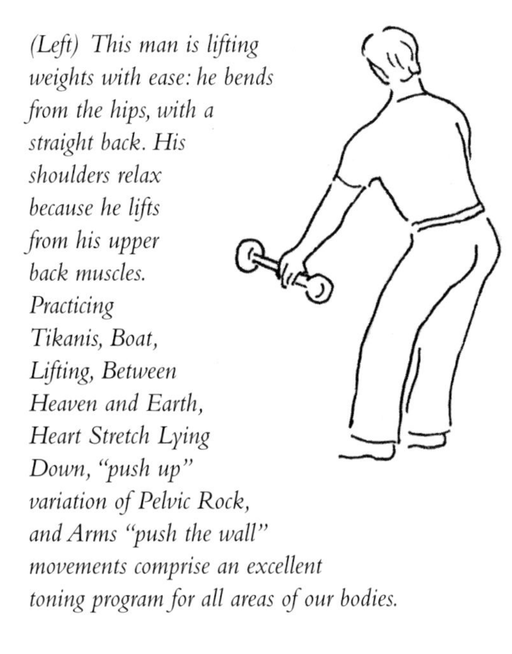

(Left) This man is lifting weights with ease: he bends from the hips, with a straight back. His shoulders relax because he lifts from his upper back muscles. Practicing Tikanis, Boat, Lifting, Between Heaven and Earth, Heart Stretch Lying Down, "push up" variation of Pelvic Rock, and Arms "push the wall" movements comprise an excellent toning program for all areas of our bodies.

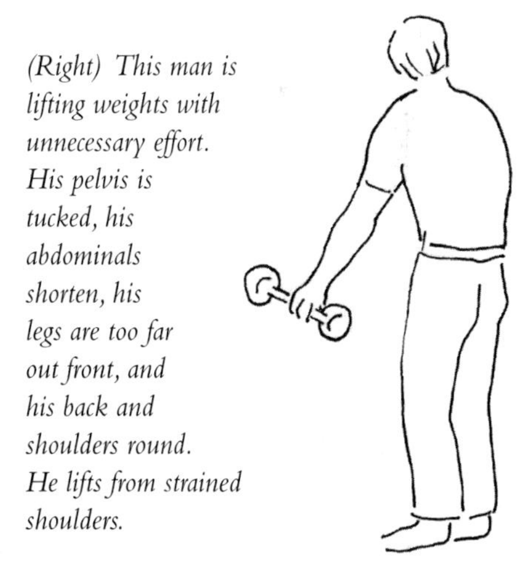

(Right) This man is lifting weights with unnecessary effort. His pelvis is tucked, his abdominals shorten, his legs are too far out front, and his back and shoulders round. He lifts from strained shoulders.

11. Lifting

PREPARATION. Place a small chair in front of a long mirror. Stand in profile to the mirror and just behind the chair. Practice Elemental Placement.

A. Place your hands on your pelvic crests and bend slightly forward from the hips. Allow your knees to bend, while keeping your hips level, your abdomen relaxed, and your shoulders and rib cage dropped.
   Place the palm of your left hand onto your lower back to sense straightening in your back as you ground (relax) the pelvic muscles. Keep most of your weight in your heels. Check to be sure your neck is in line with your spine, and center your hips with the chair so that you do not twist your pelvis or back.
B. While bending forward, Grounding yourself, notice that weight (pressure) spreads throughout your sacral area. Your legs will feel stable. *Sense a big "pulling" (both lengthening and contracting) sensation in the hamstring (back of the thigh) muscles.* Let your back straighten.
C. Contract your shoulder blade muscles, keep your bent elbows close to your body, and begin to lift the chair. Sense contraction in your upper back muscles and slight pressure in the top of your buttocks. When you lift a heavier object, you will also sense abdominal muscles working. Lift the chair for the duration of several yawns.
D. Ground yourself as you get ready to set down the chair so that optimal placement of the weight of the chair is distributed mostly through your sacral and hip area—the important pelvic center of mass in the body. Stay relaxed; let the buttocks muscles *stretch away from your torso*. Notice that you can remain in balanced Elemental Placement while you hold the chair and *sense all pelvic muscles working. Savor your feelings of comfort and strength*. Set down the chair. Rest so that your body can make readjustments.
E. When you are lifting a heavier object, bring it *close to your pelvis* and keep the object close to your body.

BENEFITS: The most significant benefit of Lifting in comfortable balance is that overstretched/shortened (strained) upper back, shoulder, lower back, pelvic, and leg muscles can relax and gently lengthen. Likewise, appropriate weight-bearing pelvic, upper back, and upper arm muscles regain strength and harmonious function. Lifting is also the easiest way to let your back, neck, and thigh muscles get a full stretch that brings long-lasting elasticity. Lifting is both strengthening and limbering for your body. Always *center your belly-button and hips with the child or object you wish to lift*, to prevent any twisting in your pelvis or back.

HELPFUL HINTS: Prevent rounding/arching your back, twisting any part of your back/pelvis and tucking, or tightening your buttocks/abdomen—all of these will lead to strain and unnecessary effort. It may take a few months of practice before your

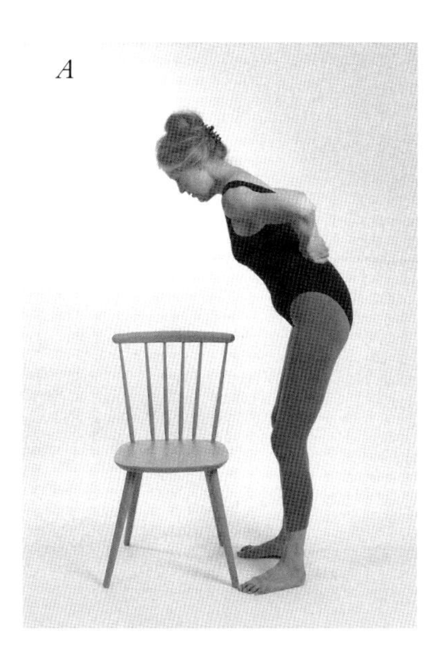

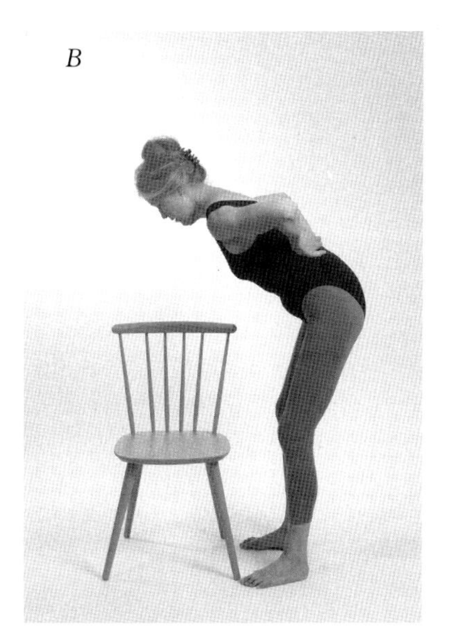

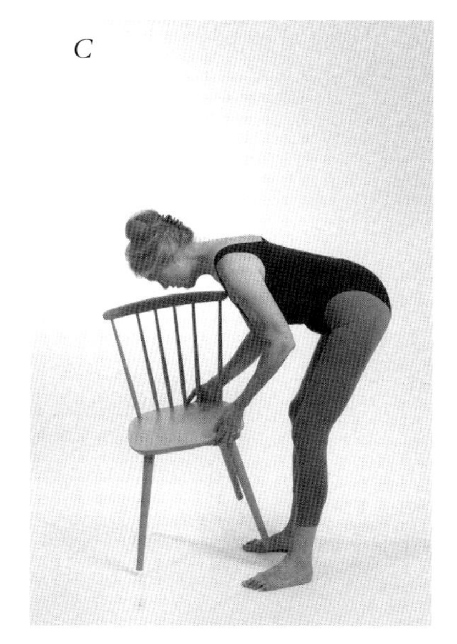

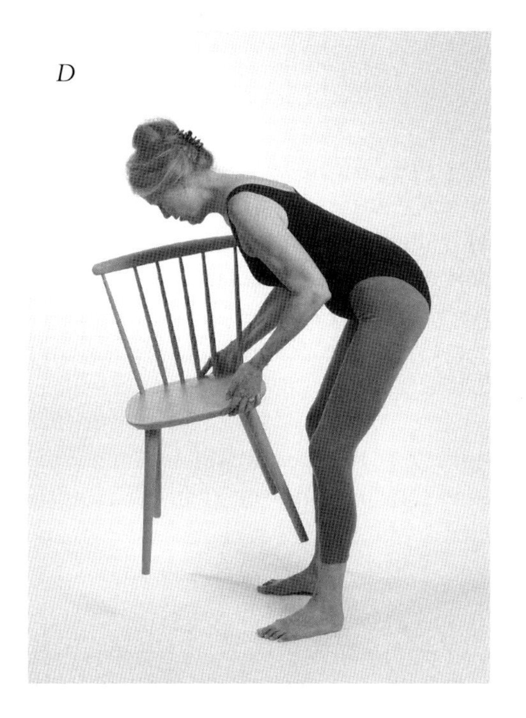

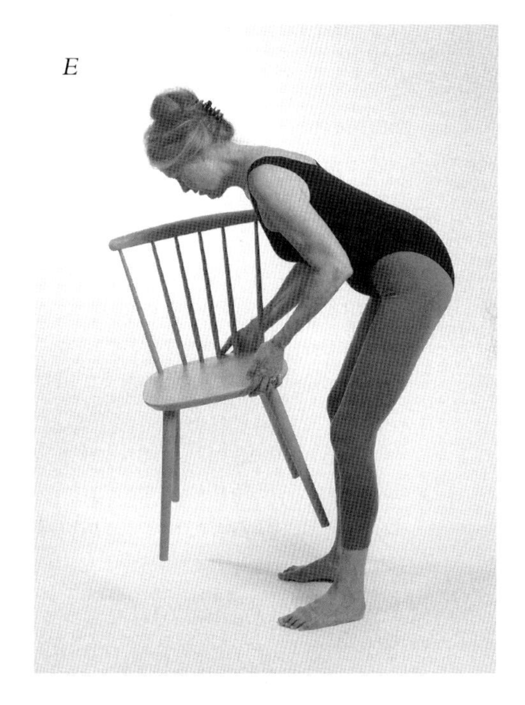

LIFTING

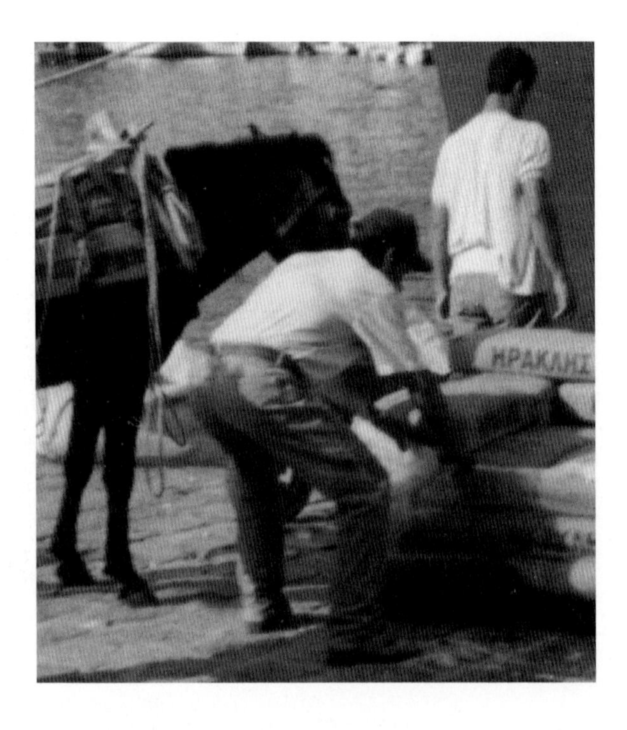

9.1. This Greek man lets his pelvis stretch out behind him for counterweight; his back straightens as he lifts the heavy cement bag from his upper back, upper arms, and pelvic muscles. The weight of the bag will be assimilated mostly in his sacral/hip region.

hamstrings, pelvic muscles, and back muscles are elastic and strong enough for you to lift in comfortable balance. Be very discerning with *how many* pounds you are lifting and for *how long*. (Note: if your doctor has cautioned you, follow his advice.) Begin with lifting lightweight objects; ALWAYS start with Elemental Placement; center the object with your body; only lift objects or children that are appropriate for your body weight or history of injuries; lift an object or child as close to your body as possible. Even people with great physical ease rest a moment before and after Lifting. Practice Tikanis, Arms Hug (and Push) the Wall, and Boat before Lifting is helpful.

VARIATIONS: Have fun Lifting with *lightweight* exercise weights. When you integrate Lifting with *pushing* furniture, wheelbarrows, or lawnmowers, you will experience similar toning in your pelvic and back muscles.

Chore to Pleasure

The ways we move profoundly influence how we experience everyday life. Over many decades, I have observed people in Greece, Honduras, Mexico, Morocco, Brazil, Portugal, and Spain moving with smooth balance. They bend from the hips with straight spines, relaxed shoulders, limber hips, anteriorly slanted pelvises, and strong buttocks and back muscles (see Figs. 9.1–9.2)[2]. Likewise, in Latin America and North Africa, I have seen people squat with straight backs and angled pelvises to play cards or to "sit." I have not seen any of these people who move with smooth balance lift heavy loads

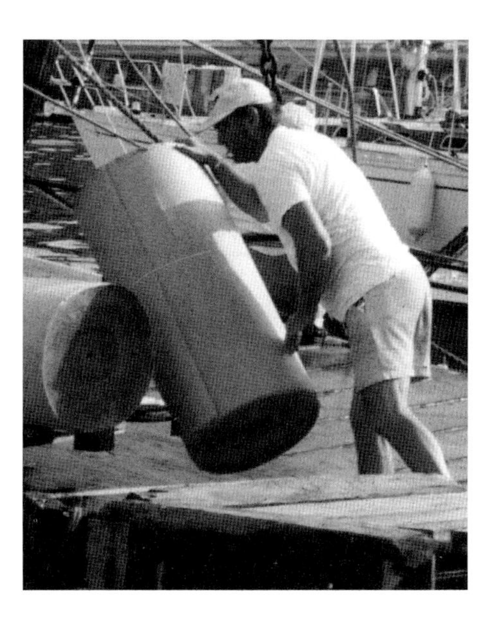

9.2. Notice how easily this Greek man is lifting and rolling the large container. When we lift with a grounded (anteriorly slanted) pelvis and straight back, the activity feels stimulating because it tones and stretches our bodies into pleasurable ease.

in the position commonly taught in highly industrialized countries: semi-squatting with a tucked pelvis and/or tightened abdomen. People lifting with optimal balance illustrate conservation of mechanical energy as they bend forward from the hips and lift with the naturally slanted, relaxed pelvic placement. Women carrying toddlers straddled on their sacrums bend forward with the same anterior pelvic slant to "seat" the child on the pelvis and to pick up a heavy basket.

When we lack centering, balancing gestures in our ordinary activities, we can expect discomfort or stiffness. Many activities may then feel like burdens or seem boring and mechanical. One reason for this is that early on in our lives, we often learn to bend, lift, sit, or stand in ways that provoke unnecessary strain. Such stressful motions, when repeated over many years, result in a familiarity with distress that decreases our sensory awareness. When we pick up a heavy casserole, we may not notice that we are bending forward with a tightened lower back, tucked pelvis, rounded shoulders, and rounded upper back.

Some habitual actions exhaust us physically and psychologically. We tend to think something is "off" with our body when ordinary motions feel cumbersome (i.e., sitting and lifting) [Figs. 9.3–9.6]. Yet by incorporating KENTRO guidelines into our "chores," even lifting an object becomes a pleasurable, strengthening movement. When we lift with centered, balanced placement, our bones can bear optimal weight, which in turn allows the main weight-bearing muscles—the buttocks and back muscles—to lengthen, expand, and contract with ease and minimum effort.[3] Such optimal balance requires the natural anterior placement of the pelvis.

We particularly see the anteriorly placed pelvis in top figure skaters, acrobats, jockeys, and dancers (see Vignette 5, *Activities in Balance*, p. 68). However, most people habitually stand with a tucked pelvis (to "stand up straight") and habitually sit with a rounded back; as a result, they will automatically bend with a tucked pelvis and rounded back and will semi-squat for lifting. Sometimes guidelines for keeping a straight back in bending forward *also* include flattening the sacrum as well as the belly, which constrains the pelvis. Following such "modern, correct" postural directions pushes the legs and pelvis forward into a posterior angle (See *Setting the Stage: Postural Movement in Highly Industrialized Countries*, pp. xvii-xxii). This decreases bone support; in turn, pelvic and

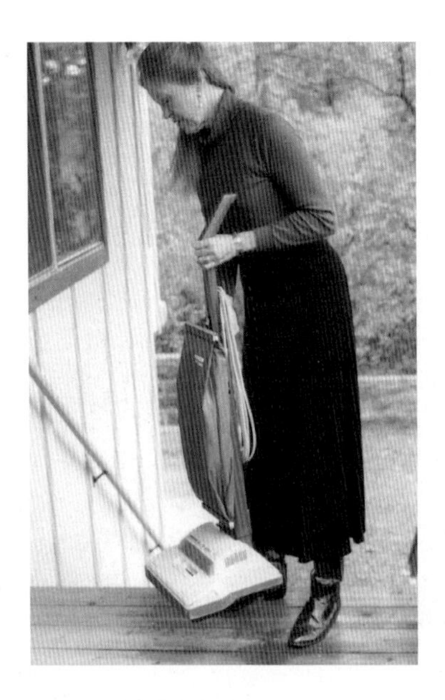

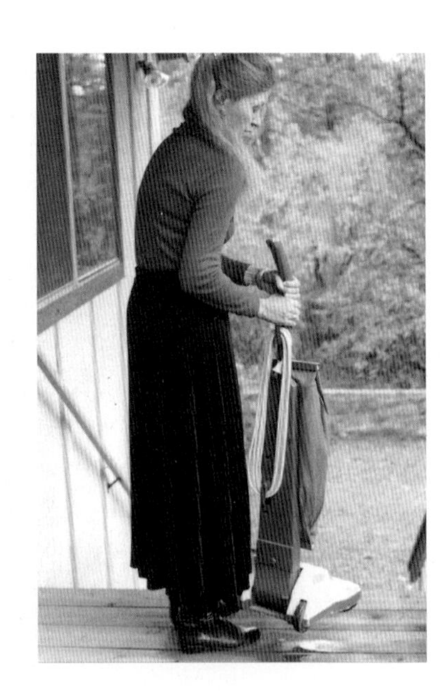

(Top left) 9.3. I am easily lifting the vacuum cleaner with my upper back muscles: My pelvis (anteriorly slanted) stretches and the weight of the vacuum cleaner is transferred through my sacral/ hip region. My back is straight and my shoulders are dropped. I feel toning in my upper back, upper arms, abdomen, and pelvis.

(Top right) 9.4. I am lifting the vacuum cleaner with unnecessary effort: My pelvis (posteriorly slanted) tucks, my abdomen shortens, my back rounds, and there is too much weight in my straining shoulder muscles, in the front of my thighs, and in my wrists, back, and neck. I feel weak in my legs, abdomen, buttocks, back, and arms.

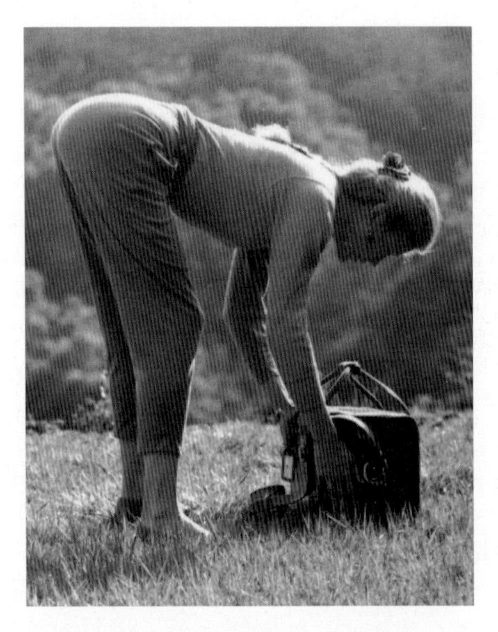

9.5. Over time, when the hamstring (thigh) muscles become resilient enough, we can bend easily from the hips and lift easily from the upper back, upper arm, thigh, abdominal, and pelvic muscles with an anteriorly slanted pelvis; the sacral—hip area resembles a weight-absorbing bridge. I feel most weight (pressure) in my pelvis. My back and whole body feel strong.

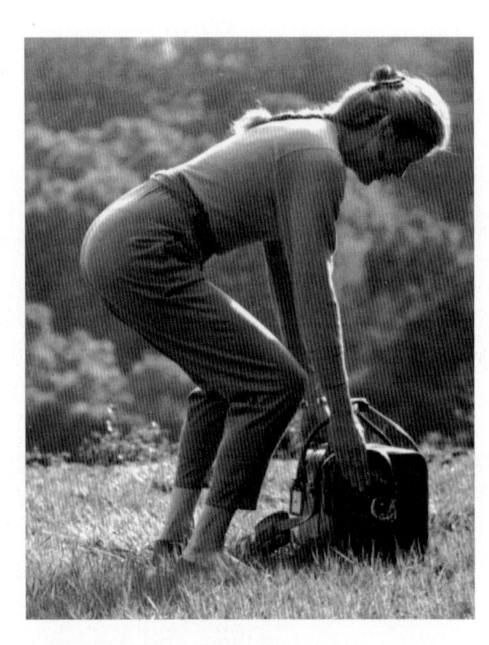

9.6. When the pelvis is tucked and in a posterior slant, we automatically have less bone support (from strong pelvic and thigh bones); bending and lifting then strain and weaken abdominal, pelvic, thigh, back, and shoulder muscles. I feel most weight (pressure) in my knees, lower back, and shoulders. My pelvic position resembles a fallen bridge. My back and whole body feel strained.

abdominal muscles must compensate (i.e., tighten) continually to support the spine and prevent the abdomen from weakening and "pouching out front." Tightening the pelvis requires constant effort, which decreases body elasticity. As long as tucking the pelvis is seen as the means to "protect" our pelvis and back from injury, we find ourselves in a vicious cycle of placing increasing strain on an already stressed region of the body.

Mainstream conventional posture guidelines are in accord with KENTRO guidelines on important basics such as viewing the pelvis as the core (most important) area for motion, keeping the hips and shoulders level, and avoiding too much curving in the spine or neck. However, as long as flattening of the pelvis is prevalent, we are missing out on moving freely from the pelvic main center of motion and support. Conventional "neutral" spinal alignment discourages excessive arching or curving of the spine and tucking of the pelvis. Yet, as long as neutral is accompanied by the dictum "flatten your belly and tuck the buttocks," the abdominals, buttocks, and thigh muscles will tighten and shorten, the legs will slant forward, and the pelvis will become more posteriorly slanted. The legs, pelvis, and spine remain on hold—in a state of muscular over-contraction, limiting our pelvic mobility and strength. Centered, relaxed, balanced expression cannot happen. Significantly, our bodies are so *superbly adaptable* that we can lift objects with this strained bearing; over time though, our bodies complain, and lifting becomes an increasingly risky process.

Both the KENTRO method and conventional methods recommend keeping a straight back and using the legs. Yet they differ significantly in *how to incorporate* these recommendations. By applying KENTRO centering and balancing guidelines, we can feel most body weight balanced (distributed) through the main center of bone mass: the pelvis. Perhaps the explanation for this sensation is that, in bending forward with centered balance, the pelvis is at the natural *anterior* angle, in a position in which it may act as an arch. The weight of the torso can transfer from the sacral promontory to the femoral (hip) joints via *the two iliac bones, which form a strong weight-bearing arch with the sacrum*. This arch directs the body weight (and the load we lift) to the femurs (thigh bones), the strongest and longest bones of the body; and the line of gravity passes through the center of the hip joints—which can optimally balance body weight [Figs. 9.7–9.8].[4] The powerful pelvic arch supports body weight similar to the architectural bridging of an open space. Regardless of a mechanical explanation, the more anteriorly placed pelvis is at the heart of the centering, balancing movements because it allows the back to straighten naturally, without effort, and it allows the pelvis to become more resilient while in motion. As we bend from the hips with KENTRO guidelines, the pelvis moves back and we feel the buttocks muscles stretching further back (which cannot happen with a tucked pelvis). We feel more weight (pressure) in the buttocks and this counterweight allows the pelvis to counterbalance the weight that we are lifting. This advantageous body placement and motion may be similar to the mechanics of a teeter totter. While we are lifting, there is no muscular holding in the pelvic-abdominal area. In this situation, we do not have to consciously pre-set, tense the abdominals to "protect" the back, because with centered, balanced motion,

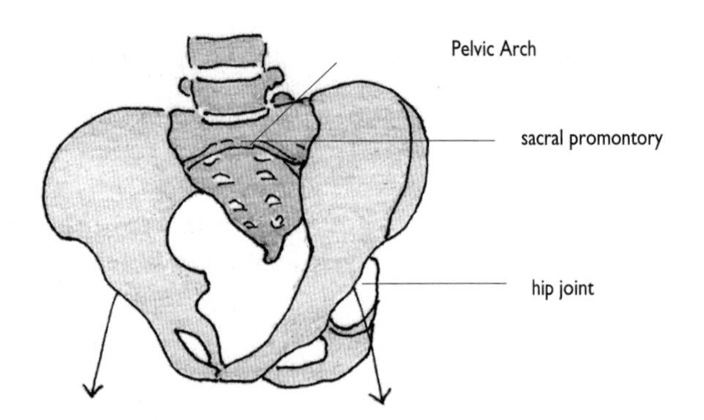

9.7. **Optimal Pelvic Arch**
In this drawing (based on the portable model used in KENTRO classes) the anteriorly placed pelvis allows the optimal slant of the pelvic arch, for optimal weight bearing function, similiar to the architectural bridging of an open space. The weight of the torso (and of a load) is smoothly tranferred from the buttocks (the strongest muscles) and sacral promontory to the hips (the femurs are the strongest bones) via the iliac bones (see the arrows),

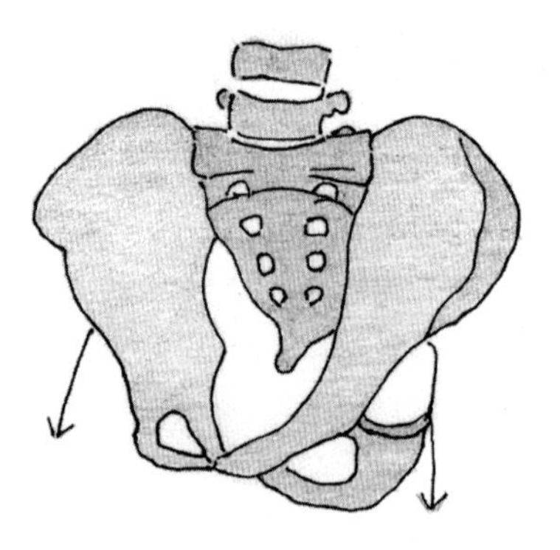

9.8. **Limited Pelvic Arch**
In this drawing of the same model, the posteriorly placed pelvis decreases the horizontally inclined slant of the pelvi arch, thus decreasing its weight bearing function. With this tucked pelvic placement, the sacral promontory is less like a platform and more vertically inclined as the sacrum flattens and the iliac bones as well as the hip joints move out front. The weight of the torso (and of a load) is probably stressfully transferred too far forward of the body (see the arrows).

all appropriate muscles will naturally keep the body strong and safely aligned. We feel a workout throughout the thigh, buttocks, abdominal, and back muscles.

When we follow conventional guidelines, we bend from the knees and hips but do not ground the pelvis into a more anterior placement or center the legs (with most weight in the heels). The pelvis is tucked, which decreases the slant of the sacrum and diminishes the pelvic arch (which becomes less bridge-like and more vertically inclined). The abdomen tightens and shortens, the back rounds, the shoulders strain; we feel a workout mostly in the *front* of the thighs, and too much pressure is on the knees and lower back. The pelvic and other muscles in the body are not at their optimal length for most efficient function, and lifting becomes more difficult [Figs. 9.9–9.16].

With careful practice (see suggestions below), you will gain confidence and enjoy sensing the difference between supple versus strained approaches to lifting. Before you try out the Lifting exercise, you need to have understood and practiced the basic KENTRO attitude and principles. Read Chapter 6: *Keys to Effective Practice*; Chapter 7: Elemental Placement; Chapter 8: Elemental Movements, and Chapter 9, Movement 5, Bending, and Vignette 5, *Activities in Balance*. If you have a history of joint or muscular problems caused by lifting (even if you find that the KENTRO approach to lifting does not provoke your symptoms), be cautious and consult your doctor.

The KENTRO Approach to Lifting with Ease

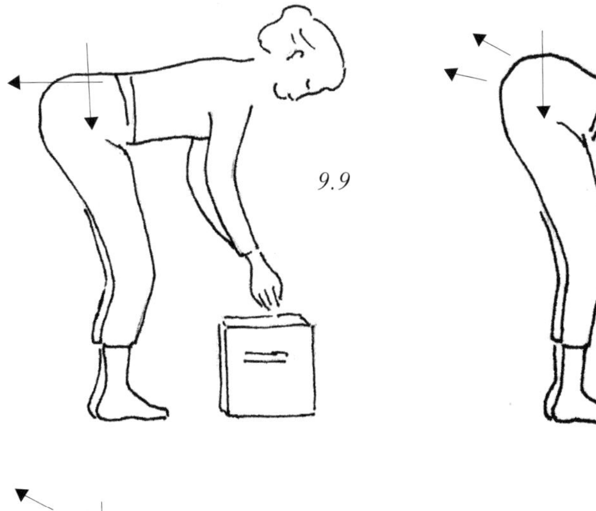

9.9. Bending the knees and bending forward from the hips with the anteriorly placed pelvis creates the optimal bridge-like slant of the pelvic arch, and lets the back straighten. There is no muscular holding or compensating. Pressure is sensed mostly in the pelvis, suggesting that weight is mostly distributed through the sacral/hip arch region (and through the buttocks), for counterweight. The arrows indicate main weight distribution and the buttocks stretching further back—with ease.

9.10. The anteriorly placed pelvic arch is the most effective placement for optimal weight distribution. The strongest muscles—the buttocks—stabilize the spine and contract powerfully for lifting. The buttress-like legs are strong and allow the buttocks/pelvic/abdominal muscles to stretch and shift weight away from the torso. Back muscles lengthen and strengthen the back, and the shoulders relax. There is no strain as long as the the hamstrings have become flexible enough. Lifting tones the legs, abdomen, pelvis, back and upper arms. The arrows indicate probable main weight distribution and the buttocks stretching further back—with ease.

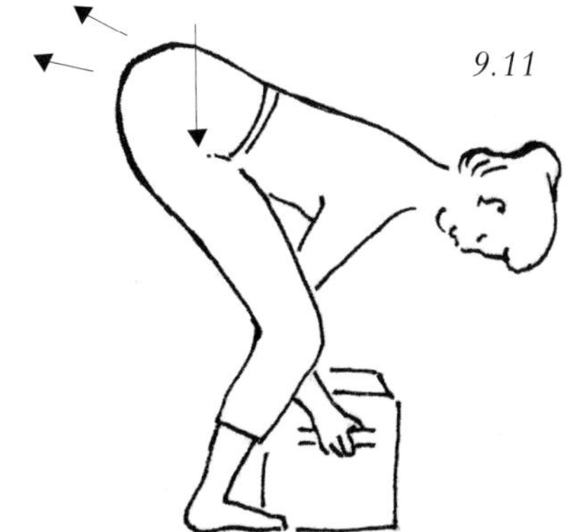

9.11. If your hamstrings are not supple and for lifting a heavy object, bend your knees more, and place the load close to your body—for ease.

Here are some suggestions that will help you to contrast how you lift presently with the KENTRO approach:

- First and foremost, carefully avoid tucking the pelvis. This alone will help you to bend forward in more carefree, comfortable balance.
- If you believe that pelvic tucking is necessary for lifting, then you will keep on unconsciously tucking your pelvis, and strain your body.
- Practice KENTRO *Bending* hundreds of times to help your back straighten easily and to allow your thigh, back, and buttocks muscles to stretch gently and progressively—to create the strong pelvic slant required for safe lifting.
- Initially, practice *Lifting* with only light objects to release strain and to tone your back, pelvic, abdominal, leg, and arm muscles.

- For additional strength, practice the KENTRO *Boat* and *Heart Stretch Lying Down* movements, for your abdomen, pelvis, back, and legs.
- Develop your awareness of postural differences by comparing people with strained motion to children and adults with supple motion.
- By integrating KENTRO movements into your *repetitive* actions at home or work, you learn to distinguish comfortable movements from taxing ones.
- Over time, your overstretched and shortened muscles become more resilient.
- Regained ease allows you truly to avoid tucking or straining muscles, and, therefore, to avoid deep-seated habits of pushing your body into fitness.
- Mopping the floor or carrying groceries with centered balance stretches and strengthens your upper backs, upper arms, buttocks, and legs. Routine actions become delight-in-action.

Be Sure to Avoid These Compensations

9.12. If you bend forward from the hips and deliberately stick out the buttocks (instead of simply letting your torso bend farther forward and letting your pelvis stretch farther back), the pelvis tightens, the abdominals weaken, the lower back tightens, overarches and bears more weight; the upper back rounds, and the shoulders tighten and bear more weight. Body weight is too far forward and lifting is difficult. The arrows indicate strain.

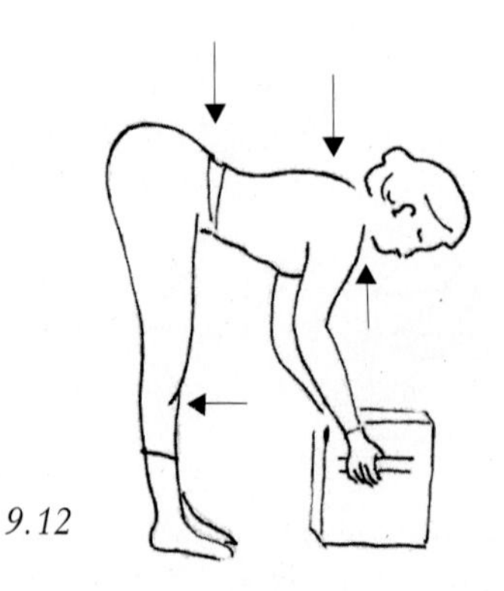

9.12

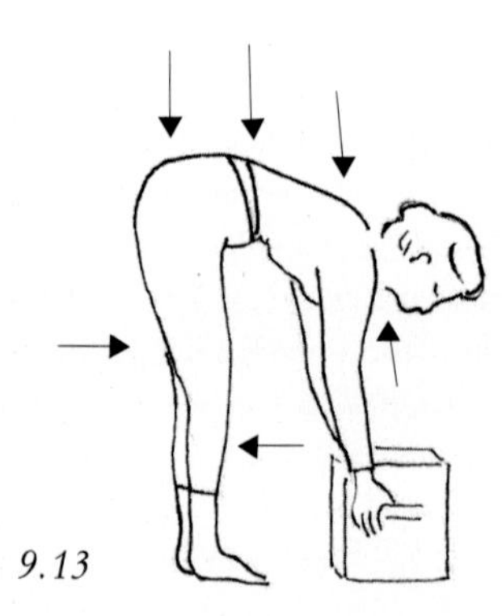

9.13

9.13. If you bend forward from the hips and tuck the pelvis, the pelvic muscles will tighten and over-stretch and weight falls forward. As a result, there is hardly any counterweight of the pelvis stretching away from the torso. The abdominal muscles are in a less functional position because they are shortened, and the back and shoulders bear more weight. The entire back rounds, and there is undue strain on the vertebrae because they are over-compressed on the front side of the spine and over-stretched on the back of the spine. The back and the shoulder muscles tighten and bear more weight. Body weight is too far forward and lifting is difficult. The arrows indicate strain.

The Common Approach to Lifting involves Strain

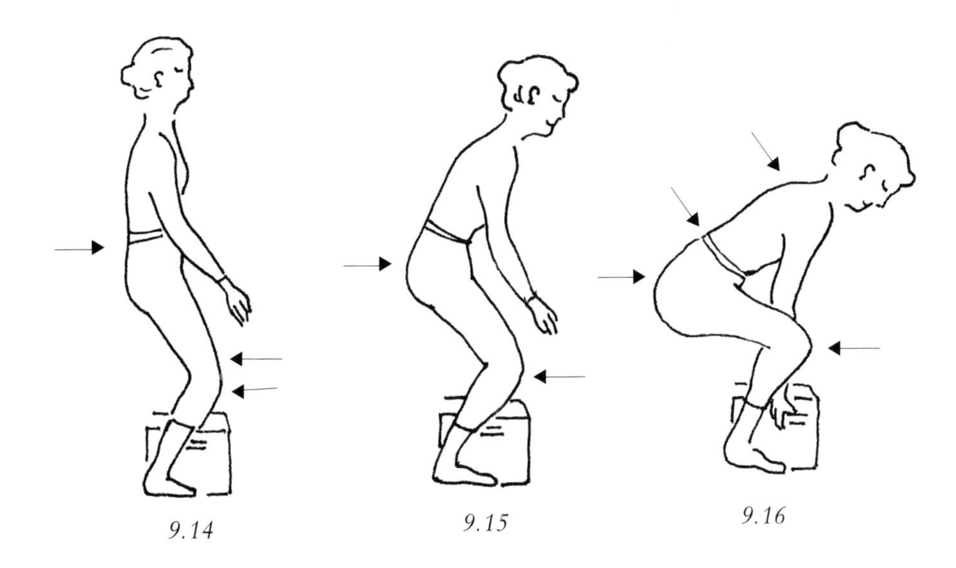

9.14. Bending with the more posteriorly slanted pelvis, tucking the buttocks, and tightening (shortening) the abdominal muscles. The sacrum flattens, the pelvic arch decreases (inclines more vertically), weight moves forward toward the front of the thighs, knees, feet, and shoulders. Arrows indicate strain.

9.15. Bending the knees and keeping the tucked posterior placement of the pelvis keeps shifting more body weight to the balls of the feet, knees, front of the legs, abdomen, top of the back, shoulders and neck. The upper back becomes heavier and the shoulders tend to move out front. The arrows indicate strain.

9.16. Continually keeping the tucked posterior pelvic placement significantly decreases the pelvic arch, and limits pelvic counterweight. The upper spine and shoulders automatically have to round, to reach the object. The hip joints and body weight shift even farther forward. Even though the object to lift is placed close to the model, the abdominals, pelvis, legs and back are weakened, so lifting strains many joints and muscles. The abdominals/buttocks are kept tight to "protect" the back; however, the spine is already in a vulnerable placement, increasing the likelihood of injury. The arrows indicate strain. In contrast, lifting with Kentro guidelines (figures 9.9–9.11), generates a deep experience of a "neutral" spine without compensations, and additionally, is a dynamic, active spine—supple and strong.

Observations (The Kentro Approach to Lifting)

Sensations of weight (pressure)

- — Through the top of the sacrum
- — Through the hips and thighs
- — Through the heels (the line of gravity goes through the arches of the feet)

Feelings

- — Strength (in the pelvis, legs, back, and upper arms)
- — Stability
- — Limberness
- — Comfort
- — The pelvis a broad, supportive and mobile "bridge"
- — The legs like strong buttresses

Bones

- — The pelvis is in optimal arch-like placement (maximum weight transfer through the strongest bones—the femurs and heels)
- — The spine straightens of its own accord
- — The small 'natural' arch between the fourth and fifth lumbar vertebrae (the small of the back) lengthens of its own accord
- — The pelvic-abdominal area is spacious

Muscles

- — All muscles are in naturally appropriate tension
- — The buttock and lower abdominal muscles stretch away from the torso (for counterweight) and contract of their own accord to lift
- — The upper back and upper arm muscles contract of their own accord to lift
- — All thigh muscles (front, back, and side) get a workout

Observations (The Common Approach to Lifting)

Sensations of weight (pressure)

- — through the base of the tucked sacrum
- — through the front of the thighs and knees
- — through the front of the feet (the line of gravity goes through the balls of the feet)

Feelings

- — Stress in the pelvis, knees, and shoulders; weakness in the back, arms, abdomen, and legs; pressure (weight) only in the front of the thighs
- — Lack of stability
- — Tightness
- — Discomfort
- — A seemingly small and immobile pelvis
- — Legs struggling to stay bent for lifting

Bones

- — The tucked pelvis decreases the pelvic arch (diminished weight transfers through the strongest bones—the femurs and heels)
- — The upper spine rounds and bears too much weight; the shoulders are too far out front and bear too much weight
- — The natural arch between the fourth and fifth lumbar vertebrae and the lower back bear too much weight
- — Pelvic-abdominal space decreases

Muscles

- — Major pelvic, abdominal, back and leg muscles are not functioning optimally, so other muscles must compensate
- — The buttocks and lower abdominal muscles are tight and do not stretch away from the torso (for counterweight)
- — The upper back and upper arm muscles *over*-work to lift. The upper back (lower trapezius) muscles over-stretch and the shoulder (upper trapezius) muscles shorten and tighten
- — The quadratus muscles in the front of the thighs over-work (over-contract) to lift
- — The knees strain and are vulnerable to injury

12. The Prayer

PREPARATION. Get on your knees on a mat, soft carpet, or blanket. Practice Elemental Placement.

A. Spread your knees a foot apart, level your hips, and relax your belly. Place your hands on the crests of your pelvis and slowly turn your thighs outward to align your hips and knees into comfort. *Sense slightly more pressure (weight) on the outside of your knees than toward the inner side of your knees.*

B. Bend forward, placing a hand on your lower back to *sense lengthening (straightening) in your back.* Place your hands on the floor, level with your knees. Spread your fingers. *Sense agreeable spaciousness and stretching between your fingers.* Remember to keep your neck in line with your spine. Move your torso slightly back. *Sense weight off your shoulders and shifting into your sacral/hip region.*

C. With your shoulders down, simultaneously let your arms stretch out in front of your head as your pelvis stretches out behind you, away from your torso. *Sense the resulting two-directional stretch: muscles in your lower back lengthen toward your head, while muscles in your pelvis stretch away from your torso. Sense a straightening of your entire back.* If you are uncertain of what is happening in your back, use your hand to check for an even groove in your back. Your thighs will be in a slight diagonal position. *Keep sensing most weight in the sacral region.*

D. When the underside of your arms is tired, bend your elbows, bring your arms toward your head, put one hand on top of the other, and place your forehead onto your hands. You can stay in this placement as long as you wish.

BENEFITS: The *Prayer* KENTRO movement is extremely *relaxing* and allows the easiest, fullest stretching in your back and pelvis, simply by placing your body into balance and centering your torso and pelvis. This two-directional stretch fosters releases and limbering of tight tissues or chronic aching—(by lengthening your back toward your head, while your pelvic muscles lengthen away from your torso). The increased spaciousness in your lungs promotes fuller breathing.

HELPFUL HINTS: Prevent tightening your shoulders or belly. Arching your lower back or rounding your upper back will constrict the anterior (front) side of your upper spine and tends to tuck the pelvis. Neither of these moves (conventional Pelvic Tilt) will create equal space between each vertebra, as is typical of a resilient spine; nor will they smoothly balance the back or pelvic muscles. Practice Pelvic Rock and Leg Rotation before Prayer.

VARIATIONS: Place a pliable wedge/pillow under your ankles and forehead.

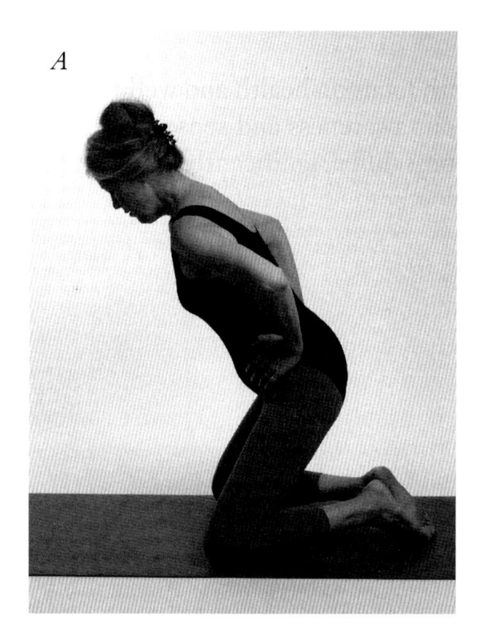

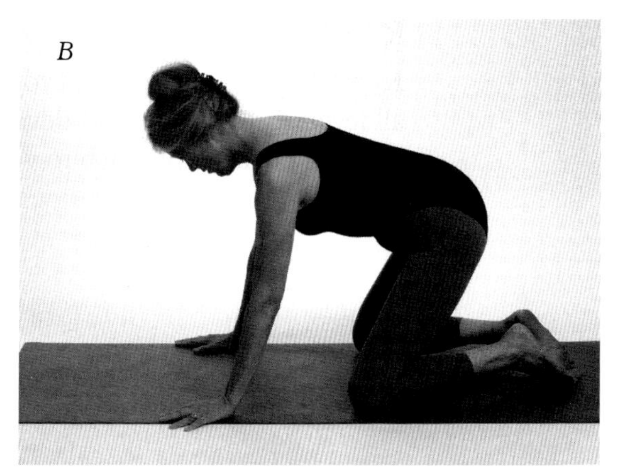

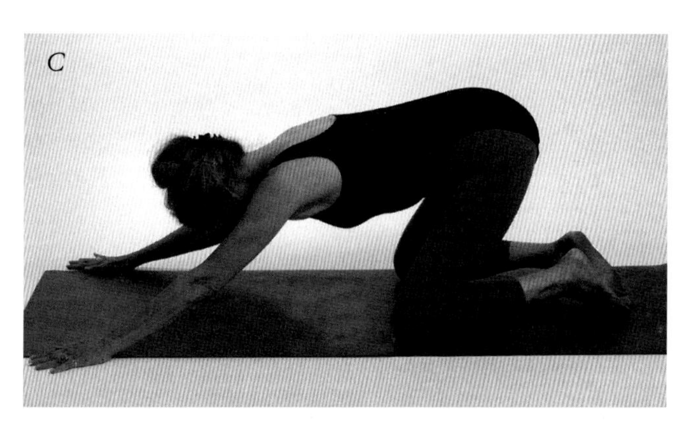

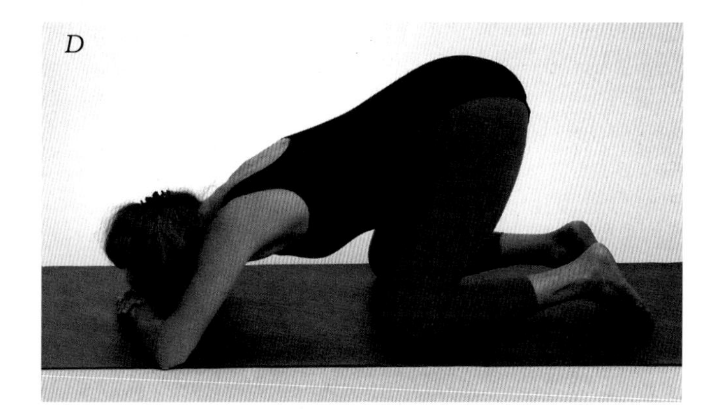

THE PRAYER

KENTRO and Yoga

KENTRO Body Balance and yoga both focus on health and well-being. They encompass all levels of our being and develop our awareness and sense of quietude. Although the background and approach to wholeness differ significantly between KENTRO and yoga, practicing KENTRO guidelines for centered balance will enhance yoga postures.

A glance at the historical origins of yoga reveals the complementary relationship between the KENTRO method and yoga. Yoga, a Sanskrit word meaning "union," is an orthodox system of Indian philosophy and mysticism. It was developed thousands of years ago for the disciplined practice of monks, who most likely moved with ease. The early classical writings on yoga, collected in the *Yoga Sutras* (aphorisms), were written around 200 BCE by the revered yoga master, Patanjali. These principles are described in four books, *On Concentration*, *On Practice*, *Supernormal Powers*, and *On the Self-in-Itself* (or *Liberation*). In *On Practice*, Patanjali outlines the eight pillars of yoga. One of these, *hatha* yoga, describes specialized physical postures called *asanas*.

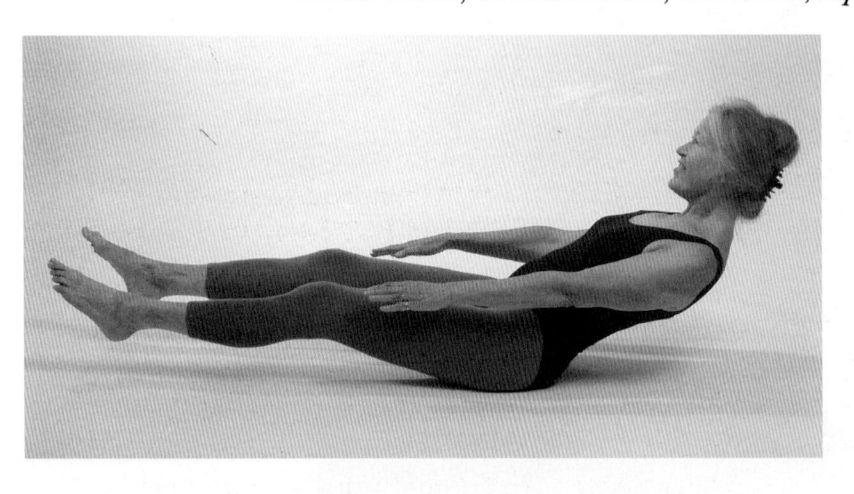

Try out this full-body toner only after many months of practicing the Boat *(p. 90) and other back, pelvic, and abdominal* KENTRO *strengtheners. Avoid tucking your pelvis, shortening your belly, or pushing forward your shoulders. Drop your shoulders, and relax your entire body while you are in this* Boat *variation, which is akin to a yoga* Boat *pose.*

In Sutra 46, Patanjali focuses on the fundamental qualities of *asanas.* Swami Prabhavananda translates this *sutra* to read: "Posture [*asana*] is to be seated in a position which is firm but relaxed."[5] Swami Hariharananda Aranya likewise carefully translates these qualities as the "Motionless and Agreeable Form [of Staying]."[6] We later read that "the spine has to be kept erect" in all yogic *asanas.*[7] In this *sutra,* we learn the importance of positioning our pelvis—the core-seat area of the body for unified posture. Patanjali suggests that even while standing, bending, or lying down, we have to look for a steady, smooth sense of "seat," settling into a posture and allowing the pelvis to support the torso so that the back straightens. He elaborates on his soothing approach to *asanas* in Sutra 47. "*Asanas* are perfected," Swami Hariharananda Aranya translates, "by Relaxation of Effort and Meditation on the Infinite."[8] We are instructed that, after sitting, "the whole body should be relaxed, taking care at the same time that the body does not bend." Likewise, "the habit of keeping the body always at rest and effortless helps the practice of Asana."[9]

Stability, centering, relaxation, and comfort are actually the principal feelings generated by KENTRO practice, beginning in the pelvic area and echoing throughout the entire body. However, unlike *hatha* yoga, there are no postures or philosophical requirements in the KENTRO program. All that is necessary is a willingness to caringly practice specific movements, which shift us into ease during our activities. Elemental Placement prepares the way for each KENTRO movement, focusing on continuous placement of our pelvis into centered balance so our torso can be erect without taxing the body. Students report that, over time, the pelvis begins to feel like a mobile, steady seat while they are standing, bending, and sitting down.

KENTRO guidelines were developed over a period of fifteen years. Balance (defined as optimal bone support and weight distribution of the body), interwoven with centering (experienced as release of strain in the soft tissues), influences all areas of our being, as our bodies reshape themselves into spirited posture and free movement. This suppleness can be incorporated into yoga postures to embody the ancient belief in freedom from physical exertion for spiritual development described by Patanjali.

I first noticed the relationship between agreeable balance and hatha yoga postures when I tried to sense balance in the yoga postures I learned at the Paris Iyengar and Aplomb Institutes. At the time I was not yet familiar with Patanjali's aphorisms, and I did not feel even an inkling of relief from stiffness while practicing these asanas. Because I had already begun to sense dynamic peacefulness in my everyday actions, I believed I could somehow blend this quality into formal postures.

What Patanjali describes as stable, enjoyable postures I later recognized in ancient Indian sculptures and miniature paintings depicting men, women, gods, and goddesses in balanced asanas during ordinary activities. I saw the same poise in contemporary Indian films and photographs.

Little by little, as I transformed my body, I was able to discern when a yoga student struggled or moved softly into a stance. I noticed Indian yoga instructors who became frustrated because they could not communicate their physical flexibility to Western students with excessively tightened musculature. However, the dedication to yoga I found in many Western students inspired me to revisit certain yoga poses, this time with the intent of merging asanas with comfort and centering movement.

I gradually developed a series of movements that were helpful for yoga postural placement. I encouraged yoga students to *sense* their movements and rest their bodies into placement instead of rigorously imitating their teachers. Yoga instructors who studied with me commented that even simple bodily shifts, such as bending the knees instead of locking them while bending forward, increased their plasticity.

Contemporary Western hatha yoga instructors honor Patanjali's writings whenever they emphasize the supportive placement of the pelvis and encourage students to slow down their motions. In general, however, the principles presented by Patanjali have become significantly abstracted from yoga practice, since most of us who explore yoga move out of *comfortable, centered* balance. Certain yoga postures and even prolonged sitting and bending during daily occupations may feel like chores because we feel stiff and uncomfortable.

As in dance or the martial arts, yoga students rely on their teachers to instruct them in the right placement of asanas. Many well-known contemporary hatha yoga masters, who have reflected on and respect the complexities of yoga, interpret the words of Patanjali according to their own experiences and language. There are a myriad of approaches to posture found in hatha yoga.

Hatha yoga instructors vary from being reassuring to being exacting in their approaches, but all instructors systematically teach the same postures, which do not vary structurally. They incorporate breathing techniques and are practiced in a quiet space. The yoga student can choose which of the many approaches to yoga she prefers, but she will have to conform to the basic form of every *asana.* The *asanas* tend to be progressive and sequential.

Yet how can a yoga student who experiences physical distress—and who is already struggling to position her body "correctly"—apply these yoga principles and integrate Patanjali's empowering recommendations? It is difficult for her to do so if she does not see comfortable physical balance in the instructor. Even if the yoga instructor moves in fluid balance, students may have trouble experiencing less tension because there are no traditional, specific hatha yoga guidelines that sharpen the senses, enabling them to distinguish strain from ease and to dissolve years of stressful postural patterns.

The KENTRO approach to well-being sheds light on how we can move with resiliency:

- There is no concept of effort.
- There is no discipline; there are no *should*s.
- We focus on enlivening the senses, expanding our perceptions, and enjoying our gestures.
- The vital ingredient for KENTRO practice is an affectionate relationship with the body.
- By celebrating our nature, we celebrate all nature.
- KENTRO guidelines can help yoga instructors and students approach postures in a relaxed manner, moving toward Patanjali's description of comfort.

Basic aspects of the KENTRO program can be smoothly integrated into hatha yoga practice, even when students have hurried and complex lives. Yoga students can then honor the ancient, highly structured *asana* patterns that aim at both progression and unity, while learning how to avoid forcing their body into a superficial, fixed form. By moving safely into a challenging posture, postures will be flavored by releases.

Centering guidelines prepares students to experience yoga postures in a completely new and creative way, embodying Patanjali's descriptions of postures without constraint. Balancing actions feel like expansive, gentle stretches. When yoga students integrate such feelings into a physical stance, they perceive the structured yoga pattern in a freer way.

There are no advanced KENTRO movements; all are equally valuable. With practice, the movements are felt on a deeper level as the benefits broaden. By practicing KENTRO, the students' concern over slow progress will be replaced by a subtler perception of yoga—that of enjoying even simple *asanas*.

Attentiveness to our automatic inhalation and exhalation improves our ability to amplify a muscular stretch. In Sutra 49, Patanjali advises us that, "When Asana is Perfected, Regulation of the Flow of Inhalation and Exhalation [results in] Pranayama (Breath Control).[10] Postural quality precedes breath control in yoga. The KENTRO emphasis on regaining physical spaciousness promotes smoother breathing—useful preparation for yoga breathing techniques combined with gently balanced postures.

Physical mobility entails increased volume in the rib cage and abdomen, as well as improved functioning of basic life systems, such as respiration. The torso broadens; muscles become more elastic. Breath becomes a natural component of an expanding and lengthening stretch in the torso (see Vignette 14, *Breathing Up Your Back*).

There is no particular sequence of KENTRO movements because (a) we can decide which area of our body we wish to limber and strengthen; and (b) the activity (e.g., sweeping the patio) itself defines which movements we will experience. Such common sense concepts can help yoga students confidently choose yoga postures that feel appropriate for home practice.

In turn, postures will not be forced or static because the students will feel more flowing motion. They can then experience the "motionless staying," described in Sutra 46 as continuous, tiny bodily readjustments that create robust relaxation.

KENTRO practice does not require a secluded place because *all* activities—sorting laundry or doing construction work—are places for practice. The resulting limberness in our repetitive gestures allows gentler balancing in yoga postures; leisurely daily movements develop into soothing daily *asanas*.

KENTRO movements offer vital benefits to those who practice yoga postures; they generate the formless, sensuous release that Patanjali describes as fundamental to yoga postures. As our body lets go of tension, it can reshape itself without mental discipline or unnecessary physical effort. Instead of striving and pushing our body to conform to "correct," idealized, or superficial poses, we can gently feel our way into any occupation or *asana*.

Everyday posture extends into *specific* yoga postures. KENTRO guidelines can be thought of as yoga for daily life, in which we focus on harmony in humble, repetitive actions. Our powerful creative core then generates a lovely ease.

Centered balance in everyday and specialized activities alters how we experience our bodies. Agitated movements become more restful, soulful movements. When we feel such exhilarating shifts, yoga postural forms act as a fine guide, not a rigid boundary. By sensing flow in ordinary gestures, we gradually expand into the flow of a posture.

As we move from the inside out, at our own rhythm, we can find in each *asana* a hospitable, unifying shelter.

13. Arms Hug the Wall

PREPARATION. Stand about one and a half feet away from a wall, facing it. Shift your body into Elemental Placement with at least a foot of space between your feet.

A. Place the palm of your right hand onto the lower back (with your fingers on the spine) and the palm of your left hand onto the left buttock. Begin to bend forward from the hips, keeping most weight in your heels. *Sense straightening, lengthening in your back, and an expansive grounding stretch in your buttocks.*

B. Keep your shoulders down, your hips level, and your neck in line with your spine. Bend your arms while, and place your hands (at the level of your shoulder) on the wall. Relax your body. Slowly—inch-by-inch—move your hands up the wall while your pelvis stretches slowly—inch-by-inch—away from your torso. This *bi-directional* stretching of your back and pelvis is the essence of this KENTRO movement. *Sense that your arms move up the wall by muscular action in your upper back.*
Now and then, place a hand on your lower back to feel *it straightening*; *sense a lightness (weightlessness) along your back and pelvis*. There is no goal in Arms Hug the Wall: you are simply *allowing* releases to happen. Place your hand back onto the wall.

C. As you continue moving your hands slowly up the wall with gentle pressure of your hands "hugging" the wall and you continue to *Ground* your pelvis away from your torso, keep relaxing your body, and keep your shoulders down. If you feel your shoulders move up (toward your ears), you have raised your arms too high: lower your hands a little so that your shoulder muscles once again soften. You can be in this placement for a few minutes. Keep bending your knees slightly, and keep your neck in line with your spine; periodically check your back for straightness.

BENEFITS: This relaxing, limbering placement relieves you of stiffness and easily straightens the spine while expanding and realigning the pelvis.

HELPFUL HINTS: Prevent tightening your back and pelvis by raising your arms but keeping your pelvis immobile (or worse, pushing it toward the wall). Prevent arching your neck and lower back, pushing up your shoulders, sticking out your buttocks, or locking your knees as you bend forward. Practice Bending Forward, Tikanis, before Arms Hug the Wall.

VARIATIONS: Try Push the Wall, a *strengthener* for the upper back muscles. Practice the guidelines for A and B, but keep your hands level with your elbows and no higher than your shoulders. *Sense your upper back muscles contracting as much as possible (for toning)* as your hands "push" the wall. Keep your shoulders down and avoid arching the lower back.

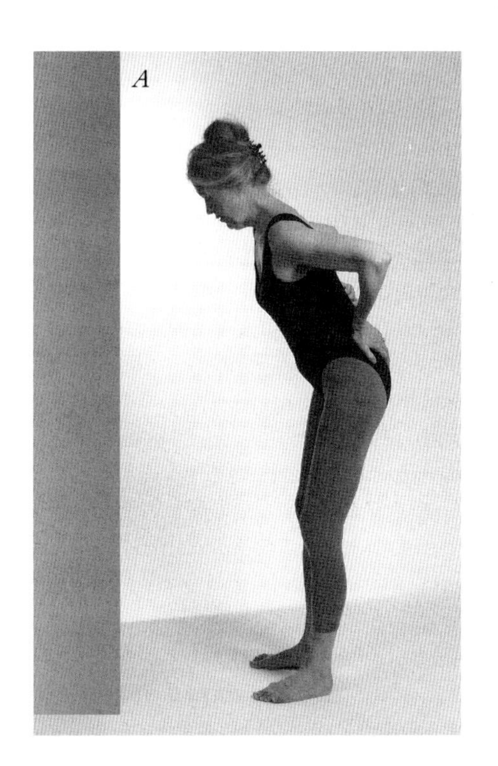
A

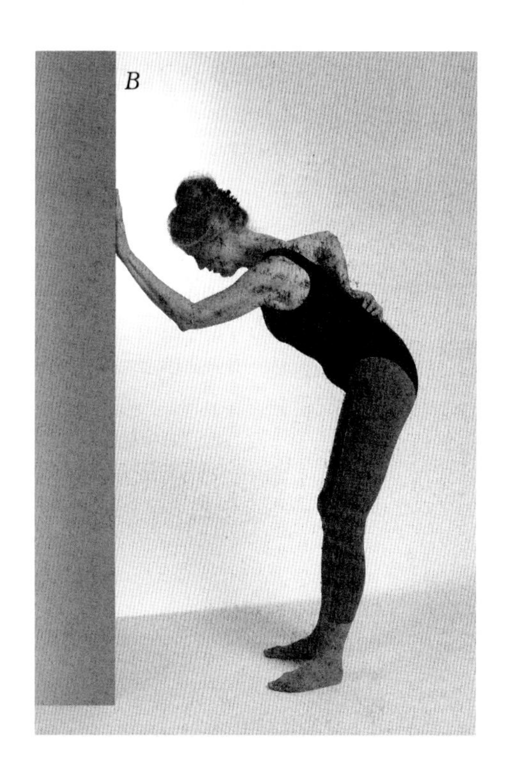
B

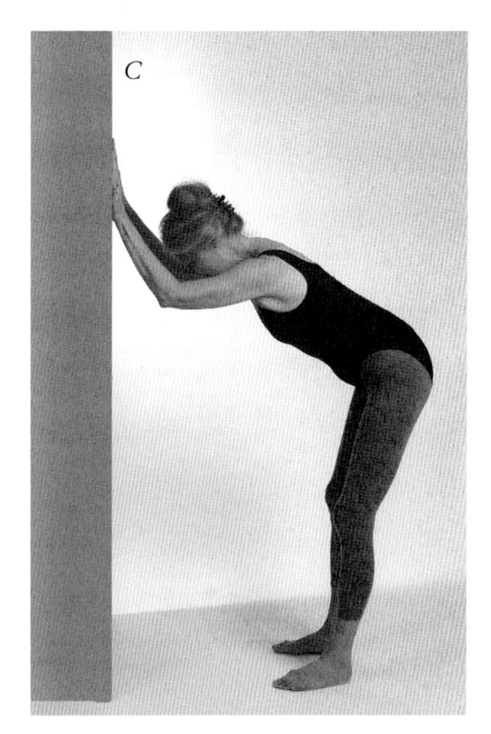
C

Arms Hug the Walls

Images for Your Artist

Our bodies are inherently resilient. Pleasing depictions of agile women and men can motivate us to reshape ourselves into limberness. Such images nourish our love of expansive movement. Many travel magazines and magazines from other cultures as well as U.S. historical images are filled with uplifting scenes of ordinary people who reflect physical comfort. Some devotional images and much art—French Impressionist paintings and sculptures, Indian miniatures, ancient Greek frescoes, and Greek, Indian, African, and Asian sculptures—convey physiological fluidity. Certain television programs document everyday life in these regions and show people constructing furniture, harvesting crops, or lifting objects with ease.

Yet, in highly industrialized countries, the magazines, movies, and even charts at doctors' offices represent "good" posture as a flattened, tucked pelvis with the shoulders pushed back from a rounded back.

When we have consciously or unconsciously struggled into "right" posture, strained motion becomes habitual. As a result, we are likely to try to *force* our bodies into the posture shown in illustrations of mobile people. By avoiding a goal, and simply perusing these images as indicators of our bodies' potential for comfortable action, we will have a clearer vision of how optimal bone support allows well-proportioned, unique

Savor the expansive gesture of this ancient Greek sculpture of the god Poseidon (National Archeological Museum, Athens). Notice the even groove down his back, as well as his strong back, buttock, arm, and leg muscles. Notice, too, his angled pelvis, the relaxed angle of his head, and his relaxed shoulders. He conveys strength and ease. In contrast, the young man on the left has a tucked pelvis and strained shoulders. He conveys stiffness and lack of ease.

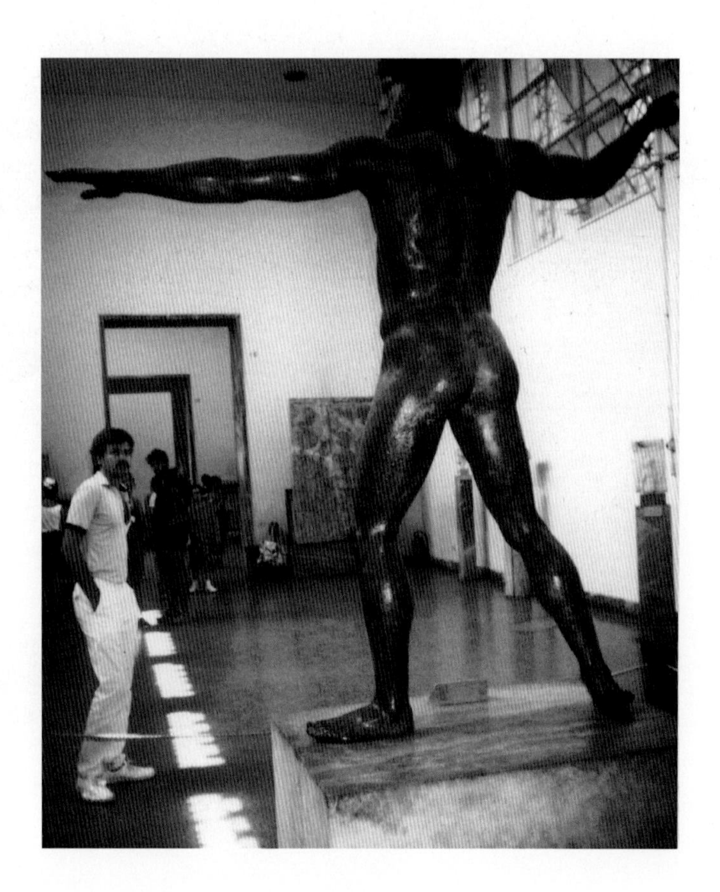

shaping of our muscles. This transparent understanding of our kinetics engenders an affectionate, aesthetic approach to our posture. Our imagination is then freed into boldly picturing ourselves with supple bearing.

Focusing on enhancing photos and artwork of limber people sharpens our sense of physical flexibility. As our centering movements surge from a deeper level, there will be a fulfilling exchange between the viewer and the subject.

Our inner artist can sculpt our flesh and instill our every action with a fluidity that was already present, at the quick of our malleable bodies. By dwelling on how we wish to look, instead of how we *should* look, we prepare the way for winsome ease.

Soon after I began practicing KENTRO I felt I had a 'secret.' I learned how to walk and stand powerfully without fatigue, bend and stretch with grace, and awaken without pain in my back. The brilliance of Angie's work as a healer is that she gently awakens dormant energy lying in the body and gives it a natural, soulful expression. I am ignited by her confidence in my ability to listen to and find my own centered body balance. I continue to discover and explore new ways of comfort and joy in my movements. In this arena I have found no equal to Angie as teacher, guide and healer.

–Lin Steers, Registered Nurse, Massage Therapist (Oregon)

14. Lying Down

PREPARATION. Place a pliable, thick pillow for your head on a comfortable mat. Stand on the mat (facing the foot of the mat) and practice Elemental Placement and Bending Forward.

A. As you bend, open your inner thighs for pelvic mobility and place one hand on the mat to help you sit down on the mat.

B. Keep at least one foot space between your knees and lean your torso back onto bent elbows. Relax your body; *sense weight (pressure) on the base of your buttocks.* Slowly hike your elbows toward the pillow, especially relax your entire body and especially your belly and lower back. *Sense that your lower back muscles soften and lengthen.* Picture your lower back like a little "hammock"—to undo arching in the lower back—without tucking your pelvis.

C. When your elbows have moved up as close as possible to the pillow, place your fingertips in the occipital grooves (small indentures at the base of your head) with a slight upward pressure as you place your head on the pillow. Let your shoulders touch the base of the pillow to allow comfortable placement of your head, neck, and rib cage. *Sense the upward occipital stretch releasing and lengthening the back of your neck, while you bring down your chin. Sense that your face, especially your jaw, can relax.*

D. Place the inside of your hands on your pelvic crest and let the Little Moon extend your legs, one at a time: To straighten your left leg, put downward and outward pressure onto your left pelvic crest, and rotate your left thigh outward (six to eight inches) as your leg straightens. Let your right hand put enough pressure onto the right crest so that your pelvis stays centered. *Sense release and expansion in your left hip, groin, and sacroiliac areas*. Straighten your right leg. Extend your arms beside your body. *Sense Grounding—your pelvis stretches away from your torso, your torso stretches toward your head. Sense more of your lower back on the mat than when you lie down quickly and your mid-lower back remains arched and off the mat.* Over time, you will only have space to slide a hand under the small natural arch area—between the fifth and third lumbar vertebrae.

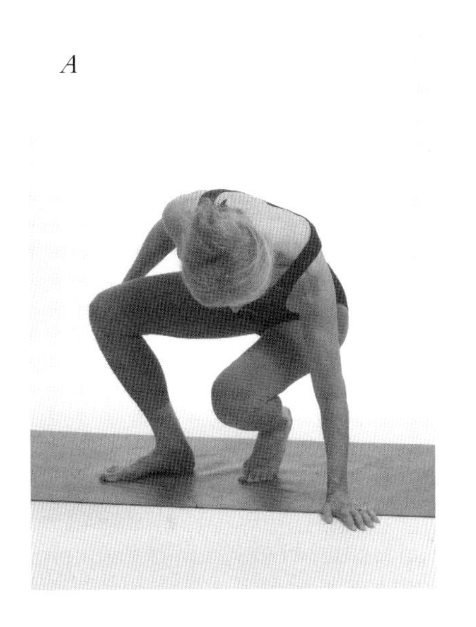

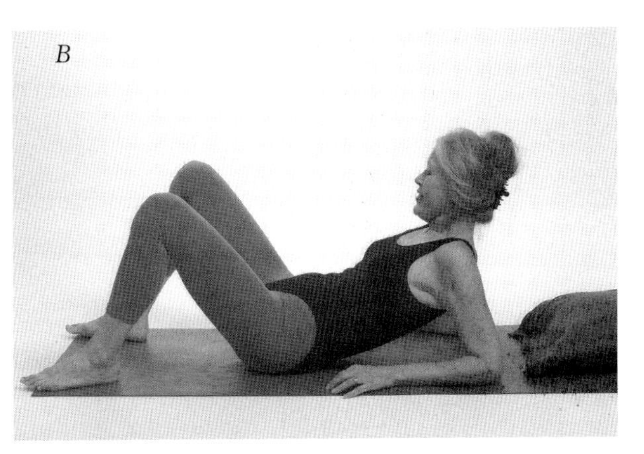

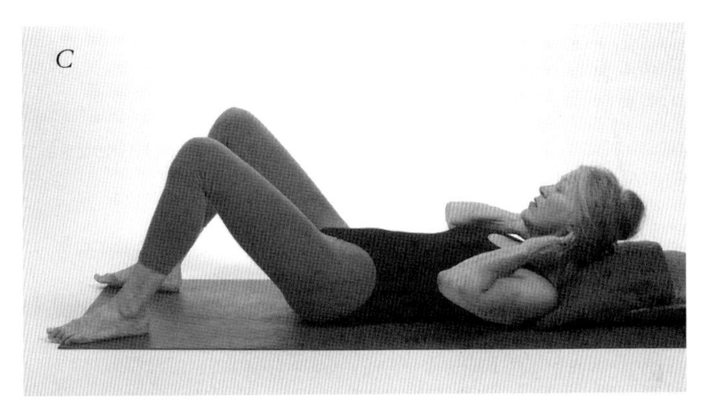

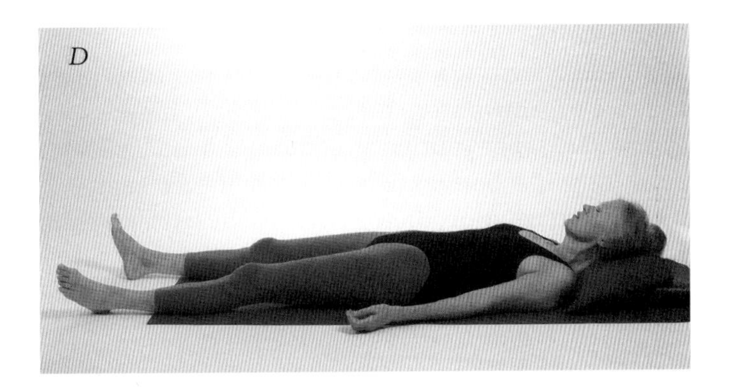

LYING DOWN (A-D)

E. Let your buttocks contract slightly, just enough to roll over to your left side, with your knees slightly bent and your torso and pelvis rolling over *as one unit*, to prevent stressful twisting in your back. Rolling over in this supple balance is toning for all pelvic muscles.

F. Place your pelvis into Elemental Placement; *sense that pulling the pillow slightly forward will straighten your neck and spine.* Extend or bend your legs as you like. *Sense Grounding—your pelvis lengthening and expanding away from your torso.* Bend both or just one leg, as you wish. Placing a pillow between your knees is helpful if you have a hip or knee symptom.

G. To rise in smooth balance, start with raising your torso off the mat with weight on your left forearm for support.

H. Keep raising your torso from left upper arm muscles, and then raise your pelvis up off the mat using strong buttocks muscles (as though a little string on your sacrum is lifting you up). Keep one foot of space between your knees; center your hips and legs, as you straighten your torso. Use these guidelines to lie down and get up—always beginning the action from your pelvic area.

BENEFITS: Taking a moment to stretch out comfortably and expansively as you lie down is the most practical and relaxing placement for tiny readjustments and releases to happen. Likewise, *Lying Down* alleviates stressed shoulders, overarching in your neck and lower back, and congestion in your thorax.

HELPFUL HINTS: Choose a resilient mattress. Pillows that are too narrow, or hard, or foam pillows with indentures may risk fixing, straining, or overarching your neck. Prevent tucking your pelvis, arching your neck or lower back or rounding your shoulders and upper back. Even if you are used to sleeping on your back, try resting on your side to get the benefits of Lying Down. Lying on your belly may overarch and tighten your lower back and neck.

VARIATIONS: Lying Down is the most propitious placement for letting your breathing enhance expansive stretching in your back muscles (Chapter, 9, Vignette 14, *Breathing up Your Back*). For your neck, slide your head back and forth on the pillow while your head "draws" a horizontally inclined "figure eight": "draw" a circle to the right and, without interruption, draw a circle to the left. Integrate the Executive or Pan with your leisurely Lying Down.

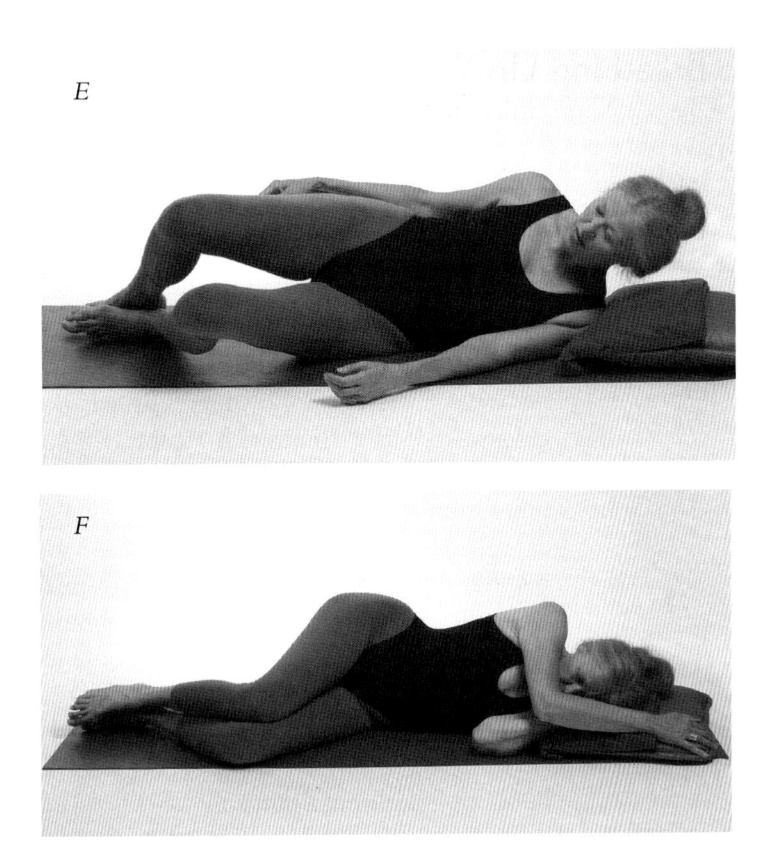

E

F

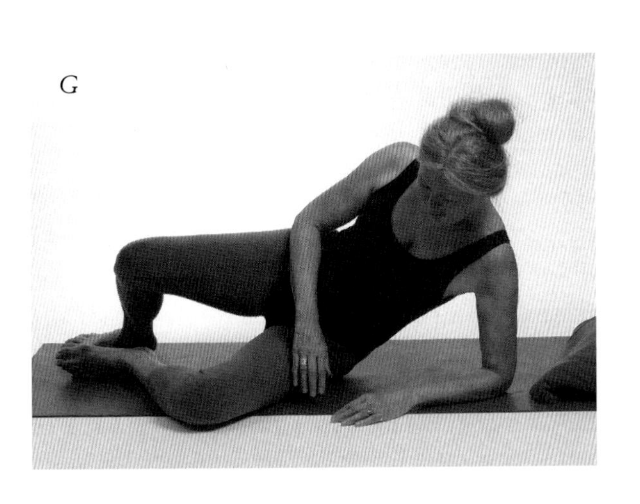

G

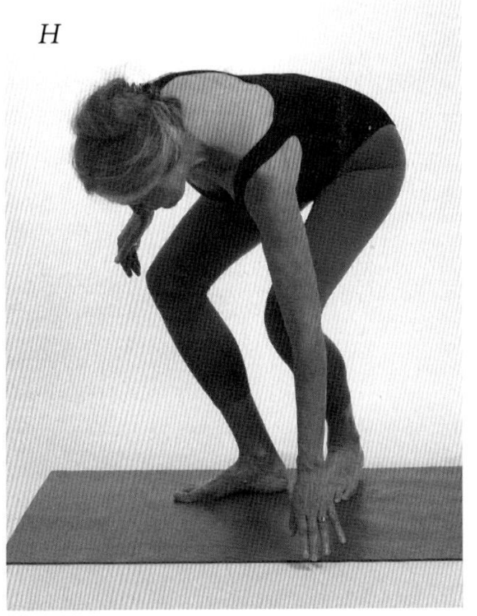

H

Lying Down (E-H)

Breathing Up Your Back

Breath is life. Inhaling fresh air and exhaling used air is the mysterious dynamic that keeps us alive. The root of the word "breath" is *spirit:* a vital force that has a rhythm of its own. By practicing centering and balancing guidelines, our bodies become spacious. Our ability to breathe deeper and more naturally is restored, and we feel fuller expression in our actions. When our natural capacity for breathing and our rhythm of breathing are enhanced, breath can invigorate each cell of our porous bodies, regardless of our activities.

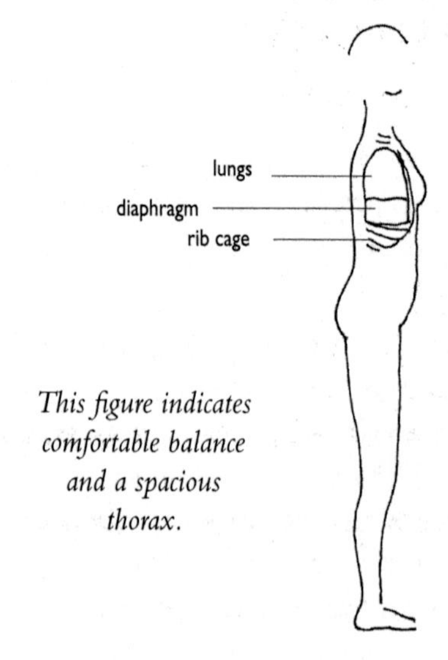

This figure indicates comfortable balance and a spacious thorax.

The essence of our respiratory system is to provide us with as much air as possible; the more volume there is in our lungs the more our body is oxygenated. As we breathe in (inspiration), our diaphragm muscle flattens as it presses on our abdominal organs, thus increasing the volume of our lungs, allowing air to fill the lungs. Many lower and mid-back muscles, as well as ten muscles attached to the ribs, all aid in inspiration. When inspiration is complete, pressure rises in the lungs, and respiratory passages diffuse air out of the body—facilitated by the relaxed, dome-shaped diaphragm, pushed up by the abdominal muscles.

Muscular resiliency is necessary for optimal vertical lengthening and lateral expansion in the torso while we breathe. Gray calls this "ordinary, tranquil respiration."11 When we need active strength for running or dancing, abdominal muscles work as well; Gray refers to this type of breathing as "forced respiration."[12] Stressful posture—the legs too far out front, a tucked pelvis, a distended or tightened abdomen, a shortened (arched) lower back, and an over-stretched (rounded) upper back—all limit muscular elasticity and reduce the volume of the thorax (upper torso). As a result of these compensations, the diaphragm muscle is less flexible and the abdominal muscles shorten or weaken. We may push up our rib cage in an effort to breathe deeper, yet physiologically, this effort does not increase the volume in the thorax.

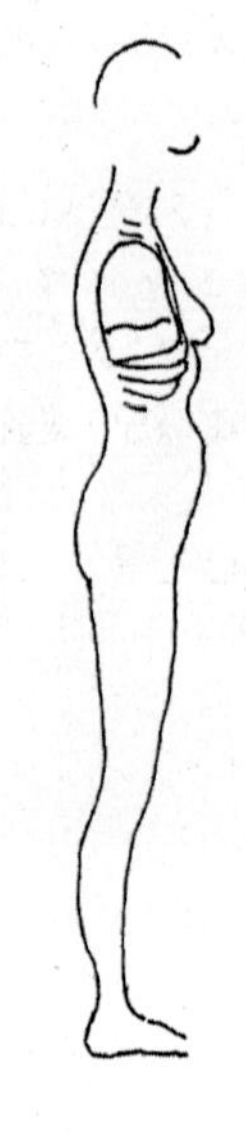

This figure indicates strained balance and a restricted thorax.

Centering our movements can slowly, steadily relieve shallow breathing because our tissues become more limber and our bodies more spacious when we move with smooth Balance. *Breathing up Your Back* is a KENTRO visualization that has a twofold effect: 1) it develops our ability to increase muscular pliability and 2) it heightens the potential for amplified oxygenation of our tissues. This visualization is not a breathing technique; it does not require a specific breathing pace, counting breaths, holding breath, or tightening or pushing out our belly.

When we are in comfortable balance with Elemental Placement guidelines and wish to incorporate the breath-visualization, we simply focus on assisting ample stretching throughout our pelvic, abdominal, and back muscles. There is no "doing" at all, there is just letting muscles expand whenever we feel an inhalation happening on its own. Of course, air does more than oxygenate our back muscles. Focusing on our backside helps us avoid habitual tightening/distension of the abdomen, or arching of our lower back, or pushing up our rib cage. Placing our attention on air moving up our back like a "fresh breeze" lets our back, abdomen, and pelvis relax into being stretched. Regard inhalation as similar to a sigh or yawn (which spontaneously straightens our back and enlarges our thorax); this is the most effective approach to allowing breath to extend stretching in Elemental Placement. While bending, sitting down, or lying down, place the inside of your left hand on your diaphragm and the inside of your right hand on your belly. Notice that on the inhalation, your rib cage gently stretches upward, while your belly stretches slightly downward (toward your feet). Now place the fingers of your right hand onto the vertebrae in your lower back with the palm of your hand on the muscles. When you sense air coming in, immediately visualize "breathing" starting in the small of your back; imagine that this is the only place where breath can begin to do its work. While you picture air moving up your back, notice the sensation of tiny ripples along your spinal muscles as your lower back stretches; and with your left hand sense an upward and lateral stretching in your rib cage. You can feel an enlarging stretch in the shoulder blade areas as your sternum area also broadens.

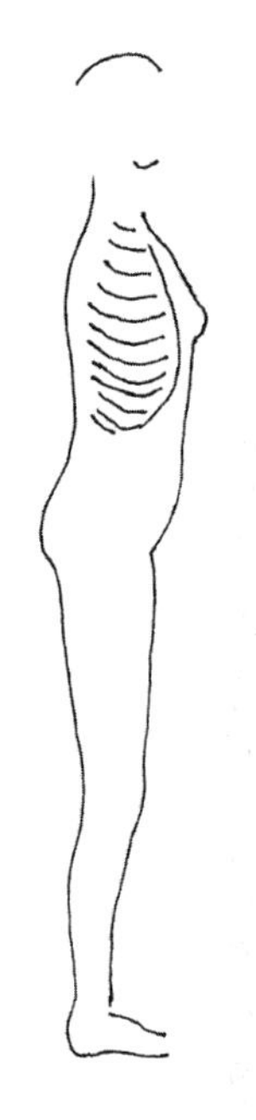

This figure indicates a straightening stretch in the back as well as an expansive rib cage, which allows costal (rib) muscles to expand easily during inhalation.

With each intake of air, your lung capacity will increase, your diaphragm and abdomen will become more elastic, and your rib cage will lift and expand without any arching in your lower back. At first, you may not sense much extension in your thorax; yet with practice, you will feel such stretching on the inhalation. When the inhalation is complete, forget about everything and just let air go out on the exhalation. Savor this whole process that corresponds to Gray's description of up-and-down tranquil breathing.

Breathing "up our back," integrated with Elemental Placement slows us down and makes us more aware of how to foster extensive stretching and to allow deeper breathing. This may also positively influence the flow of the cerebrospinal fluid, which nourishes the nerves between the brain and spinal column. Certainly, it helps us avoid tiring, forced (active) breathing with strained posture and prematurely being "out of breath" physiologically. It prepares the way for smooth active breathing during aerobic activities and smooth tranquil breathing during rest. This practice can be beneficial to singers and yoga or meditation practitioners who use specific breathing techniques. An English friend remarked that when she began to sit back on her sofa in Elemental Placement, she felt more open in her torso, and breathing "up her back" *simplified* sensing her breathing. Fuller sensing of our breathing, combined with centering comfort, enhances our conscious use of breath to relax and vitalize our body.

15. Heart Stretch Lying Down

PREPARATION: Place a mat on the floor, lie down on your back, straighten your legs, and practice Elemental Placement.

A. The Heart Stretch Lying Down starts in your upper back. Place the fingertips of your left hand onto the front of your spine and around the heart area; place the inside of your right hand on your lower abdomen. Stay relaxed. Keep your chin and shoulders down. With your attention on the heart area, slowly contract your upper back muscles and raise your upper back slightly off the mat—until you *feel toning (muscular contraction) in your abdomen*. Expect some "pulling" in your neck muscles; remember to focus on activating this stretch from your shoulder blade muscles. *Sense toning in your abdominal, back, and pelvic muscles*.

   After the duration of a yawn, recline again and rest. This is an active, toning stretch, so make the rest *longer* than the actual stretch, to give your body time for tiny readjustments. Start out with three to four stretches. You may double the number of stretches after a few months of practice.

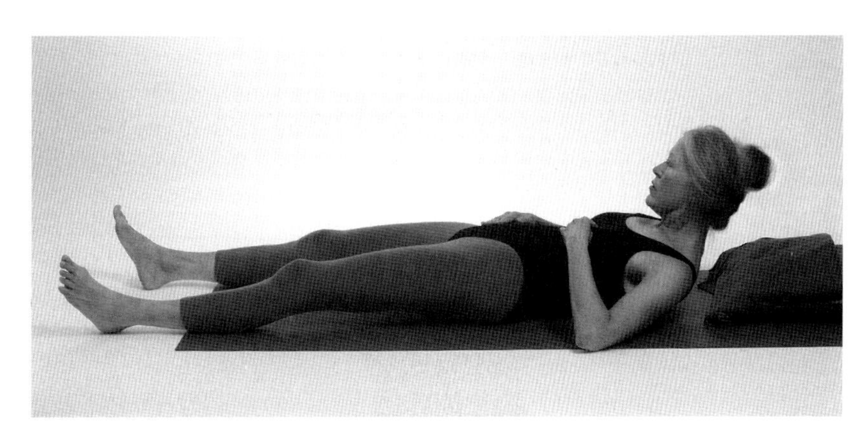

HEART STRETCH LYING DOWN

BENEFITS: The *Heart Stretch Lying Down* is highly effective because all your torso and pelvic muscles become stronger automatically, without undue effort. Your back muscles, especially upper back muscles, likewise, will obtain a favorable releasing stretch. This is a full-bodied, toning stretch for the back muscles.

HELPFUL HINTS: Forget any goal of raising up your torso as far as possible—do no push your body. The stretch is complete as soon as you feel toning in your abdomen. Notice whether you start out by tightening your belly or tightening your shoulder muscles to raise up your torso. As you get ready to raise your upper torso off the mat, from the heart area, relax your entire body, to prevent rounding your upper back straining and over-contracting your neck, pushing your shoulders out front, and tightening your diaphragm and abdomen. Practice Looking for Elbow Room, Tikanis, and Lying Down before Heart Stretching Down.

VARIATIONS: Vary this stretch by adding Looking for Elbow Room to Heart Stretch Lying Down.

Milagros Pequeños: Small Miracles

The Spanish word *milagro,* "miracle," is used to describe events that frequently include special physical changes. Big miracles are seen as direct, inexplicable acts of God. Small miracles, on the other hand, occur unpredictably but are seen as the result of a natural process that has not yet been conventionally explained. *Milagro* can serve as an empowering metaphor of our bodies' inherent mobility.

In Honduras, words with theological connotations act as bridges to secular life. A *milagro pequeño* is a down-to-earth happening. An example of a *milagro pequeño* can be seen in the recovery of a student of mine in Honduras who was partially paralyzed in a car accident. She decided to combine biofeedback with her learning to walk in smooth balance. After consistently practicing the KENTRO Pelvic Rock, Little Moon, and Pan to limber her pelvis, as well as the Grounding, Bending, and Walking movements, she unexpectedly stopped limping.

Another Honduran student felt she had a *milagro pequeño* when, following diligent practice of Little Moon, Grounding, Leg Rotation, Gliding, Walking, and Sitting, she could stand and sit with increased ease. She had been injured by polio many years earlier, and her KENTRO practice had produced significant muscular improvement in her damaged leg muscles.

Such outcomes are possible when we view our motions as more than mere mechanical function. Practiced playfully and with an organic view of our body, centering and balancing movements can renew physical expression. This realization helps us avoid quick, fix-it therapies and healing techniques that do not encompass sound anatomical principles. A shift in attitude or perspective can invite an as-yet-unknown limberness to suffuse our every gesture and change a "hopeless" state into a hoped-for reality—satisfying physical shifts.

The base of the word *miracle* is *mirari,* "to wonder at," and *mirus,* as "wonderful." KENTRO guidelines emphasize the importance of developing our sense of wonder. We can become aware of and welcome the physical and nonphysical aspects of our fluid posture through affectionate, artful attention to our body as it signals timing and rhythm for a harmonious movement.

A tender view of our bodies dispels demeaning thoughts about our posture, and allows our bodies to craft us into joyful resiliency, guiding us toward a life-enhancing way of seeing ourselves. It is a small miracle that after perhaps thirty years of unnecessary physical distress and strain, we can regain vital comfort and suppleness in our standing, bending, sitting, and lifting. We can experience wonder when repetitive gestures at home and at work feel soulful and enlivening.

KENTRO practice awakens our trust in nature.

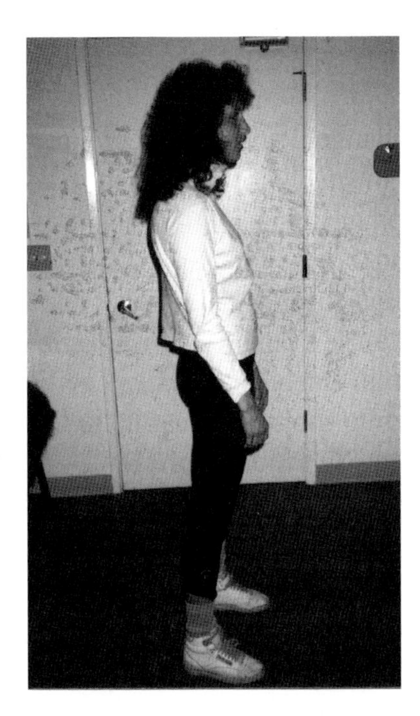

Helene, a physical therapist, already exercised on a daily basis but wished to increase her flexibility and abdominal strength.

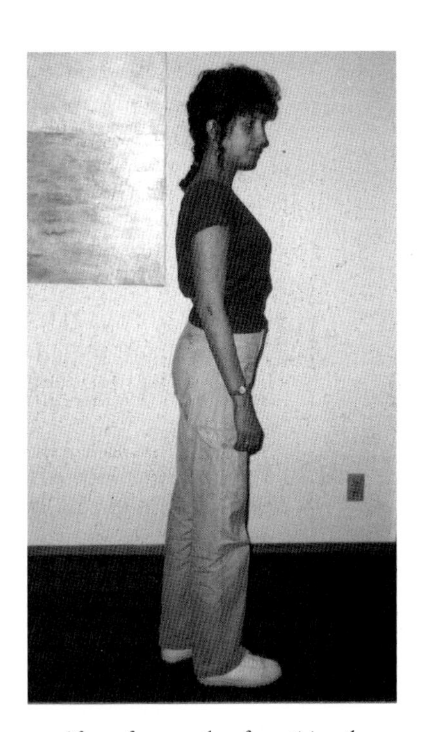

After a few months of practicing the KENTRO method, Helene's postural expression shifted into more supportive neck, spinal, pelvic, and leg alignment; stronger back and abdominal muscles; and a fuller range of movement.

16. Walking

PREPARATION: Start out by facing a long mirror; practice Elemental Placement.

A. Place the inside of your hands on the top of your buttocks and slowly shift your weight from one leg to the other to keep your hips level. Shift your weight into your left leg. Practice Grounding and relax your right buttock (which corresponds to the *resting* aspect of walking), while you consciously contract the left buttock (which is the *active* aspect of walking). Take a moment to *sense expansion/contraction in your buttocks muscles*. Alternate.

B. Stand with your torso slightly forward (for easy Grounding) *in profile* to the mirror. With your arms at your side, shift weight onto your left leg, while keeping your left hip in line with the front of your heel. Slowly bend your right knee and raise your foot. Ground your pelvis, keep level hips. *Sense that your pelvis feels like a "seat," as though you are sitting "standing up."* This is the resting, starting point for walking.

C. Keep your hips level and knees relaxed throughout the guidelines C, D, and E—"taking a step apart:" the dynamic aspect of walking. Take a step by combining three rapid motions into one movement, as shown in C, D, and E) Contract your left buttock muscles, and as you extend your right leg, keep them contracted so that they can propel your torso forward; b) the moment you set down your right heel on the ground, your left leg extends out back, and, for a second, you will *sense equal weight in both feet*. In this transition, let the momentum (push off) from your left buttock carry through, so that c) your weight shifts into your right leg.

D. As soon as you set down your entire right foot (and your right leg becomes your supportive leg), *Ground* your right buttock and simultaneously let your left leg bend slightly and swing up front.

E. Let your left buttock follow through as you swing your left leg out front; *sense suppleness in your left leg and stability in your right leg. Ground* your pelvis: your step is completed. Notice that your stance here is similar to B.

   Practicing steps A through E many times—in this patient, slowed-down manner—will help you understand and *feel the sensuous balancing within walking* and will allow you to incorporate the *Walking* guidelines into your natural walking rhythm. Over time, you will *sense a continuous flow and smooth balance when you walk*.

BENEFITS: *Walking* in centered balance is a delightful, comprehensive exercise for your body. With increased *Grounding* and symmetry in your hips, the buttocks and legs become toned and limbered. Walking results in more ease of movement. Your knees and ankles can become more resilient, and the soles of your feel get "massaged" and stretched because with each step, the heel of one foot and toes of the other foot touch the ground. Walking also helps you to confidently shift your weight into a supporting leg and at the same time ground and relax the muscles of that leg.

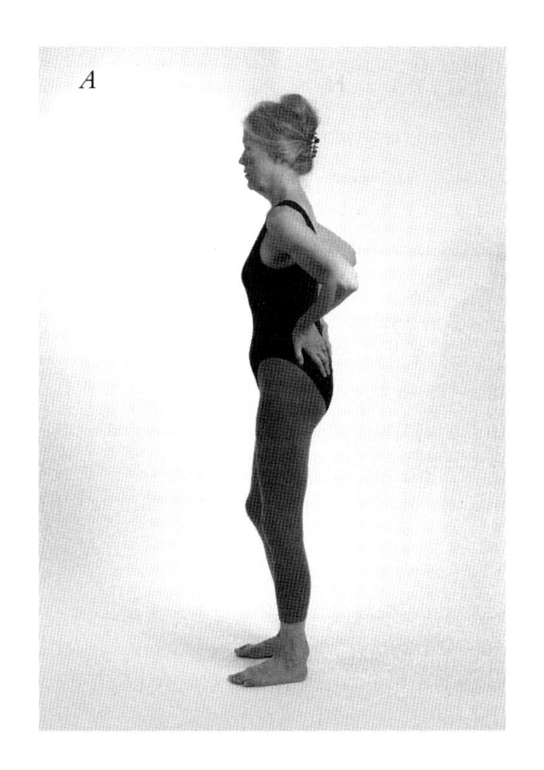

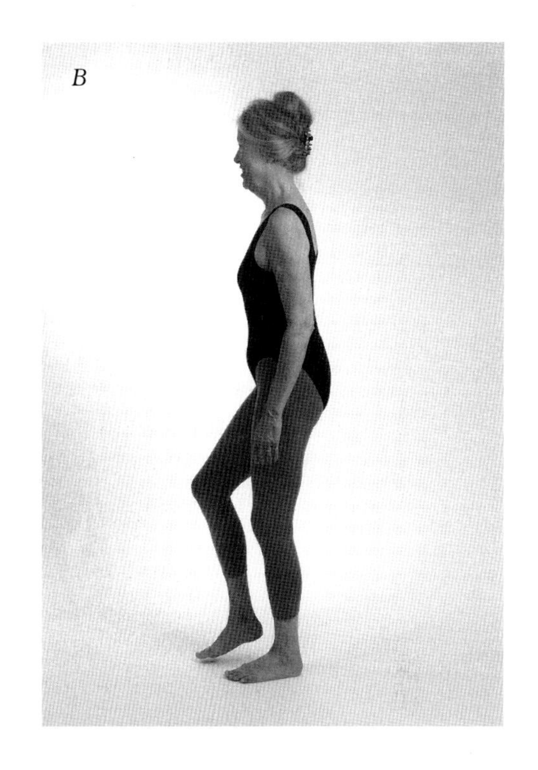

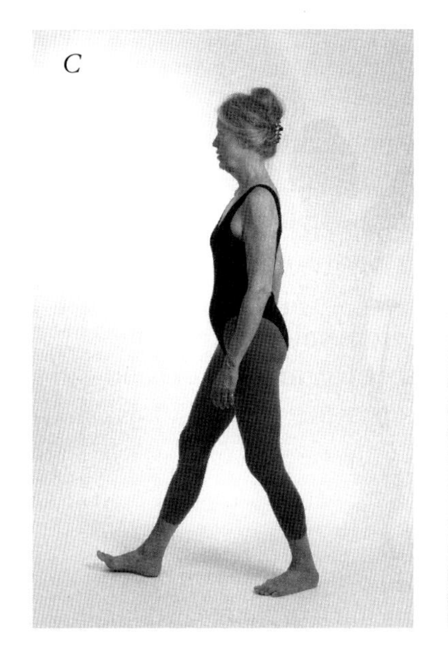

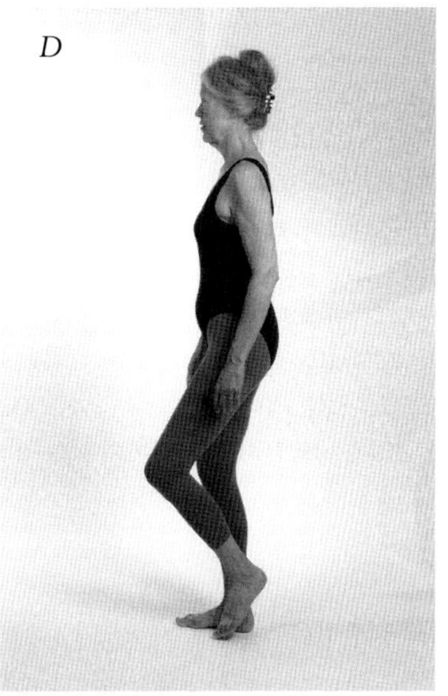

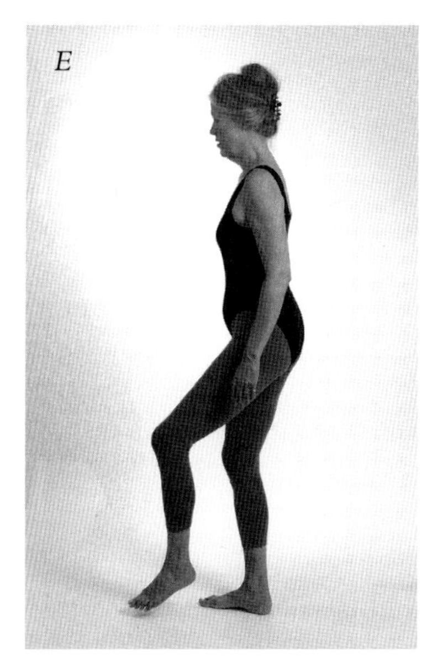

WALKING

HELPFUL HINTS: Prevent the following stresses:

- taking a step with a tightened abdomen or locked knees
- tucking your pelvis, which pushes your pelvis and legs up front
- placing one foot in front of the other, which misaligns your pelvis
- twisting your back or pelvis, or raising one hip higher than the other
- placing too much weight on the outside or inside of your feet
- lunging forward from your head and shoulders
- raising up your chin and rib cage, or pushing back your shoulders.

Over time as your pelvic and thoracic muscles become more elastic, you can be very *Grounded* and more upright for smooth Walking. Energetic strides require more pelvic and thigh muscular action. *Exaggerate* the grounding/dynamic aspects of walking to fully *sense* Walking. Practice Leg Rotation/Extension before Walking.

VARIATIONS: In Greece, we are likely to see people taking lively, lengthy steps, whereas in Honduras, people glide and flow along with small steps. People vary in how they place their feet: a pronounced upward slant, or the foot parallel to the ground for the front foot; a full extension through the toes, or letting the toes flex for the back foot; or even walking flatfooted, which is unsuitable for us because it requires extremely elastic leg muscles.

When you hike uphill, bend your knees more and lean your torso forward to allow weight to be assimilated in the hip/sacral area.

If you have to run, incorporate *Walking* extensively to prevent tucking, twisting, or tightening your body.

For *Walking* with an object on the head, begin by placing something light (such as a medium-sized telephone book) on your head to prevent muscular holding, overarching, and over-compression in your neck and back. Hold on to the object with a hand as you walk; *sense that when you take a step, your pelvis grounds and your spine lengthens to absorb the weight of the object on your head.* While hiking with a backpack, the shoulder straps of the backpack can actually help your shoulders to drop and relax, as long as they are ample straps; your spine can lengthen easily, and your pelvic muscles expand and *Ground* you. Slowed-down walking meditations can be an exquisite manner of expanding centered *Walking*.

Posture in Rhythm

Hondurans use the word *ritmo*—rhythm—as a compliment: a person who has *ritmo* exudes lively, graceful movements in dancing or ordinary occupations. As a young child, I saw many people moving in a dance-like fashion as they prepared food, built a house, or gardened. When I was a teenager, I danced to my heart's content at parties: *al ritmo de cha cha cha.* Nobody talked about posture.

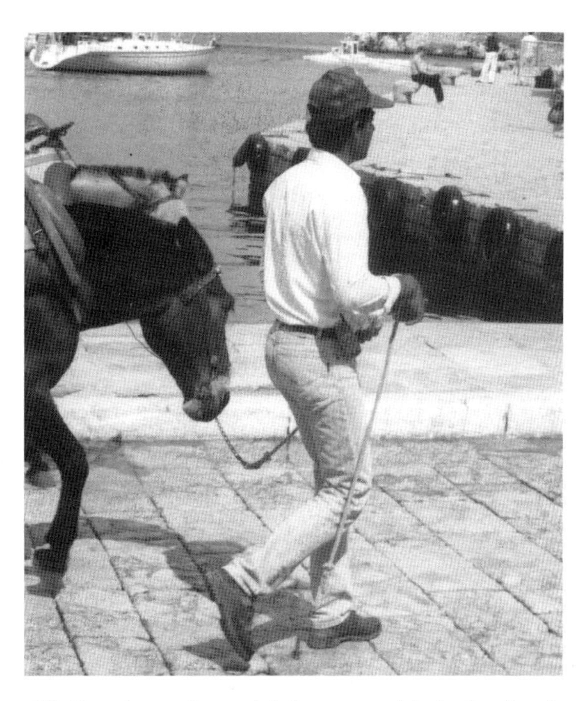

Fluid motion and smooth balance: a straight back, relaxed shoulders, and a grounded pelvis describe this Greek man's walking.

At home, nobody talked about rhythm. Instead, I was constantly reminded to suck in my belly and tuck my buttocks. My Honduran girlfriends heard no such comments at their homes, where posture was not an issue. I became ill at ease with my looks. When, at age thirteen, I traveled to the U.S. for further schooling, "correct" posture was a serious topic of conversation. Years later at the Paris Iyengar Yoga and Aplomb Institutes, the word *posture* still carried stressful connotations for me. It was only when I started to create gentle balancing stretches, integrated with centering movements, that my actions and rhythm became interwoven. Rhythm pulsated into my bodily expression.

Posture is a richly textured word that is defined as "an attitude of mind," as well as "the position of the body or of parts of the body; carriage; bearing." I began to view posture as *how we move* through space with our unique bearing and personal expression. Our physical attitude, or stance, defines the quality of our movements. Our gestures are in intimate connection with the cadence of our physical systems—respiration and circulation—and of our psyche and subtle feelings.

R*hythm* is defined as "flow, movement." In art, *rhythm* is an aesthetic relation of part to part and of parts to the whole; the rhythm of a picture, of a statue. We could extend this to also mean the flow of an activity, or our every movement.

Some years ago, articles in *Nature* described the unique gait of women in Kenya who "can carry heavy head-supported loads of up to 70 percent of their body weight with significantly less mechanical work (muscular effort) than trained or untrained people in group control studies."[13] The secret of the Kenyan women's maximal efficiency is that they do less work (energy expenditure/muscular action). This results in a pendulum-like, more complete transfer of energy during each step. They have more potential (stored) energy and thereby a greater release of kinetic (active) energy as the leg rotates forward and actually takes a step. Over many years, I have observed that people who traditionally carry heavy loads on their heads move with the optimal balance which is similar to the KENTRO guidelines for Elemental Placement, Carrying, and Walking: straight backs, slanted pelvises, and relaxed shoulders. We see this bear-

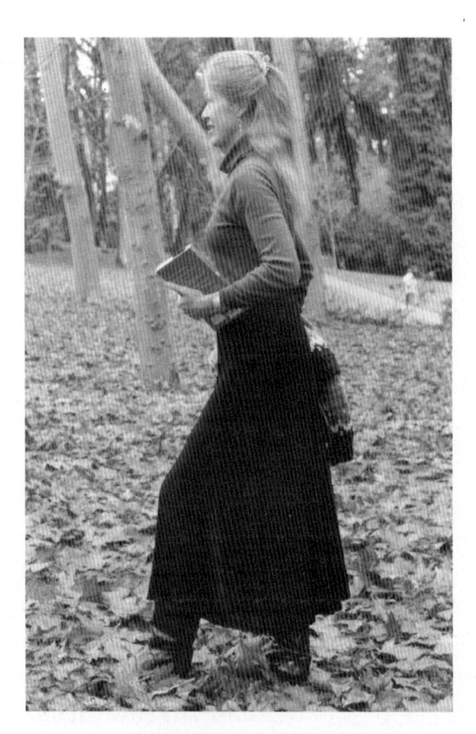

While I practice Walking, I forget about posture; I savor a grounding, restful stretch in my buttock muscles as I shift weight to my right leg, before taking a step with my left foot.

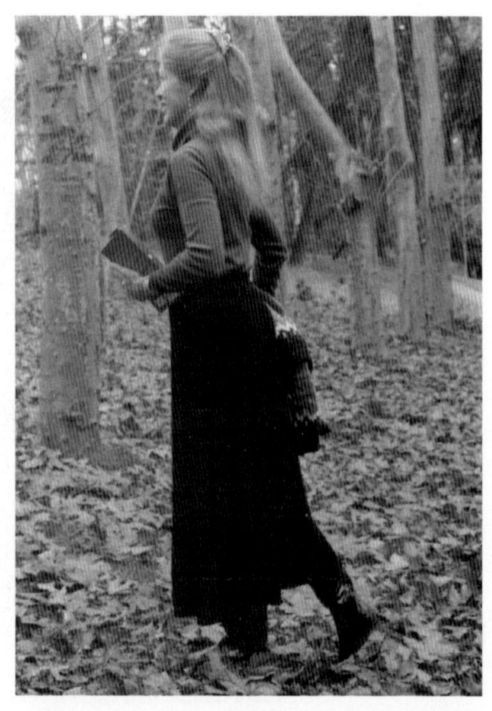

While I contract my right buttock muscles to take a step with my left foot, I feel a rhythm inherent to walking, as my body is dynamically propelled forward. As I take a step with my left foot, my right leg is momentarily extended out behind me before it quickly moves forward—and I ground myself as weight shifts to my left leg.

ing in a photo and a drawing of an African woman in a *New York Times* review of Dr. Heglund's article.[14] This bearing is also apparent in toddlers whose heads are naturally very heavy in proportion to the rest of their bodies. There appears to be a parallel between the KENTRO restful grounding aspect of walking and stored potential energy as well as between the KENTRO active step and kinetic energy. The KENTRO emphasis on the optimal anterior pelvic slant, with the legs and the weight in the feet shifting *back* (into vertical alignment with the spine)—allows the legs to support the pelvis; the pelvis itself then becomes more flexible. Most weight transfers through the sacral/hip area. The pelvis can then support the back weight-bearing muscles without effort. In turn, the buttocks muscles can relax and a flexed leg is already out front, in preparation for taking a step (see B in Walking). The rested buttocks (stored energy) can then contract well and propel the leg farther forward with an extensive swing, so that in the moment of taking the step (active energy), most weight is again distributed effectively through the sacral/hip region. There is a smooth, clear transfer between the potential and kinetic aspects of walking. However, in conventional walking there is less mobility in the pelvic center of mass and less swing in the forward rotating leg: the leg drops down sooner and thereby decreases forward speed. When the pelvis is tucked into a posterior slant, the legs and pelvis move out *front*, causing pelvic and leg muscle strain, and causing most of the body weight to move toward the ligaments in *front* of the thighs and toward the *front* of the feet. The buttocks, too, lose some elasticity. There is less of a forward swing to the leg that takes a step, and the other leg does not instantly flex and come forward—it "lags" behind. Probably, the transfer from potential to kinetic energy decreases. Compensatory muscles struggle to "put on the brakes" to prevent the falling forward of the head, shoulders, and torso. In contrast, walking with centered balance fosters an entirely different experience: there is a grounding, "sitting back" and suppleness in the pelvic region.

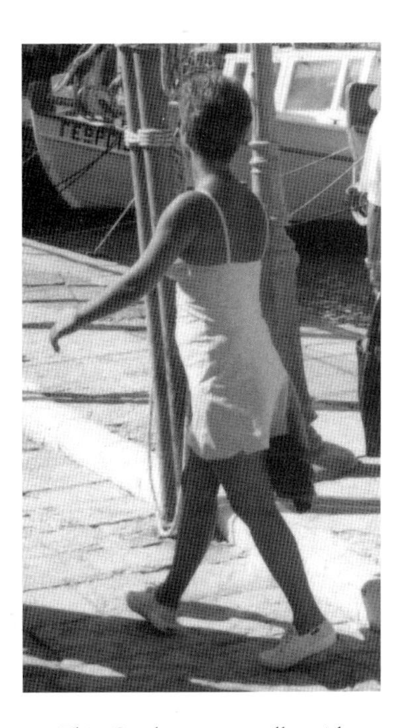

This Greek woman walks with relaxed shoulders and level hips. The weight of her shopping bag is in line with her hips. Her profile conveys a lengthy (neither shortened nor protruding) abdomen, angled pelvis, and straight back, as well as a great range of movement in her hips and shoulders. She has taken a step and, momentarily, both feet are on the ground; she is in the most dynamic-kinetic stage of walking.

KENTRO students report that when they practice *Walking* guidelines, they feel relaxed yet toned and that they can sweep across a room with three strides instead of half a dozen. Walking can become our favorite exercise, especially when it feels like a leisurely, dashing dance.

As we move with more ease, we can sense harmonious motion and toning in all our repetitive actions. Over time, we perceive the difference between monotonous rhythm and enjoyable, endlessly varied bodily rhythms engendered by our centering and balancing motion.

There is a lovely kinship between the words *pleasure* and *please*: both stem from the Old French *plaisir*, with *pleasure,* meaning delight, and satisfaction; and *please* (from the Latin *placidus* and *placare*) meaning to soothe, to give pleasure, and to wish, or to will. When we choose to balance and center our movements, agreeable, tranquil feelings and gentle stretches throughout our bodies is exactly what we experience as we walk, sweep the floor or clean the windows. Postural fluidity generates pleasurable rhythmic gestures in tune with our daily activities.

17. Carrying

PREPARATION: Stand beside a lightweight chair (preferably a folding chair) in profile to a long mirror. Practice Elemental Placement. Bend forward and lift the chair (see Lifting), *centering it with your bellybutton while you lift it and while you carry it.*

A. Keep the chair close to your body, and slightly contract the muscles in your shoulder blade area (without pushing your shoulders back), to carry the chair easily. Keep your elbows as far back as possible tucked close to your body. Keep weight mostly in the heels of your feet while relaxing your knees and belly. *Feel weight (pressure) shift off your shoulders and into your buttocks-sacral area, upper back, and upper arms. Sense that your abdomen is getting a workout. Sense stability.* Look in the mirror and observe your Elemental Placement. Continue to Ground yourself while you carry the chair back and forth for the duration of a few yawns; keep your belly-button centered with the chair. *Sense your strong sacral, upper back, and upper arm muscles contracting.* Set the chair down in front of you and take a moment to rest.

B. For contrast, briefly pick up the chair with tucked buttocks, feet together, and lifting from your shoulder muscles. Notice how distressing this *feels*, compared to lifting the chair with smooth balance.

C. Lift the chair again and face the mirror to notice whether your shoulders stay down, your hips stay level and your pelvis stays Grounded. *Sense stability*.
Look in the mirror as you move your feet to the left, bend forward, and set down the chair (to your left). This will allow you to verify that *your pelvis remains centered with the object at all times*. Alternate sides—setting down the chair to your right. Rest.

D. Fold the chair and pick it up with both hands. Hold it lengthwise in your left hand, close to your body. *Sense* pressure (weight) in your heels and sacral area. *Feel a "work-out" in your "carrying" muscles—pelvis, upper back, and upper arms.*
Carry the chair back and forth for the duration of a few yawns or as soon as you feel your muscles getting tired. Unfold the chair, set it down, and rest.

BENEFITS: *Carrying* in smooth balance is a highly effective means of strengthening your appropriate weight-bearing muscles, especially in the buttock, upper back, and upper arm areas. Abdominal, core pelvic and lower back muscles also get toned when you carry a slightly heavy object. With practice, you may actually look forward to Carrying because the toning in your muscles will feel energizing. Using your naturally appropriate weight-bearing muscles generates gentle strength.

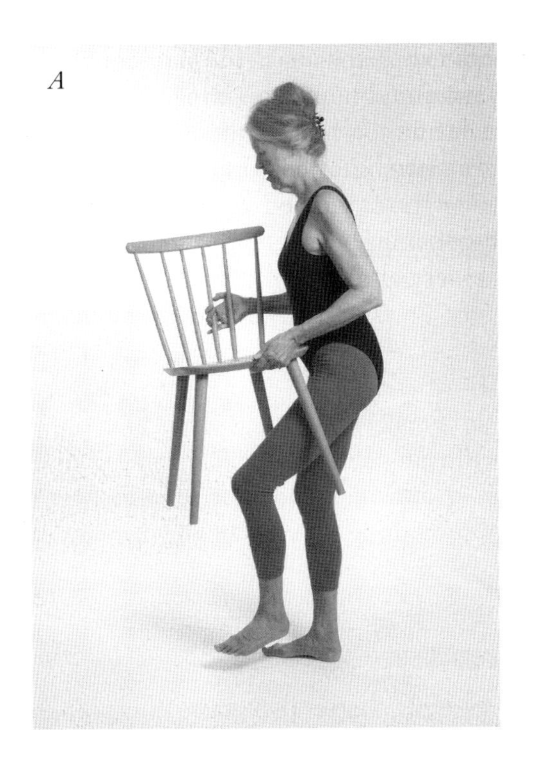

A

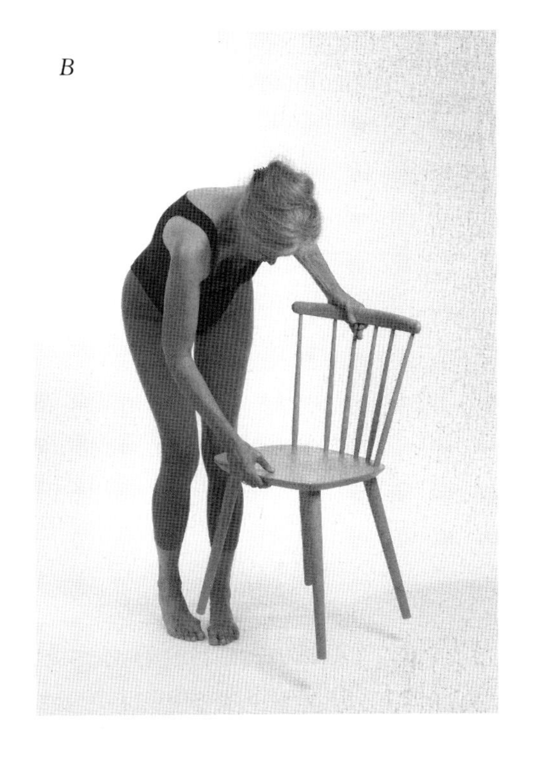

B

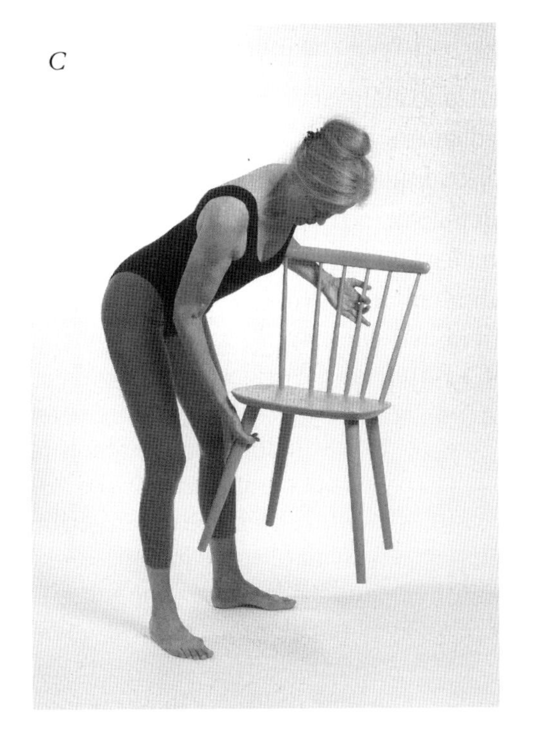

C

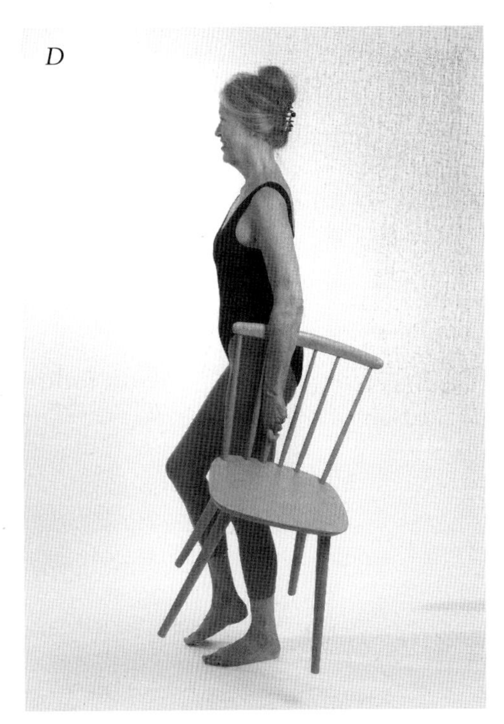

D

Carrying

HELPFUL HINTS: Always discern *how much* weight is suitable for you to carry—in proportion with your height, shape, weight, history of injuries, lifestyle, and KENTRO practice—and *how long* you can carry comfortably without taxing or pushing your body. Pause frequently whenever you are carrying. If you gasp or feel pain, the weight you are carrying is too heavy. If your doctor has cautioned you about lifting or carrying, heed those warnings. Prevent twisting, tucking, tightening, locking *any* part of your body, and rounding or arching your back or pelvis. No matter what you are carrying, place it *as close as possible to your sacral/hip area.* Practicing Arms Hug (and Push) the Wall, Tikanis, and Boat are helpful before Carrying.

VARIATIONS: If you are strong, you may try carrying something on your shoulders or your back—in small increments of time. Start out by Carrying your casserole, books, and groceries. Your muscles will need time to become extremely relaxed and strong before you can attempt to carry something on your head without arching your spine and straining your tissues.

Work Becomes Play

For four years during the early eighties, I attended classes on pre-Columbian Indian societies at the Paris Sorbonne University. I was intrigued by the philosophy of these Indians who—with the exception of the Incas, Aztecs, and Maya—had self-designated chiefs who wielded no coercive power over the members of their tribe. Everyone, including the chief, spent most of his or her time in games, relaxation, and storytelling. Play was an important aspect of daily life. When a problem arose between neighbors, the chief resolved the conflict by telling an uplifting story about ancestors who lived peacefully with one another. If people grew tired from working in the field or at home, they would take frequent breaks to sing or nap. Work was interwoven with abundant relaxation.

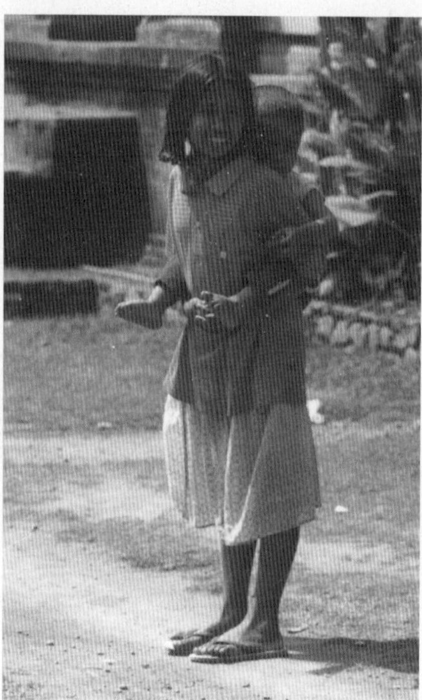

With her legs comfortably aligned with her pelvis and back, this young Nepalese girl can carry a toddler on her sacrum without muscular strain.

Shifting our approach to work is an essential component of the KENTRO program: a subtle blend between action and rest, which we can observe in people who carry things in smooth balance. The more relaxed our practice, the more we will notice new strength and comfort. It may seem difficult to include a note of leisure in our work if we are tired or stressed. However, we can be inspired by images of children at play. Young children move

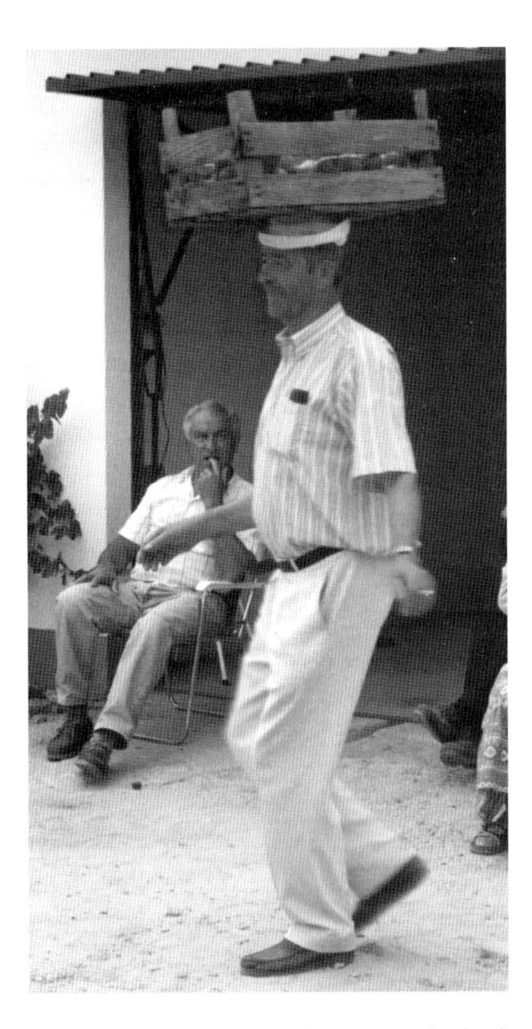

Dancing with a heavy crate of tomatoes on his head, this strong and limber sixty-five-year old Portuguese man displays a grounded pelvis, straight back, broad torso, and relaxed shoulders.

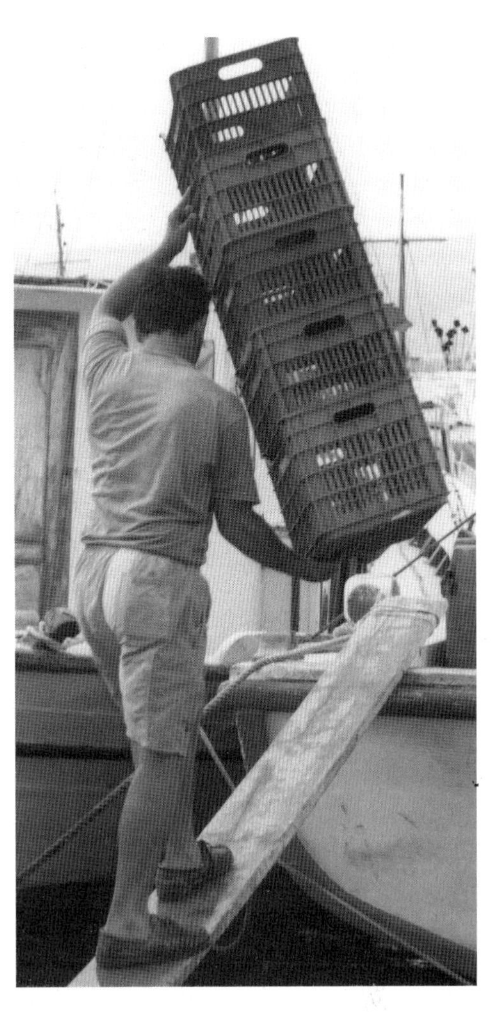

Notice the straight back, level hips, and limber pelvis and legs of this Greek man carrying a stack of crates. There is no twisting in his strong back or grounded pelvis. His shoulders stay down and relaxed while his torso bends slightly forward from the hips. The weightof the crates can be assimilated mostly in his pelvis and hips.

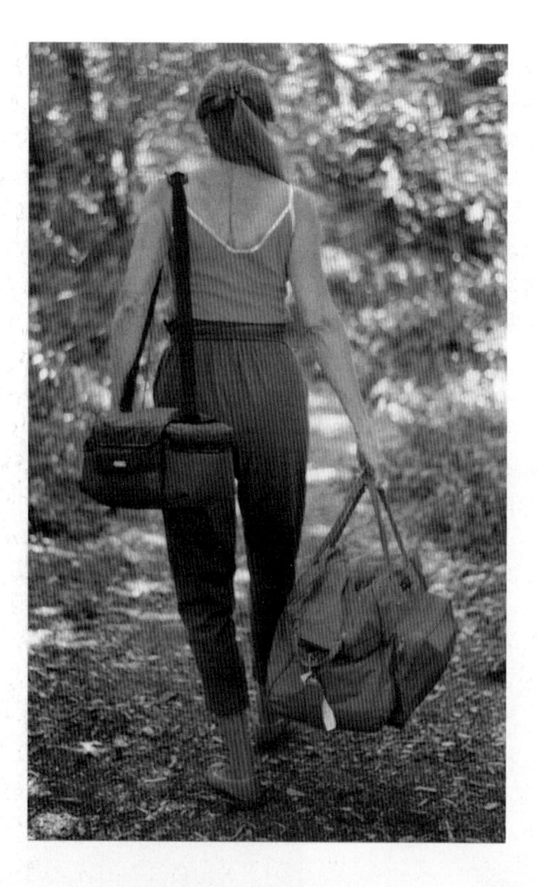

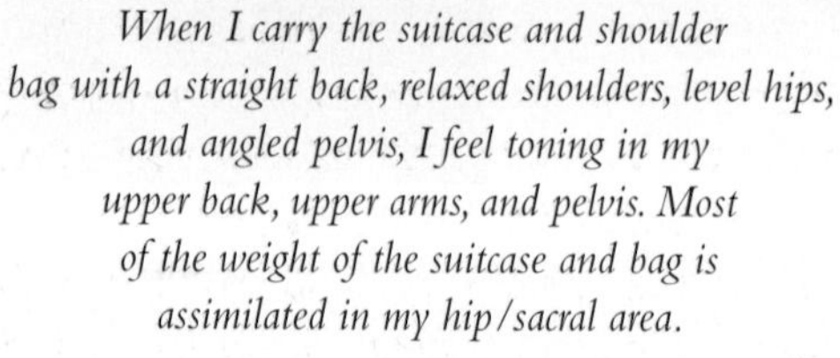

When I carry the suitcase and shoulder bag with a straight back, relaxed shoulders, level hips, and angled pelvis, I feel toning in my upper back, upper arms, and pelvis. Most of the weight of the suitcase and bag is assimilated in my hip/sacral area.

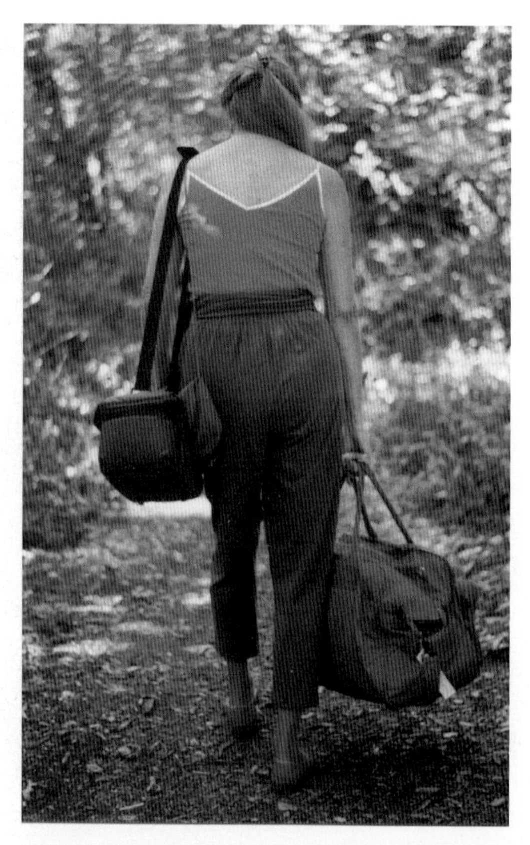

When I tuck my pelvis, round my back, or shift the weight of the suitcase and bag forward onto my shoulders and belly, I feel much discomfort.

in rhythm with their activities and their mobile little bodies are wholly engaged. They are focused and at ease. We, too, can integrate such dynamic relaxation into our adult lives.

When I give workshops for people who sit at computers, I include music in the lesson. I invite the participants to imagine they are playing a musical keyboard as they type, to feel the rhythmic quality of their movements. Students have reported that such an *aesthetic* approach to their KENTRO practice helps them shift from feeling stuck in their bodies to a childlike connection with their work, enabling them to sit, bend, lift, and carry comfortably.

There is a lovely sense of warmth in the word *play*, which has its origin in the German word for "taking care of," *pflegen*. By centering and balancing our movements at work, we can cheerfully participate in our activities.

Our work then becomes a valuable grounding base in our life because we bring along our lighthearted self. Thanks to physical resiliency, we expend less effort while getting more done. Our lively gestures connect us harmoniously with our work place, whether it be the home, office, garden, school, or clinic.

My introduction to KENTRO was through a patient of mine who suffered from chronic and unstable low back pain. After several weeks of KENTRO instruction, her pain virtually disappeared. I now use these simple, gentle, yet incredibly effective movements myself. Angie has amazing insight and is a great teacher of this innovative work.
—Cynthia Wright, D.C., Chiropractic Physician (Oregon)

18. Pelvic Rock

PREPARATION: Place yourself on "all fours"—on your knees and hands—on a mat or simply on your living room carpet. Practice Elemental Placement.

A. Allow at least one foot of space between your knees and between your hands. Spread your fingers and slightly open your inner thighs outward to further realign your hips and knees. *Sense more pressure (weight) toward the outer edge of your knees.*
B. Relax your entire body and shift your weight off your shoulders and onto the top of your sacrum by stretching your pelvis away from your torso until there is a slight diagonal slant in your thighs. *Sense some pressure in the sacral area and hardly any pressure in your shoulders and wrists.* You are now ready to move your pelvis slowly, with gentle rocking-like movements, in an almost circular pattern.
C. Keep your hips level as much as possible, and keep your torso fairly stationary. Focus your attention on your left buttock muscles and let them stretch away from your torso, out behind you. You will *sense expansion in these muscles.*
D. Let your stretch shift slightly toward the center of your pelvis and then let your right buttock also stretch out behind you. Detect *similar expansion in the right buttock as in the left buttock.* Your *Pelvic Rock*-arc is completed: it feels *subtle and wave-like.*
   Without interruption, continue to practice several slow *Pelvic Rocks*, counterclockwise or clockwise, as you like. Rock your pelvis without actively stretching your torso out front; just allow your torso to move along with your pelvic motions. You will *sense releases in the hip/buttocks/sacral area.* You can gently rock for a few minutes, as this stretch is very relaxing.

BENEFITS: The *Pelvic Rock* is a very relaxing stretch. It frees tight and strained tissues in the hip, buttocks, and sacral area while aligning your hip and sacroiliac joints into more comfortable, spacious articulation. This stretch also develops your sense of Grounding.

HELPFUL HINTS: Minimize the rocking motion for a vulnerable hip area. Prevent weight in your shoulders, tightening your belly, tucking your buttocks, twisting your pelvis, pushing your hips out (to the side of your body), arching your lower back, rounding your upper back, or tightening your shoulders. Practicing the Leg Rotation, Turning, and Prayer before Pelvic Rock is helpful.

VARIATIONS: Try the Pelvic Rock with your torso moving up front—becoming an integral part of the circular rocking movement. For deeper releases in your sacroiliac joint area, let your buttocks "draw" a *horizontally inclined* "figure eight" configuration: "draw" a small (up and outward turning) circle to the left with your left buttock and, without interruption, "draw" a small (up and outward turning) circle to the right with your left buttock; repeat with your right buttock. Rest and repeat several times.

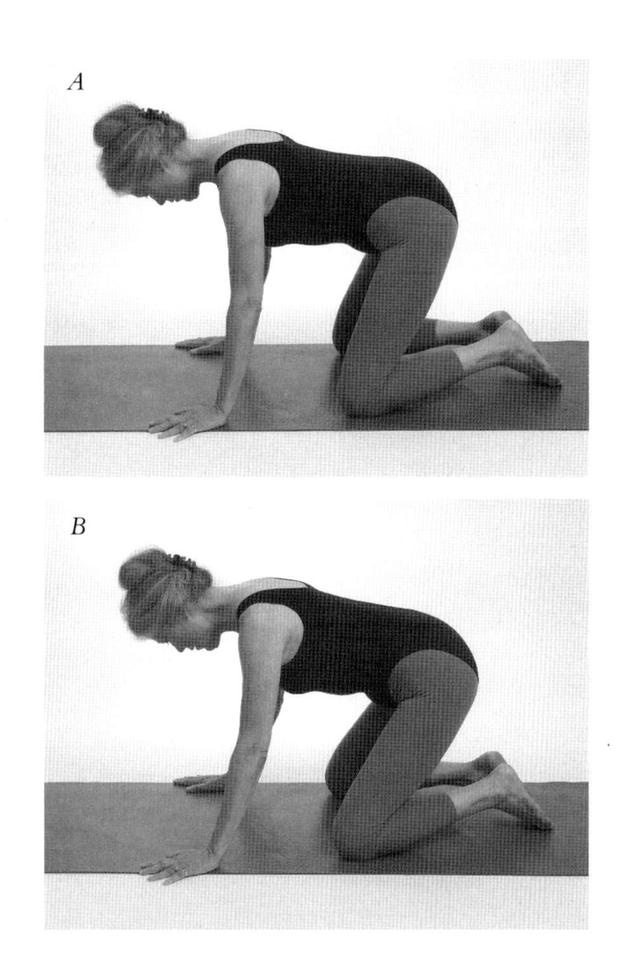

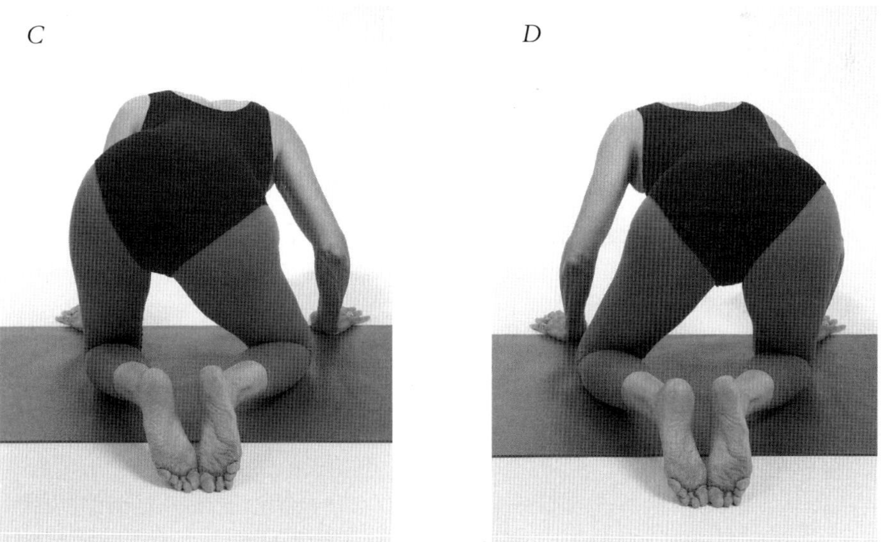

PELVIC ROCK

Resting into Your Own Current

During one of my trips to Brighton, England, to teach KENTRO workshops, I contacted Berkeley, my homeopath and osteopath of some years ago. He was surprised to discover that I no longer needed his treatments due to my centering and balancing practice. He became intrigued and desired to study with me to experience the new suppleness he observed in my movements. After a series of private classes, he remarked on the kinetic and emotional benefits he and his patients gleaned from practicing the KENTRO movements.

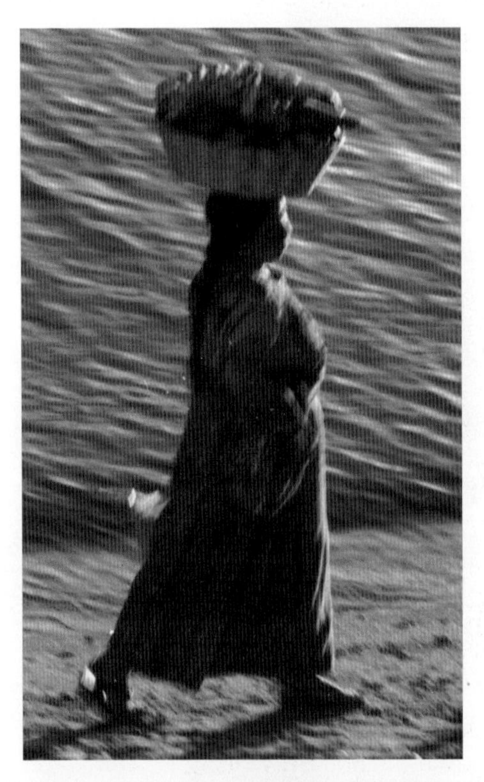

Even though she is walking in soft, uneven sand, this Guatemalan woman is carrying the heavy basket on her head with smooth, balanced motions. The weight of the vegetables is centered through her spine, sacrum, and hips. Notice the relaxed angle of her head, which keeps the basket centered as she walks. With each step, there will be a tiny forward/backward rocking motion in her pelvis.

When Berkeley learned of my plans to move to the United States, he warned me that it would be difficult for me to interest people in the KENTRO method because North American's conventional definition of "correct posture" requires tucking and tightening the pelvis and abdomen. My techniques would "go against the current" because KENTRO does not back up the belief that posture has to be either "coped with" or corrected.

I reflected on Berkeley's statement, and that night dreamt I was drinking from a fountain. The following morning the inspirational words: "going *with* my own current" welled up and settled within me. Trusting my personal experience of increasing resilient expression sparked me to teach centered balance with confidence and enthusiasm.

A few years later, after arriving in California, I went on meditative walks and decided to direct all my energies into creating KENTRO classes, which was challenging, yet truly vitalizing.

Some years later in England, while visiting a friend, a beehive taught me more about the importance of slowing down before taking action. I slept in a room that had a large window facing the garden. The window had a small glass panel that was permanently open, which was frequently accessed by a colony of bees that had decided to make a hive in a closet near the window. Since I was accustomed to painting fields of French lavender while swarms of bees buzzed around me, I felt fine about sleeping in a bee-room.

The bees flew busily back and forth between the closet and the garden. Most of them bumped into windowpanes and fell to the floor, then struggled again before successfully reaching the garden. A few bees, however, popped out of the closet and fluttered about a foot's distance from the window, pausing in mid-air to survey the space. On the first try, these bees found the small opening that led to the garden. Their "time out" had prepared the way for effortless flight.

A brief break goes a long way. Women and men in Greece, Guatemala, Spain, and Portugal who carry baskets of vegetables or crates of fish on their heads would not dream of rushing into this activity. They first ground their bodies into balance and then bend forward slowly *before* their muscles contract to lift the baskets energetically onto their heads.

When our movements are agitated, it is difficult to let go of strain without a brief pause in our gestures. Letting go precedes fluid movements. By practicing KENTRO guidelines at our own pace, we can settle into savoring muscular expansion before contraction. When our muscles expand easily, they are nourished by blood, allowing them to quickly contract into limber motion. In this transition, the muscles are both soft and firm. With such smooth blending coursing our actions, we can move as we wish—fluid and strong.

I am very excited and privileged to have experienced the KENTRO body balance techniques. As a physical therapist, I have been frustrated by conventional ideas describing correct posture as a holding, maintaining process which requires a great deal of effort. Angie's techniques demonstrate a real insight into human biokinetics. Her exercise and stretch program is easy to incorporate into one's daily life without the use of expensive equipment or hours of practice. My posture is more aesthetically pleasing to me and I feel more flexible and comfortable, as well as safe and well-supported by my body. I have used her techniques on many of my patients, even in acute stages, with incredible success.

—Helene Lubben, Physical Therapist (California)

19. Looking for Elbow Room

PREPARATION: Place a mat on the floor, lie down on your back, and practice Elemental Placement, straightening your legs.

A. With your shoulders down, bend your elbows, put your hands together, and place your hands near your sternum, with your fingertips toward the ceiling. Let your upper arms slant diagonally downward, with your elbows at the level of your heart area.

B. Relax your shoulders and contract your upper back muscles to let your elbows move away from your body, without lifting your elbows off the mat. Slowly let your elbows stretch away from your body as far as possible, letting your hands separate.

   When you have stretched as far as possible, rest your elbows onto the mat and place your hands onto your thorax. *Sense much horizontal expansion in your entire upper back (and front) as well as on the underside of your upper arms*. Stay in this stretch for the duration of a few yawns. Repeat it a few times, with brief rests between the stretching.

BENEFITS: The *Looking for Elbow Room* movement is a basic limbering and relaxing stretch for your upper back to expand into spaciousness; it also helps to realign your shoulder blades (straightening your upper back) and shoulders, as well as release strain from over-stretched shoulder blade muscles and from tight shoulder muscles.

HELPFUL HINTS: Prevent raising or tightening your shoulders, raising your elbows toward the ceiling, or stretching your elbows up toward your shoulders. Practicing the Prayer and Tikanis before Looking for Elbow Room is helpful.

VARIATIONS: You can practice the Looking for Elbow Room when you sit up or sit back on a chair. Also try standing with your elbows bent and your hands on the crests of your pelvis.

A

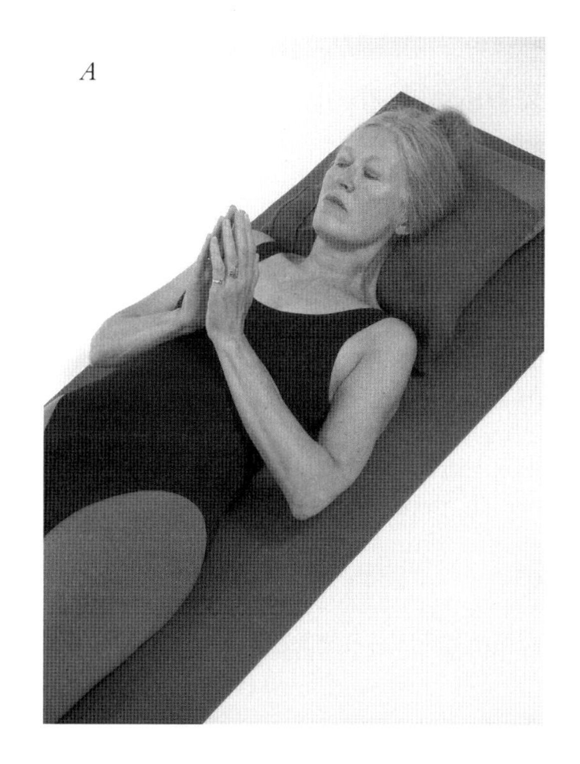

B

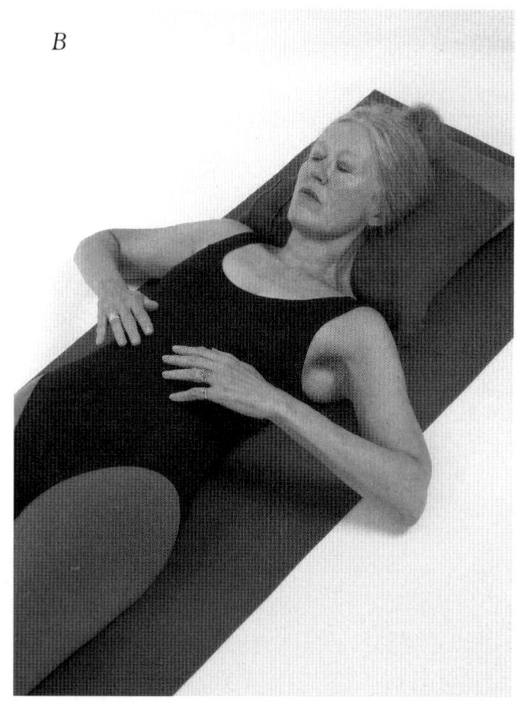

Looking for Elbow Room

Take It Personally

There is a wondrous impulse within us that generates expansive personal expression. We see this impulse reflected in our visions, projects, and also in our every day movements. Our fluid bodies shelter our individuality and, at the same time, express it through each ordinary gesture.

When we feel ease in our activities, we inhabit them; they fill us with enjoyment and satisfaction; they nurture us. We may feel springiness while sitting at the computer for an entire morning. We may feel supple standing all afternoon.

Yet in our society, we tend to abstract our posture and strain our bodies into "correct" carriage and push our bodies "into shape." Repetitive movements may seem mechanical and without charm. Such depersonalized expression engenders agitated motion which, in turn, triggers a longing to "fix" our posture and our lifestyle.

By integrating centering relaxation with balancing movements into our daily living, rigid views of our bodies are replaced by a heartening experience of our simple gestures. We broaden our sense of smooth movement and perceive our bearing as a pliable extension of our most intimate self. Such sensuousness soothes us and empowers our bodies to carry us forward into our postural uniqueness.

A charismatic Catholic nun, Sister Michaela, studied with me in Honduras in 1990. She wished to overcome pain in her knees and back. She eventually felt limber again, especially when she was on her knees, praying. Sister Michaela easily related her

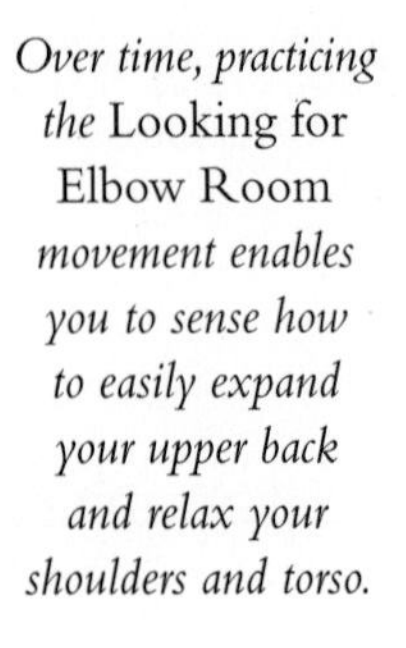

Over time, practicing the Looking for Elbow Room *movement enables you to sense how to easily expand your upper back and relax your shoulders and torso.*

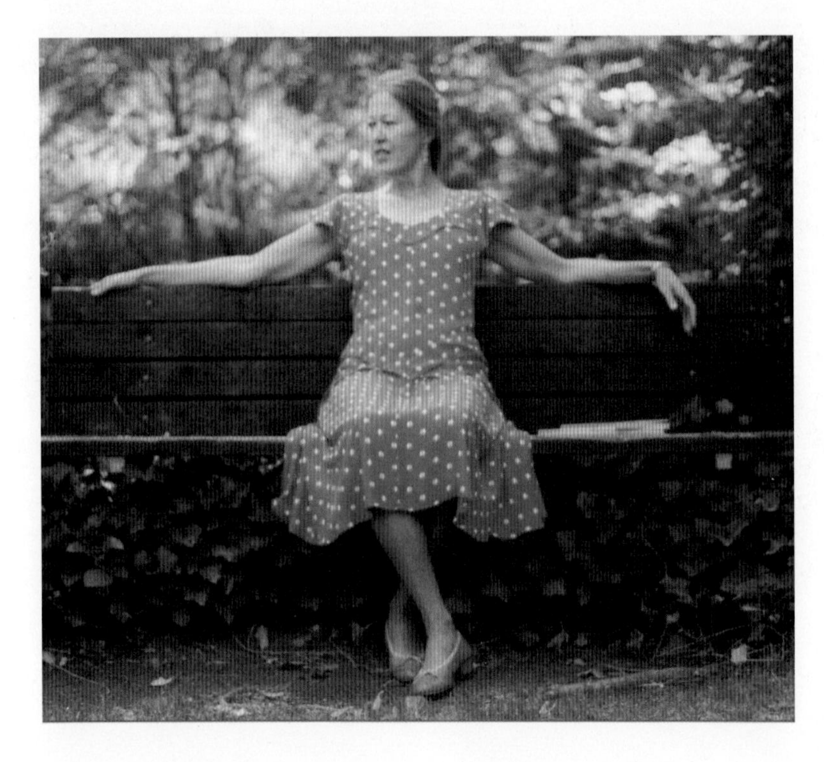

KENTRO practice to her practice of centering prayer, an approach to prayer that emphasizes an immediate and singular tie to God. There is no criticism of the ego or personality. No part of us remains excluded. We are whole, and spiritual engagement transpires through a simple wish to commune with Creation.

A gentle, caring approach to centered balance in our occupations allows our bodies to expand us into resiliency; our feelings synchronize with our movements. Cooking or sitting on a bench or dancing link us kindly with our self and our surroundings. We feel spirited by our everyday actions.

KENTRO movements are simple and gentle, yet one gets a deep workout with profound effects. At the piano, a difficult Brahms' piece suddenly becomes smooth and easy. KENTRO is not only accessible, strengthening, and enjoyable, it feels meditative. I had back pain for twenty years and tendonitis in my elbows from carrying heavy musical instruments but I don't any more. Now I can do any activity that requires heavy lifting (including gardening and backpacking) with ease. Angie Thusius is a wise, compassionate, and eloquent teacher.

—Mary Yount, Music and Voice Instructor

20. Pan

PREPARATION: Face a long mirror for easy balance and place your right hand on the back of a chair, which is to the right of your body. Practice Elemental Placement.

A. Keep your hips level, allow about one-foot of space between your toes and about eight inches between your heels, and place your left hand on your left pelvic crest. *Sense stability in your legs and equal weight in your feet.*

B. Slowly, keeping your hips level, shift your body weight onto your right leg. *Sense lightness, lack of weight in your left leg.*

   Combine a broad Little Moon movement with bending your left knee (so that your left inner thigh can rotate easily outward) and place your left heel onto your right ankle (or slightly in front of it). Relax and Ground yourself to facilitate expansive stretching and release of strained tissues

   Look in the mirror to make sure your bellybutton is centered and your hips are level. *Sense* barely any weight on your left heel, and almost all pressure (weight) on your right foot (primarily on the heel). *Feel stretching in your inner thigh, hips, and sacral area.*

BENEFITS: The *Pan* movement is an exceptionally gentle yet efficient movement that generates thorough hip/sacroiliac releases in strained tissues and realigns joints into comfortable balance and smooth articulation. Likewise, the inner thigh and knee tissues can re-stretch into improved elasticity. By contracting the buttock muscles of the hip that is being stretched, Pan also strengthens the buttock muscles.

HELPFUL HINTS:

Prevent twisting your pelvis or lower back, tightening your abdomen, tucking your buttocks, and pushing your inner thigh far out, which tightens your lower back and twists your pelvis. Move out of Pan and rest when the hip area of *the leg that you are standing on* begins to *feel* uncomfortable. This discomfort is due to tight, scarred tissues that are beginning to release—a good sign! Practicing the Pelvic Rock and Belly Dance before Pan is helpful.

VARIATIONS:

You can practice variations of Pan by sitting back in a chair (or sofa) or lying down on your back: recline in Elemental Placement, bend both knees, place your left hand on your left crest and raise your left bent leg and your left ankle just above your right bent knee. Relax your pelvis, abdomen, and thighs. Keep your hips level and your bellybutton centered. When you stay in this Pan for longer than a few yawns, you may feel some stiffness in your inner thigh/hip area, due to the strong stretching that occurs. Shift out of Pan and rest.

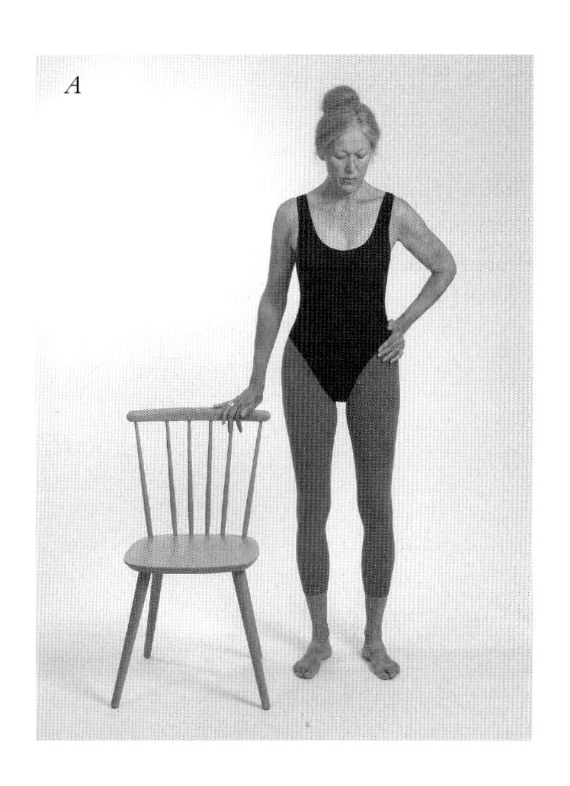

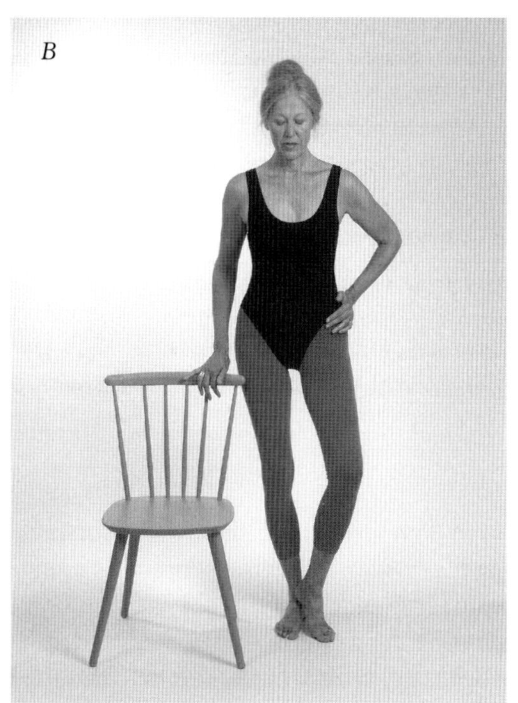

PAN

Beauty in Movement

The voluptuous body of a Navajo elder encircles a young girl, who is sitting at the loom. The child weaves, bending forward from the hips, her hands moving lightly to and fro. Her back straightens; her shoulders relax. As she works, her grandmother also bends, and her hands make slight motions in space; she moves in concert with her grandchild in an exquisite connection.

"Make it beautiful," the Navajo woman advises her eight-year-old granddaughter. Having learned the technical aspects of Navajo weaving, the girl is about to create her first blanket. "Make the blanket beautiful," her grandmother repeats. This simple message is powerful and invites the child's aesthetic sense to flow freely, encouraging her to shape the blanket without worrying about the end result—to focus only on loveliness.

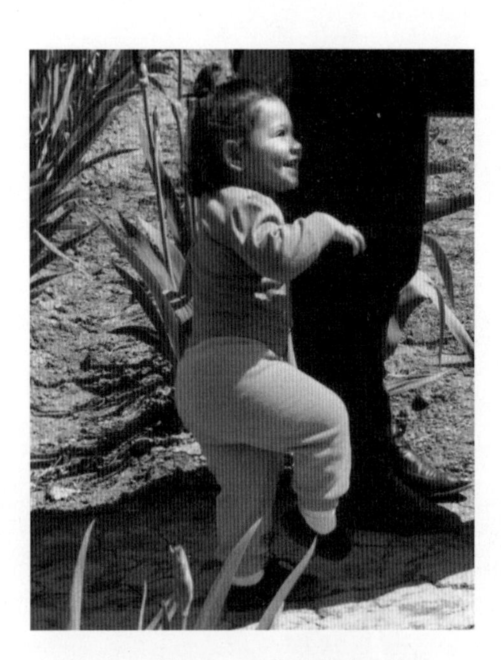

The dance-like gesture of this little Mexican girl is akin to the Pan movement. The child is enjoying the petal-like outward rotation in her leg and arm.

Beauty is defined as the quality attributed to whatever pleases or satisfies in certain ways, as by color, form, or proportion, but also by rhythmic motion, behavior, or attitude. The grandmother trusts her granddaughter will have a relaxed attitude as she crafts traditional blankets. She kindles her granddaughter's creative fire, encouraging her to weave from her heart and hands. The child's body moves rhythmically, smoothly, making the blanket beautiful, "which gives the highest degree of pleasure to the senses or to the mind."[15]

We, too, can be as the grandmother, mentoring ourselves as we weave a delightful quality into our ordinary movements.

By infusing our repetitive motions with images of beauty in nature our actions become like threads that extend from our inner nature. Focusing on the petals of a flower opening outward while we practice the Arm Rotation or Pan is a useful illustration for precise realignment of the limbs and for limbering the tissues. Likewise, starting as many movements as possible from the principal area of free motion—the pelvis—is a powerful comparison with the center of a flower. Integrating flower metaphors with daily occupations distances us from tucking our buttocks, tightening our abdomen, and pushing our shoulders back for "correct" posture. Comfortable balance prepares the way for sensuous gestures innocent of effort and control. Our senses awaken to the aesthetics of supple expression.

Centering our actions then becomes a way of life—ordinary life. It becomes the art of harmonious movement. Activities like archery, cooking, and typing all feel equal in flow, value, beauty, and fullness: in each of these occupations, our back straightens, our shoulders slant downward, our pelvis is grounded, and our limbs are flexible. We hold the bow and arrow, and chop the leeks, and type our essay from strong upper back (heart area) muscles, relaxed shoulders, and a mobile pelvis.

Such everyday ease invites pleasurable appreciation of our own bodies, belongings, and community.

After five years of KENTRO classes my spinal scoliosis has decreased and recently I was amazed at how much weight I could lift when I built a stone wall. I especially enjoy the refreshing feelings I experience throughout my body while walking. I sense that I am re-experiencing how I walked as a child, with fully felt movements, perfect presence, and exquisite balance. I am getting to know my body in a loving and cherishing way.

—Linda Thomas, Registered Nurse (Oregon)

21. Farmer's Rest

PREPARATION: Sit down on the edge of a thin wedge placed toward the front of a chair, with one foot of space between your knees and both thighs slanting slightly downward. Practice Elemental Placement. Extend one foot slightly forward of the other.

A. Slowly bend forward with the palm of your left hand on your lower back and your fingertips on your spine. *Feel an even groove in your lower back. Sense stretching and straightening in your lower back muscles.* Place your right hand on your buttocks and *sense those muscles stretching away from your torso in this grounding gesture.*
B. After checking your back, allow your arms to come out front, bend your elbows, and place your forearms onto your thighs (and close to your knees). Drop your shoulders. Center your legs by aligning the center of your knees directly over the center of your feet—the space between your second and third toe.
C. Bend farther forward with a straight back, keep your shoulders down, relax your belly, and let your neck be in line with your spine. You may drop your head to further relax your neck. *Sense smooth extension in your back and neck.*

   When your upper back starts to round and your shoulders move out front, you have bent too far; simply raise your torso, slightly. *Sense counterweight between your elbows and wrists (your main weight is in the hip and sacral area) which takes weight off your shoulders and back.*

   When you feel relaxation throughout your body, you are in *The Farmer's Rest.* Stay in this stretch for a few minutes.

BENEFITS: *Farmer's Rest* is an extremely *relaxing* movement that lets a lengthening stretch happen easily in your torso and pelvis. This placement also creates releases and more spaciousness in your torso and pelvis, particularly in your lower back/sacral region.

HELPFUL HINTS: Check whether you are rounding your back, raising your shoulders, contracting your belly, or arching your neck, all of which will prevent your body from relaxing. Practice Farmer's Rest during and after sitting, lifting, or gardening for a long time.

VARIATIONS: You can let your head hang down to allow further small, relaxing stretches in your upper back and neck.

A

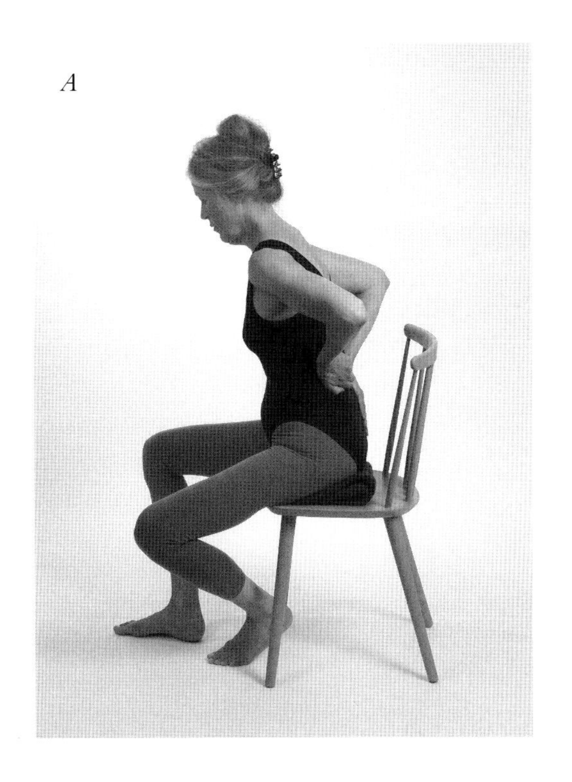

B

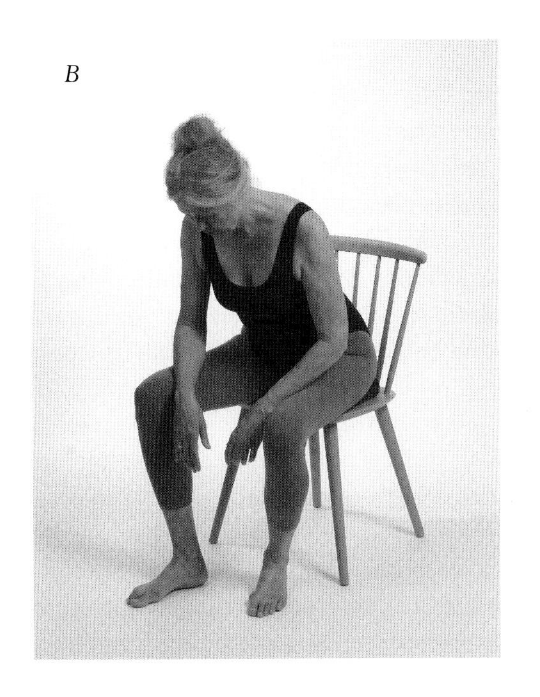

C

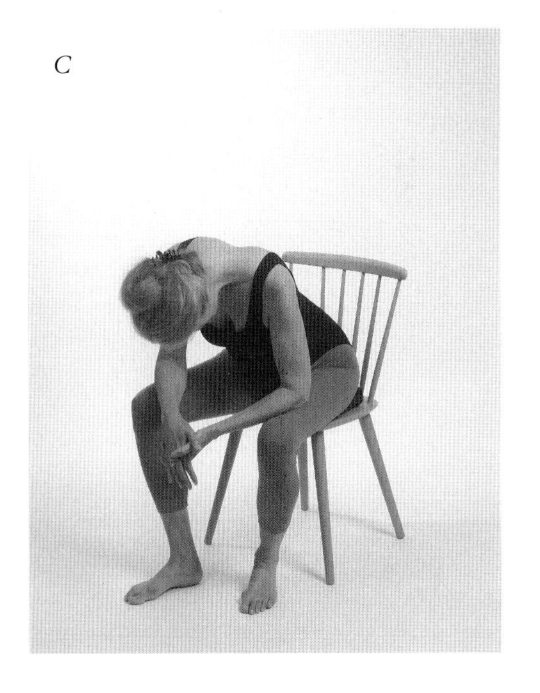

FARMER'S REST

Hearing Yourself Living: Pops, Sighs, Yawns, and Belly Laughs

Our spirits are lifted when we hear our favorite music, the voices of friends and loved ones, the rippling of a brook, or the happy gurglings of a baby. However, amidst the complexities of everyday life, we generally do not hear *ourselves* living. We are not aware of the shuffling of our feet, the thud when we sit down, or the scraping of a chair as we drag it across the room—the kinds of sound that emanate from a tired person. Practicing the KENTRO Body Balance program transforms such noise into bouncy steps and light movements. Our ordinary gestures resonate around us, not as discord but as the natural rhythmic expression of each activity. Centering and balancing our movements creates sounds that imbue our daily occupations with repose. In the process of transforming stress or exhaustion into enjoyable physical resiliency, our bodies make sounds that are reassuring signals of deep relaxation: pops, sighs, yawns, and belly laughs.

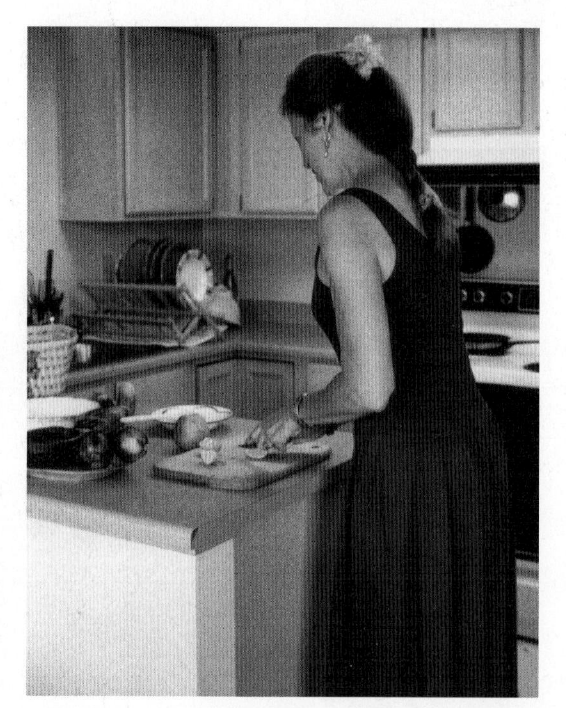

Even when we chop vegetables, we can sense the benefits of practicing Farmer's Rest*: a relaxed back, a grounded pelvis, a sigh of contentment.*

Increasing our kinetic mobility does not happen overnight, but we can experience the beginnings of deep release as we start our KENTRO practice. We sense this relief from striving and sometimes can actually *hear* it through the sighs and pops that occur in daily movements. Most of us are far more familiar with exertion than with restfulness, so it is reassuring to know that pops, sighs, and yawns are good indicators that our bodies are opening up—stretching and expanding. Instead of sitting down abruptly or chopping vegetables from tight shoulder muscles, we can prepare the way for ease by relaxing our shoulders, bending forward from our hips, grounding our pelvis, and lengthening and broadening our back into limberness. We may release a sigh of contentment. There may be a *pop* as space is automatically created between each vertebra along our back. We cannot fake natural pops, yawns, or sighs; they come from deep within and are signs of letting go.

Popping sounds in the areas that are becoming more elastic signal a decrease in undue accumulation of gases, thanks to increased spaciousness in the formerly congested area. When our bodies are placed comfortably, we can experience a long, leisurely yawn or a blissful sigh that surges out of nowhere, straightening our back and extending and broadening our entire torso. Our soft, yet firm bellies may shake as irresistible laughter bubbles forth.

These inner voices of flow and expansiveness also prepare the way for us to find fuller expression. Before practicing KENTRO guidelines, my voice used to be "caught" in my sternal area, at the top of my compressed chest. I constantly sounded out of breath—and I was out of breath. When my abdomen became more toned and my torso longer and broader, I noticed that my words seemed to originate in the abdominal area. I was on my way to a more full-bodied voice.

Madeleine Renaud, a famous French actor who was still working in her nineties, made a profound comment on the significance of sound postural expression. When an interviewer asked her what was most important to her, Madeleine replied, "Making love." What did she favor besides lovemaking? She responded, "*s'entendre vivre,*" or "to hear oneself living." With KENTRO practice, our voice and everyday actions reflect our enlivened senses. When our movements are smooth and vibrant, we are in an attuned, loving relationship with ourself and our activities.

After six months of practicing the centering, balancing movements, I felt a substantial improvement in my sleeping as my back pain went away and my lower back got stronger and more relaxed. KENTRO practice opened up my capacity for breathing and breath support. I think the KENTRO method might just revolutionize the way movement is approached by actors because KENTRO is a place where you can be as physically expressive as you wish. With centered balance, any actor can be supple, strong, and grounded. What a delight!

—Gwendolyn Overland, PhD.,
Professor of Theater, director, actor (Oregon)

22. Turning

PREPARATION: Place a wedge on the edge of a chair, sit down on the edge of the wedge, and practice Elemental Placement.

A. With your shoulders down, place your palms on top of your pelvic (innominate) bones, with your fingers spread over your abdomen. Open your right inner thigh and stretch your right leg forward, with your right foot about one foot farther out in front than your left foot. Keep about one foot of space between your knees so your hips are in comfortable alignment.

B. Relax all pelvic muscles while you bend slightly forward and slowly turn your pelvis to the right with pressure from your hands to guide your pelvis. You are simply shifting your pelvic bones; *sense gentle lateral stretching in your abdomen and buttocks.* Keep your hips level and your knees stationary. *Feel a slightly diagonal, (side) stretch in the left abdominal muscles and* sense *contraction in your left buttock.*

   Initially, you may only be able to turn your torso a few inches to the right. Resist the urge to twist your torso farther to the right. Remain turned to the right for the duration of a yawn, then bring your torso and pelvis back to center and rest.

C. Repeat Guideline B, only this time, slowly turn your pelvis to the left. Relax your abdomen and buttocks. Keep your hips level and your knees stationary. *Feel the lateral stretch in your right abdominal muscles and slight contraction in the right buttock.* Let your torso accompany the movement of your pelvis.

   Remain turned to the left for the duration of a yawn, then bring your torso and pelvis back to center and rest. Practice *Turning* several times from side to side, with rests in between. Usually, one hip/sacroiliac area is more strained than the other. If your right side is tighter, turn a few more times to the left than to the right.

BENEFITS: *Turning* while you are sitting on a chair effectively releases tight pelvic tissues and improves your pelvic range of movement. Your body is designed to turn from your essentially mobile pelvis. Turning while you are sitting down will be a limbering stretch. However, when you are standing, bending, lifting, or carrying, turn your feet (to the left or to the right), so that you *face your activity and center your belly button with it!*

HELPFUL HINTS: Prevent twisting your lower or upper back, tightening your abdomen, arching or curving your back, turning your knees inward (toward your bellybutton), or raising your shoulders. Practice Turning in all sitting situations. Practicing Leg Rotation and Belly Dance before Turning is helpful.

VARIATIONS: When you wish to turn while you are standing or bending forward, Turning is more difficult. Simply shift your feet to the left if you wish to turn to your left. *Always have your bellybutton facing the activity in which you are involved.*

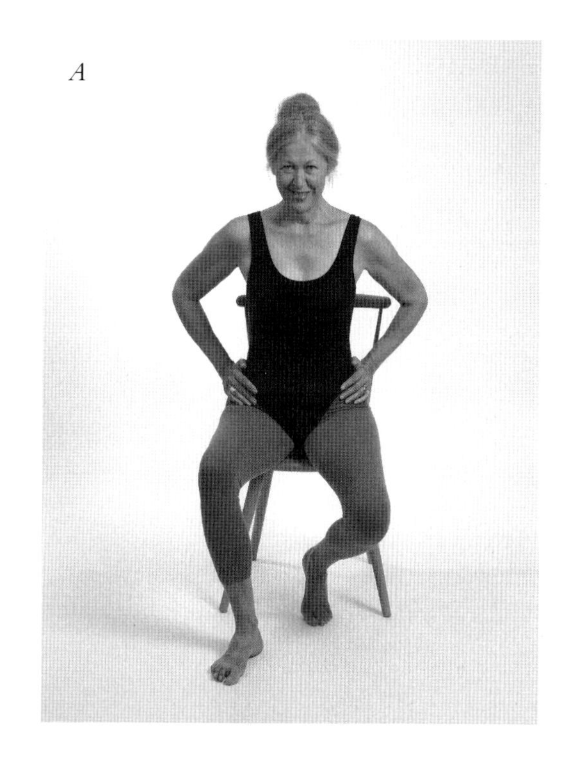

A

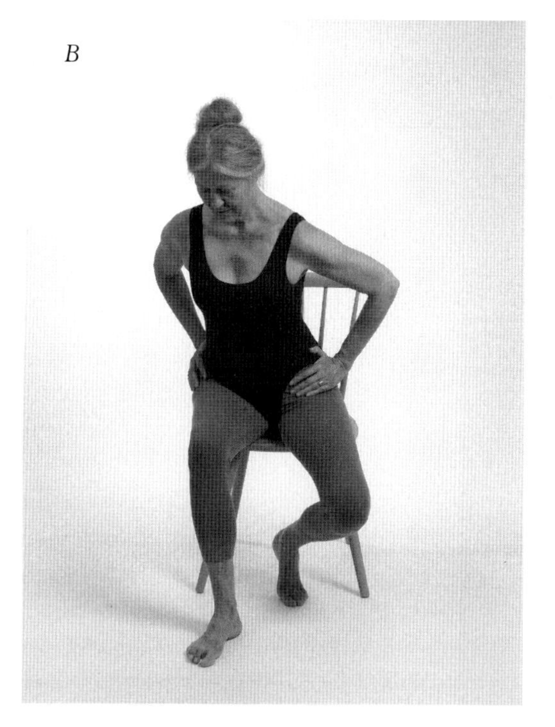

B

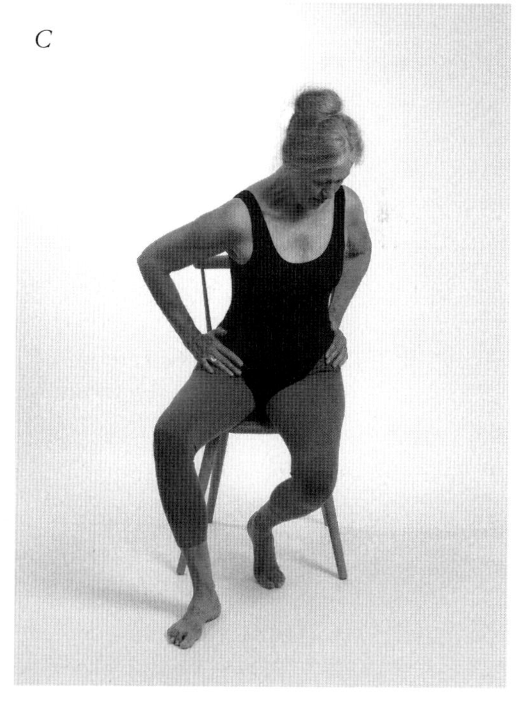

C

Turning

Peace of Body, Peace of Mind

Peace of body is a truly dynamic state.

When our bodies are relaxed, physiological systems function well and our movements feel cloaked in comfort, swathed in serenity. This state allows us to more easily discern our stressful thoughts and feelings and to replace them with enlivening ones.

Peter, a musician friend of mine, once admitted he had signed up for my classes because he liked the idea of the "gentle, balancing movements" mentioned in my brochure. He thought he would experience some light stretches. He was surprised that the slow movements powerfully transformed his back, but he was even more surprised at the new strength and feelings of physical release throughout his body. He used the word *peaceful* to describe his fresh sense of postural expression because he no longer felt distress when he played his guitar or lifted heavy equipment.

Peter equated increased mental calm with bodily comfort—not the lethargy of sitting curled up in a deep armchair, but the fluidity of movement. His comments helped me see that kinetic mobility can result from simple balancing gestures and centering movements. We can savor sitting upright in meditation, cleaning the garage, and mopping the floor without effort, feeling limber and light. Likewise, we may notice novel thoughts and images, which can inspire our actions and even our choices.

Over time, regained suppleness can become a common experience. Even though new students tend to feel odd when they first shift into an unfamiliar balance, they also begin to feel less discomfort. When there is undue strain and pressure on our bones and soft tissues from trying to achieve "correct" posture, we limit our physical pliability and automatically restrict our potential for mental quietude.

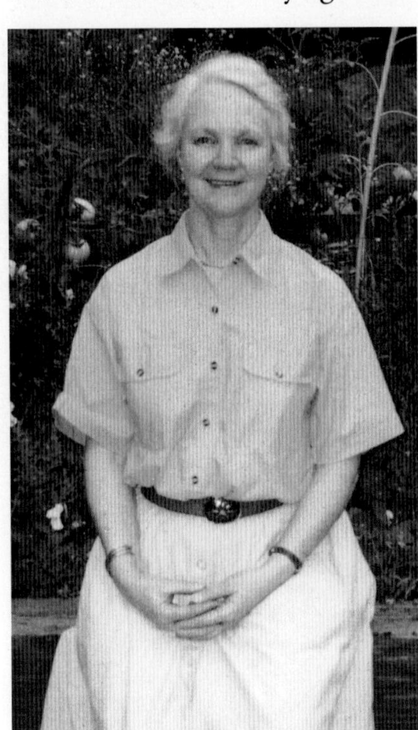

Karen is sitting up in a relaxed manner. Practicing Sitting Up *in comfortable balance enables you to turn from the hips without twisting your back.*

My KENTRO practice has been free of *shoulds* and exertion; I simply practice the movements. Galea, my healer over many years, once encouraged me to make decisions based on what *feels* comfortable. I realized my experience of enjoyable, expansive motion allowed me to discover similar places in my psyche. This helped me avoid making judgmental decisions based on what is "right," focusing instead on what felt appropriate for me. Now, when I remember to do so, I first ask, "Where is my place of comfort in this situation?" Much as an artist selects the right color—the color that *feels* right,—I try to choose spontaneously so my body and my mind stretch smoothly in various situations.

Decisions based on what feels restful and vitalizing reflect our deep wishes, which arise from the same creative place as energizing gestures. Inviting such ease allows our thoughts to broaden and become more pliable.

Resilient movements can guide us toward pleasurable mindfulness.

When I was completing the training to become a certified yoga teacher, I began experiencing pain in my right hip joint which soon worsened. I tried many things yet none of them helped. After several private sessions and about two weeks of KENTRO practice my right hip began to function normally again. Over the next year a recurring sacroiliac problem disappeared.Naturally I share body balance with my yoga students. As I guide yoga students through the steps to come into balance, I often see expressions of relief and release as the bellies relax.

—Marion Moore, Yoga Instructor, co-founder of the Ashland Yoga Center (Oregon)

23. Four Directions

PREPARATION: Sit up in a chair on the edge of a soft wedge (see Sitting Up) and practice Elemental Placement.

A. Begin with direction South: move your right leg about a foot farther out in front of the chair than the left leg (for counterweight); allow at least one foot of space between your knees.
   Relax your abdomen; keep your chin, shoulders, and rib cage down; and Ground your pelvis as you bend forward. Hold your arms lengthened out in front of you, allowing about two feet of space between your hands. *Feel your buttocks muscles stretching away from your torso, keeping you balanced on the chair.* Only stretch your arms toward the ground as long as your shoulders stay down, your back straightens, and your pelvis is Grounded. *Sense expansive stretching in your pelvis and lengthening throughout your back and upper arms.* Stay in this stretch for the duration of a yawn.
B. Continue with direction North: Slowly raise your pelvis, torso, and arms in one movement, keeping your abdomen relaxed and your chin, rib cage, and shoulders down. Again, remember to raise your arms above shoulder level as long as your shoulders remain down (even if you just raise your arms a few inches higher than your shoulders). *Sense toning contraction in your upper back and upper arm muscles.*
   Stay in this stretch for the duration of a yawn.
C. Continue with directions East and West: Keep your shoulders down, contract your shoulder blade muscles, and slowly lower and extend your arms outward (laterally) and slightly downward until your hands are level with your hips. Relax your arms and hands; keep your chin, shoulders, and rib cage down. *Feel broadening and toning in your upper back as well as toning in your upper arms.*
   Stay in this stretch for the duration of a yawn, then rest a moment before practicing the Four Directions a few more times.

BENEFITS: The *Four Directions* relaxes and strengthens your back and arms while generating a multi-directional expansive and extensive stretching throughout your upper back. Likewise, it gently stretches nerves in your upper back and arms.

HELPFUL HINTS: The Four Directions is a thorough stretch: expect some "workout" feelings. Resist doing a dozen stretches at one sitting because you may get too sore in your arms and too intense "blissful" aching in your upper back. Practice Four Directions anywhere and especially for typing or playing the piano.

VARIATIONS: Try practicing the Four Directions while you stand (bending forward for direction South) or while you lie down on your back (extending your arms toward your bellybutton for direction South). Check whether you are rounding your upper back, straining your shoulders to *touch the floor with your hands* in direction South, tucking your pelvis, or arching your back in directions North and East/West.

A

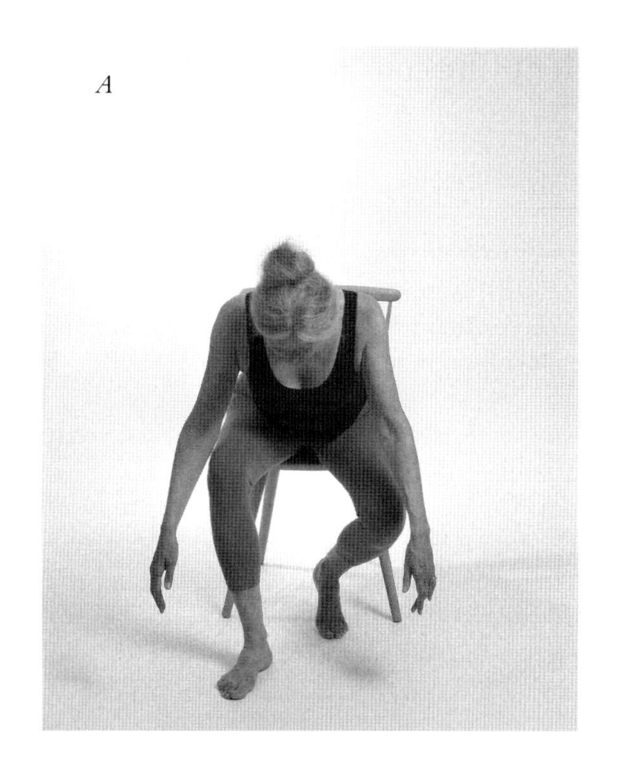

B

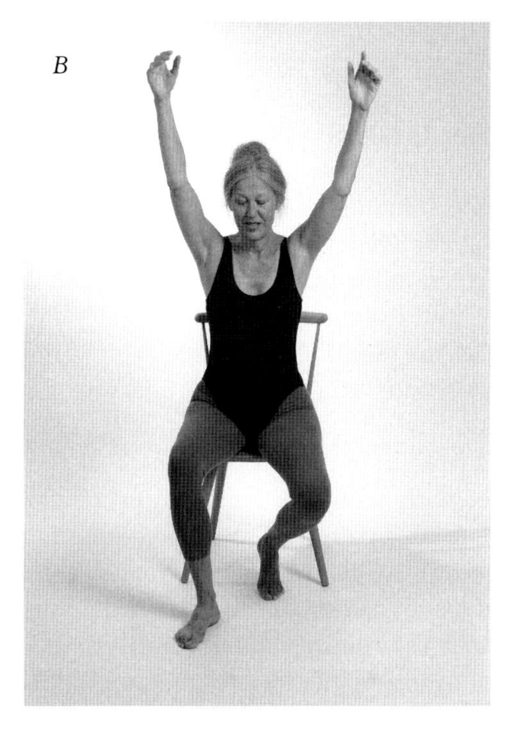

C

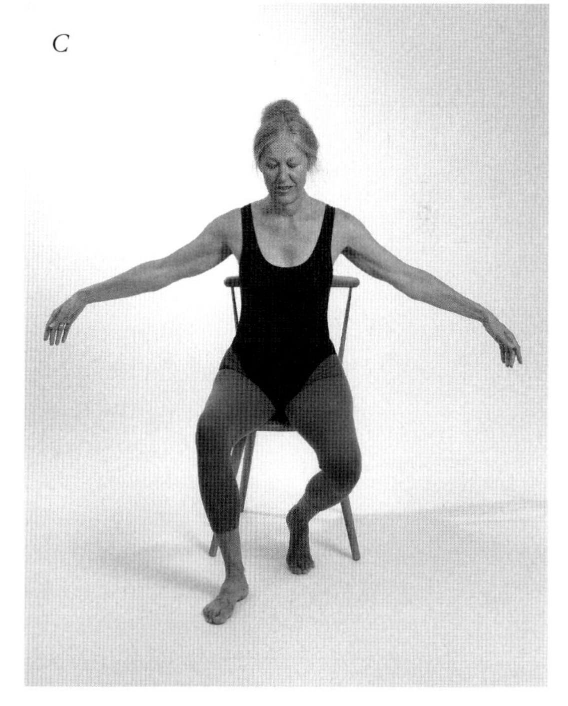

Four Directions

Ancient Rhythms for Your Heart

All of my adult life, first as an artist and later as a movement instructor, I have observed people who move gracefully in their daily actions, people who link gently with whatever they are doing, even if they are simply holding an object or cleaning a room. In my mind I can still picture a Greek woman dressed in black, making a bed slowly with dance-like movements, bending and turning without effort from her hips; two Greek teenage girls, bending forward to read a magazine, their elbows leaning on a big ice cream chest, their backs straight as arrows yet undulating and soft; an English first violinist, moving from his hips (instead of rounding his shoulders), playing his instrument as if the notes started at the pelvic center of his body. Such gestures, which inspired me to create some of the KENTRO movements, verify our inherent physical fluidity.

Listening to slow, traditional, ethnic music can amplify the rhythmic nature of our motions. Moving, stretching, and dancing to such music can help us move from within and feel in tune with every one of our repetitive gestures.

When we hear dance music that we enjoy, all of us respond from our creative core. Even if we do not get up and dance, our bodies still reverberate with the aesthetic quality of the music. We are "moved" by our feelings.

During my visits to Greece to study postural movement, I've been charmed by old men and women who are able to dance with stability and gracefulness all night long. I decided to learn Greek dance, which broadened my perception of balancing motion in rhythm. My difficulty with left/right foot coordination forced me to practice the steps repeatedly and patiently. This gave me time to explore the centered limbering that results from these dances.

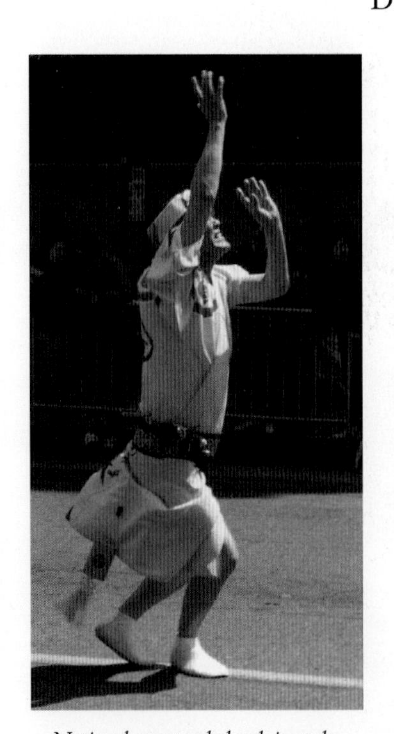

Notice the grounded pelvis and straight back of this Japanese dancer. The gesture of his arms is similar to north in the Four Directions *movement.*

By imitating and feeling the movements of my dance teachers, and taking apart the dance steps, I realized that we can move expansively without taxing our bodies. I came to understand how tissues stretch easily in the three principal rotational areas: hip, shoulder, and neck. Dance teachers and musicians illustrated how freely we can move from the pelvic and shoulder areas when the torso straightens without exertion. Above all, the feelings of grounding and vibrancy generated by the Greek dances were as new and compelling as anything I had ever experienced.

My principal instructor was Vassilis Dimitropoulos, the director of the Center for Hellenic Folk Studies in Athens. Like many of the other teachers and musicians, he danced with resiliency. He admonished his workshop participants to practice the dances patiently, for expression, instead of rushing into as many dance steps as possible. In ancient Greece, the dancer listened to inner tones, created steps for the rhythms, and *then* the musicians followed the steps of the dancer with their musical interpretations. In Vassilis' dancing I saw a subtle, momentary interval between impression (taking in the music) and expression (the danced movements). It was clear that Vassilis was not performing; he seemed to be tuning his body, accompanied by music.

I've also been inspired by dancers from China, India, Spain, Mexico, Ivory

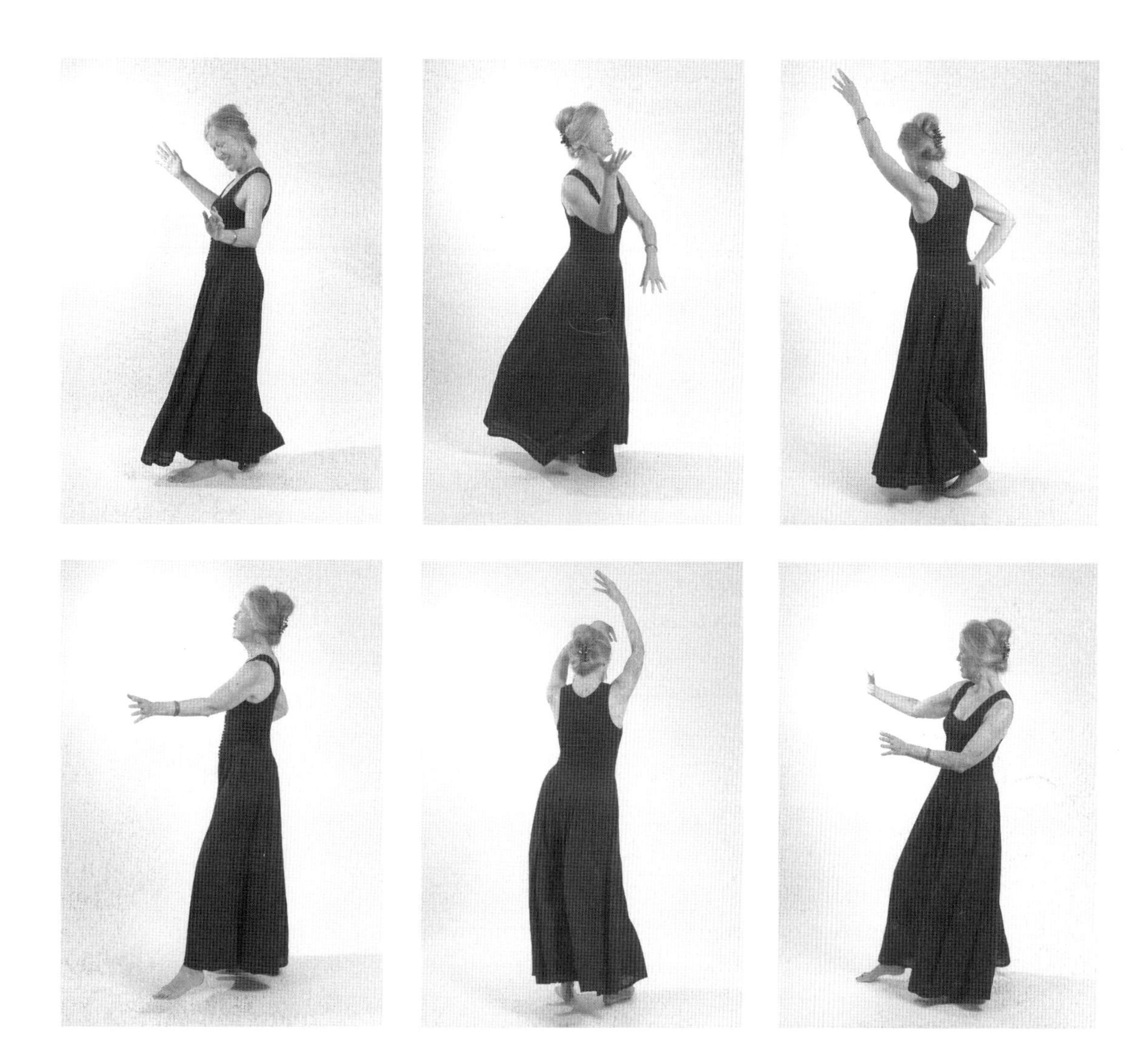

In this series of photographs, I am dancing to Greek music while I savor Four Directions, *feeling the rhythm and energy flow in this* KENTRO *movement.*

Coast, Morocco, Portugal, Japan, Senegal, Argentina, Uzbekistan, and Indonesia. The majority of these professionals moved with optimal balance. None twisted or rounded their backs; all bent from the hips. Likewise, I have heard contemporary North American cajun, Spanish flamenco, and Caribbean merengue instructors advise their students to continuously relax their pelvis and bend from their hips. The supple motion communicated by these traditional dancers also motivated me to develop KENTRO movements that, unlike a regular heartbeat cadence, generate a specific pleasurable flow in various parts of our body. When we blend ethnic music with balancing and centering guidelines, our actions can merge with the particular musicality within our responsive bodies. Cleaning a mirror may feel like a caper while we resonate with the "rhythm" of our hip and shoulder movements. Daily activities then become a sanctuary for our sensuous expression. We can move at *our own rhythm*, to our heart's content.

24. Gliding

PREPARATION: Stand facing a long mirror and practice Elemental Placement.

A. Place your hands on the top of your pelvic bones and take a broad stance with at least two feet of space between your feet, with level hips.
   Bend your torso and your knees slightly; keeping your hips level and *sense equal weight in both feet.*

B. Keep equal pressure under both heels, level hips, and centered legs, while slowly shifting your weight into your left leg (about six inches from where you started), letting your torso move evenly to the left. *Sense* Grounding *in your pelvic muscles, especially in your left buttock. Keep even weight in both feet as much as possible, even though the weight of your torso is over your left leg.* Stay in this stretch for the duration of a yawn and then center your torso with equal weight in both legs again.

C. Continue Gliding by slowly shifting your bodily weight into your right leg.
   Move your right leg slowly to the right (about 6 inches from where you started), and repeat as with the left leg. *Sense* Grounding, *especially in your right buttock, as well as mobility in your hips, toning in your thighs, and stability in your legs and feet. Sense equal weight in both feet as much as possible. Rest.* You can practice Gliding several times, as often as you like during the day.

BENEFITS: The *Gliding* stretch is very effective for Grounding and releasing strained pelvic muscles, as well as toning your thighs and buttocks. Gliding is also an excellent means for limbering and strengthening your knees.

HELPFUL HINTS: Prevent twisting your pelvis, tightening your abdomen, arching your lower back, tucking your pelvis, putting weight on the balls of your feet, or raising one hip higher than the other. Expect toning aches in your hips. Practice Gliding during vacuuming, dancing, or Tai Chi. The Pelvic Rock and Pan are helpful before Gliding.

VARIATIONS: Bend farther forward in Gliding to increase toning in your thighs. Try "front, back" Gliding, with one leg extending out behind you and letting your torso move out front or back. For easier balance, you can place your hands on a dance barre or kitchen counter.

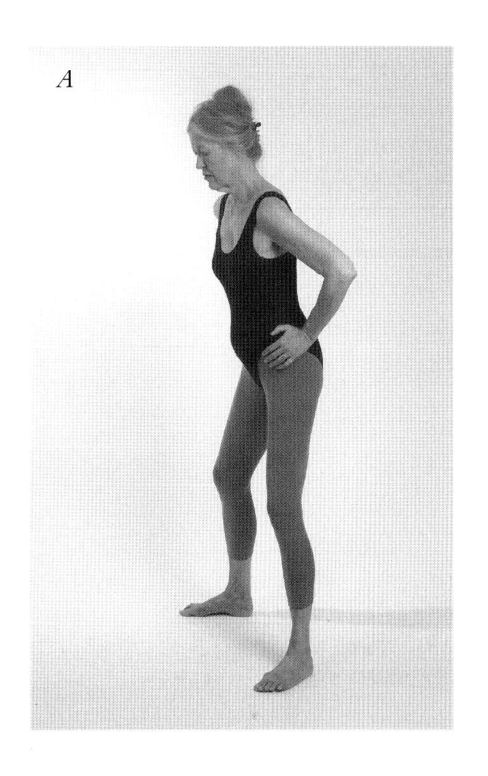

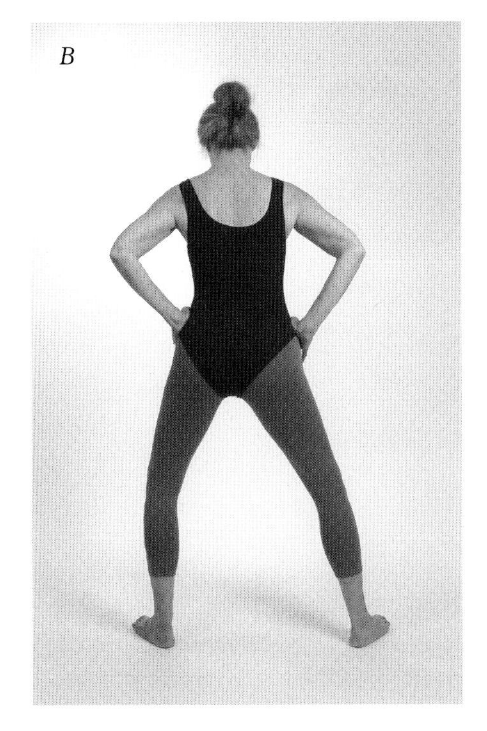

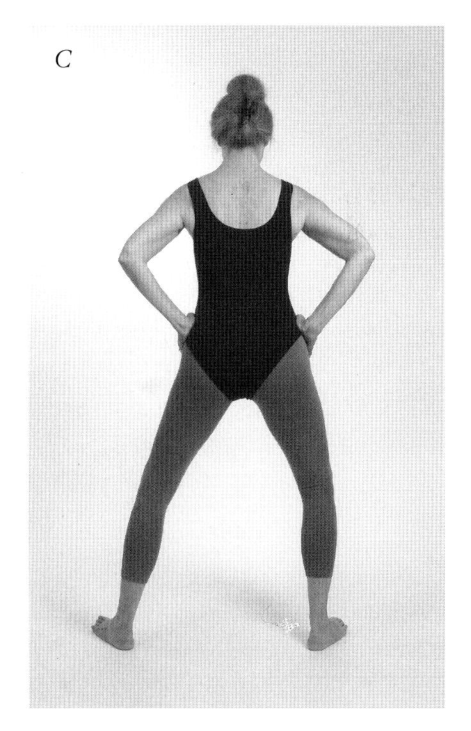

GLIDING

Standing on Your Own Two Feet

Many English expressions convey poignant physical well-being, confidence, and ease through body imagery. For example, having a "head on your shoulders" suggests both balanced head and shoulder alignment and good sense, strength, and clarity. Taking a "burden off the shoulders" implies centered, relaxed placement of the shoulders. "To stand on your own two feet" connotes a powerful whole-body image bridging physical verticality and stability with poise, strength, individuality, and presence. *Stand* has at its base "*sta,*" to stand, be placed ... stable and "to be or remain in an upright position, supported on the feet."

This comprehensive definition of "stand" accentuates the importance of *how* we stand. In our culture, standing is considered tiring, and we eagerly sink into a chair or sofa to gain relief from standing up. We do not equate standing with "a strong backbone," confidence, or relaxation. Interestingly, the phrases "to be supported on the feet" and "to be placed" suggest that standing naturally is restful. In many other regions of the world, men and women sense how to settle into standing without effort for long periods of time. In Greece, Honduras, Spain, and Portugal, we can see people at picnics and festivals standing comfortably for several hours at a time.

When we stand with stressful balance—with decreased vertical support from our legs and a reduced balanced angle of our pelvis, our whole body becomes unnecessarily taxed, as many muscles continuously contract to keep our body upright. This places us in a state of physical resistance to our environment.

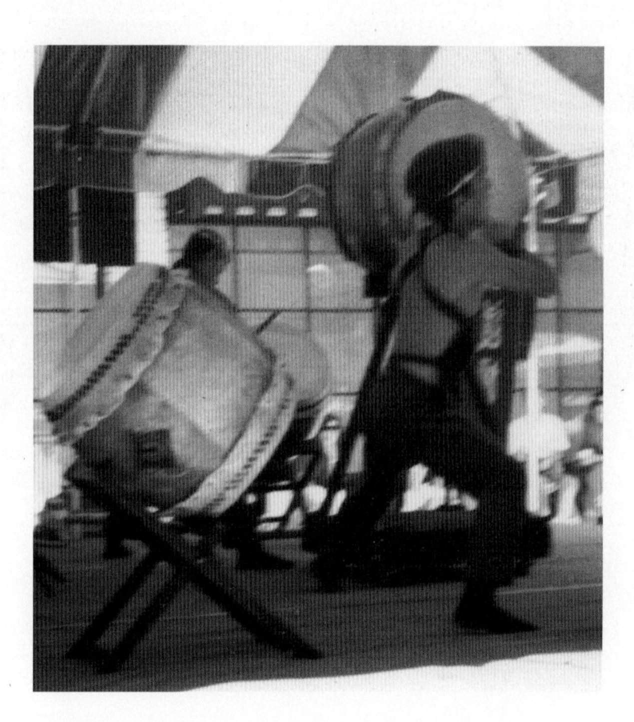

We can see poised, powerful bodily expression in the Japanese Taiko drum player. His back is straight, his shoulders relaxed, and his pelvis grounded. His stance is similar to the KENTRO Gliding movement.

We can remedy this muscular straining, these "holding" patterns. Balancing our movements from moment to moment allows our muscles to relax into centering releases.

We then feel planted, supported on our feet. Our muscles function harmoniously, and we sense a combination of grounding, stability, lightness, and ease.

Standing is at the center of human life. We give a standing ovation to outstanding performers. We stand to pay our respects to the deceased. We stand to sing in a choir.

In moments of grief and joy, we stand. We can do so peacefully.

KENTRO practice grounds us as we stand on our own two feet, helping us to "stand our ground" and "stand up" for ourselves. Such metaphors of centered, balanced standing generate full-bodied resiliency and alertness in our everyday lives, from our feet to our belly, our heart, and our head.

> The principles of body Balancing and Centering as taught by Angelika Thusius are helpful to a classical ballet dancer. Today, with the popular flourishing of many different dance forms and schools, the fundamental concepts developed over decades of classical ballet teaching have been greatly diluted and in some cases lost. A study of these methods with a corresponding comprehension of human anatomy and KENTRO Body Balance can ameliorate the "placement" of the classical ballet dancer, thus facilitating her technique. This correct placement of the body produces aligned balance, preventing strain on joints, muscles, and tendons.
>
> **—Cecile Daniker, Ballet Choreographer and Dancer (Paris)**

25. Croissant

PREPARATION: Place a wedge toward the front edge of a chair and sit down. Practice Elemental Placement.

A. With your hips level, slowly bend forward, bend your elbows, and rest your arms on your knees. *Sense* your *buttocks stretching out behind you,* grounding *you, while your back straightens evenly.*

   Drop your shoulders and slowly extend your left arm in front of your body, your elbow level with your heart area or level with your chin area. *Sense contraction in your left shoulder blade muscles.*

B. Keep your torso level, while slowly moving your left arm into a slight crescent-shape, originating from your upper back-heart area. Keep your lower back level. *Sense lateral stretching in your left upper back muscles, as well as a lengthening stretch in your lower back.*

C. Keep your lower back long and even. Let your head turn slightly to the right as your left arm continues to extend, crescent-like, to the right of your body. As soon as you *feel a stretch throughout the entire left side of your back,* you have completed the Croissant. Stay in this stretch for the duration of several yawns. Bring your left arm down onto your left knee. Rest and alternate sides. You can practice a few Croissant stretches in one sitting.

BENEFITS: Careful practice of the *Croissant* will result in a profound stretch of all the muscles on one side of your back (as long as you are in Elemental Placement)—limbering your lower back and strengthening your upper back.

HELPFUL HINTS: Prevent moving into the crescent shape from your waist area (lower back), which restricts straightening in your lower back. Notice if you are twisting your back or pelvis, rounding your upper back, straining your shoulders, or arching your neck, all of which happen when you force your left arm too far to the right of your body. Practice Croissant for reaching objects or dancing. Practice Arms Hug the Wall and Four Directions before the Croissant.

VARIATIONS:

Try the Croissant while you are lying down on your back or while you are bending forward—with one hand placed on the back of a low chair (for counterweight).

A

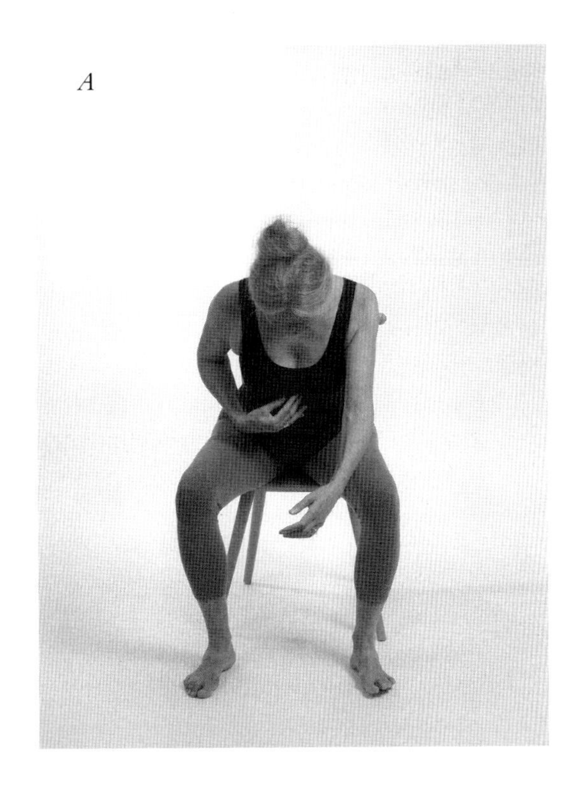

B

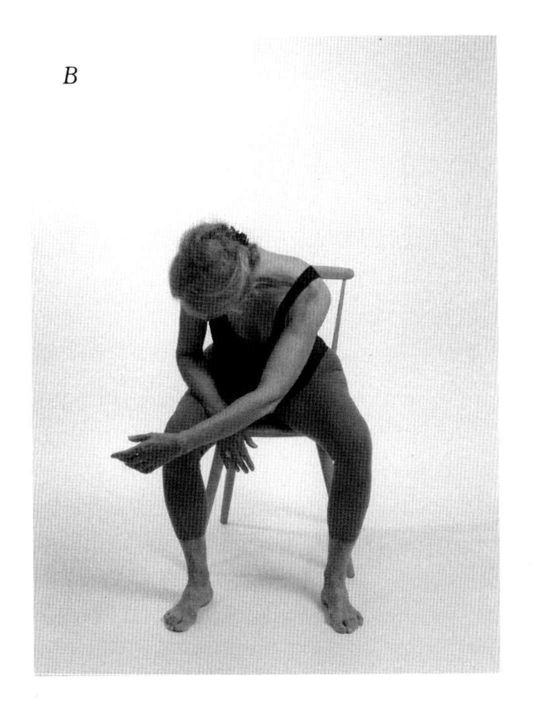

C

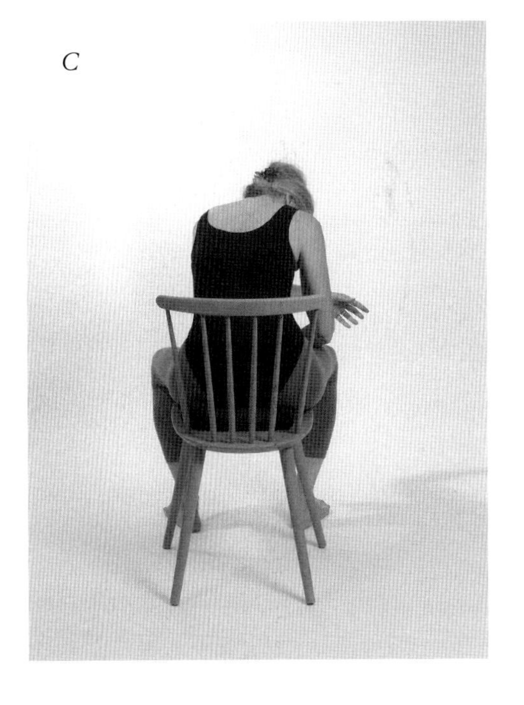

CROISSANT

Practice Makes Imperfect

Most of us are familiar with the saying, "Practice makes perfect," but within KENTRO Body Balance, "Practice makes imperfect."

The word *perfect* suggests the achievement of an almost unattainable goal. In the context of bodily placement, it implies a finished product: a fixed and ideal posture.

The verb *practice* (derived from the Greek *practikos* related to *action*) is defined as: "to exercise ... to do repeatedly in order to learn or become proficient." We practice medicine, law, piano, and painting without achieving perfection; the same is true if we practice moving with ease.

"Practice makes imperfect" frees us from judging our bodies and our progress by seeking the "right" stance. When we balance our movements, we may still seek

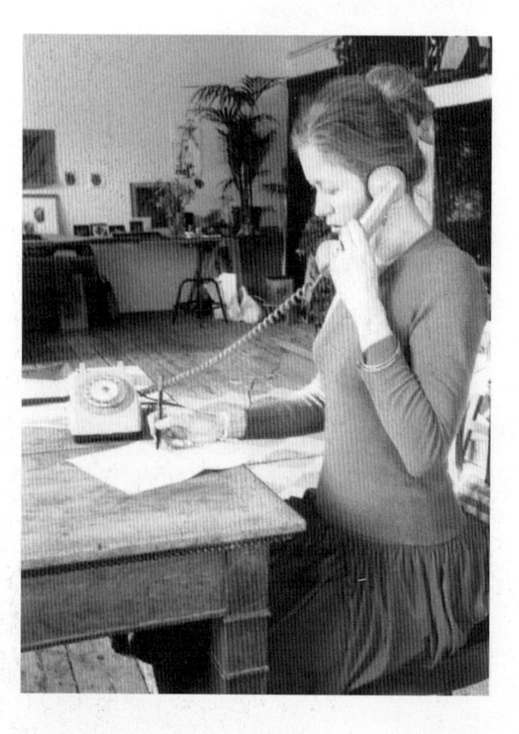

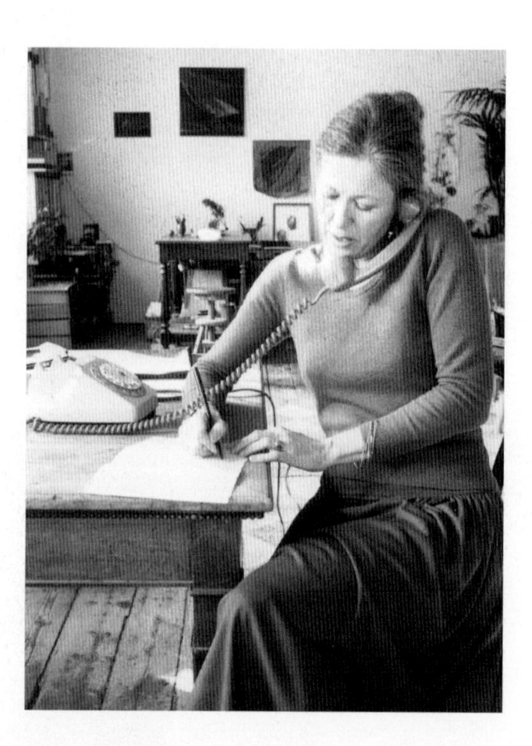

(Left). In my second year of teaching the Shoulder Roll, *I have already realigned my shoulders into more comfort; yet, my rib cage is still raised up, and my lower back is still shortened. Practicing the* KENTRO Croissant *movement thoroughly lengthens the back muscles, which decreases compensatory arching (shortening in the lower back).*

(Right). This is the way I used to sit, before practicing centering and balancing movements. My hips are cramped, my pelvis is tucked, and my shoulders are tight. When you have an urge to cross your legs, do so for a moment, and notice how it feels. Then sit in comfortable balance and notice how that *feels. Over time, you are likely to prefer* KENTRO Sitting Up *with vim and vigor.*

"perfect" back health. Yet by accompanying balance with a centering, caring attitude to our bearing, we avoid coupling failure or success with bodily shifts. The process of postural reshaping is never complete; there is only a caring enhancement of the quality of our movements. Along the way, we experience growth according to our individual nature and experiences.

Letting go of limiting goals is the most fruitful approach to regaining limberness. By releasing preconceived notions about "good" bearing and simply centering and balancing our movements, we surrender to life in its art. Each ordinary action exercises us and resolves distress from our bodies. Such physical transformation moves us into a deeper, more enjoyable extension of ourselves.

There is a lovely disorder and spontaneity to merging KENTRO movements with our daily occupations, *whenever we feel like it*. This approach liberates us from obsessing over results and activates our sensibilities.

After many years of shifting my body into increased flexibility, I forgot about physical performance, developed an aesthetic approach to kinetics, and focused only on sensing ease. As I regained suppleness—playfully and at my own rhythm—I found that a relaxed attitude yields surprising, comfortable balance in habitual movements.

It has been impossible to predict my physical shifts. For a while, I would focus on limbering my shoulders; yet my hips became more flexible at the same time, or I would suddenly feel expansive mobility in an area I had not even sensed before.

A strong *wish* to release strain, combined with incorporating balancing motions with our occupations will strengthen us without effort.

All we have to do is practice.

The unexpected pleasure of feeling invigorated by our gestures may end the struggle to model ourselves on someone else's posture. When we become impatient and want fast results, the leisurely atmosphere of our centering practice may alleviate such mental stress, replacing *"not being good enough"* with gratitude for our inherent malleability. The more we relax into our imperfections, the more we experience affinity with our ordinary activities.

> Before I started KENTRO I had battled with back problems due to scoliosis and had tried physical therapy, Rolfing, back exercises, and acupuncture, but nothing stopped my back from "going out." Yet after practicing centering and balancing guidelines, I haven't needed to have my back worked on and I actually feel that I am getting stronger each time I pick up my daughters the way Angie taught me. After twenty-five years of looking for solutions Angie's work is like a miracle!
> **—Denise Balma, Market Research Consultant (California)**

26. Wrist Warming Stretch

PREPARATION : Sit up or sit back comfortably. Practice Elemental Placement.

A. Raise your left hand and gently place the inside of your right hand underneath your left wrist to support it.
   Relax your left hand and let your right hand apply very slight pressure around your left wrist.

B. Very slowly, over two to three minutes, let the fingers of your right hand spread along your left wrist and onto your left hand, keeping slight continued pressure, especially on the left wrist. Keep relaxing your left hand. *Sense warmth and a mild lengthening stretch throughout your left wrist.*
   When the index finger of your right hand is close to the pinkie of your left hand, you have stretched far enough. Keep your left hand in this stretch for the duration of several yawns. Stay a moment in this stretch to help *sense warmth and mild stretching in your left wrist.*
   Alternate hands. You can practice the *Wrist Warming Stretch* as often as you wish.

BENEFITS: The *Wrist Warming Stretch* generates spaciousness in the wrist area; it may diminish carpal tunnel symptoms and similar wrist distress, as long as it is integrated with sitting in Elemental Placement as well as KENTRO movements that realign and limber the pelvis, back, shoulder, and neck areas.

HELPFUL HINTS: Prevent squeezing or pulling your left wrist with your right hand, rounding your back, straining your shoulders or tensing your wrist. Practice this stretch for typing and playing an instrument. Practicing Tikanis and Four Directions before Wrist Warming is helpful.

VARIATIONS: Follow guidelines A and B, and then keep your right hand around your left wrist for the duration of a yawn while you momentarily spread the fingers of your left hand for an additional release of stress. Try slowly "drawing" a horizontally inclined "figure eight" configuration with the hand you have just stretched: your hand "draws" a small circle laterally away from your body and, without interruption, draws a small circle laterally toward your body. Rest and repeat the figure eight shape several times.

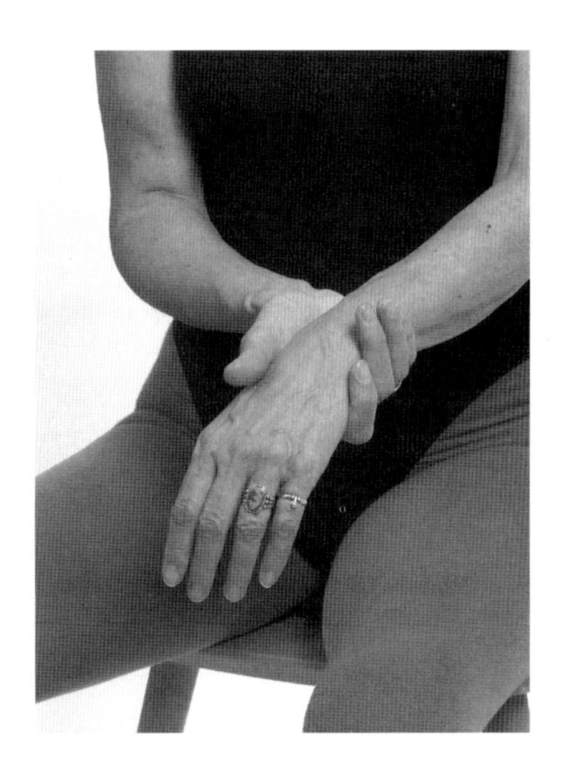

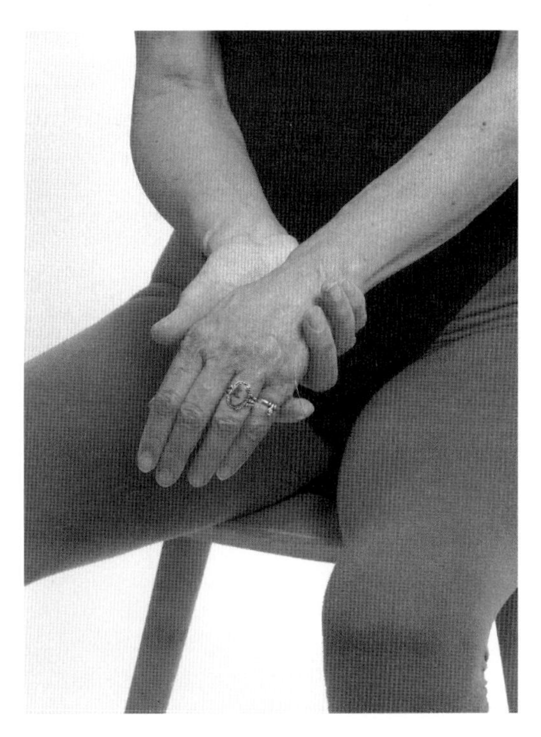

Wrist Warming Stretch

Culture in Posture

The principal definition of *culture* is cultivating—taking care of the soil, as well as refinement of the mind, emotions, manners, and taste. So, our cultural evolvement is shaped by our day-to-day thoughts, perception, beliefs, behavior, how we feel in our occupations, and how we regard our bearing. When lifting groceries feels like a chore, we believe ordinary gestures are a bore, and our day lacks luster. When making a bed feels

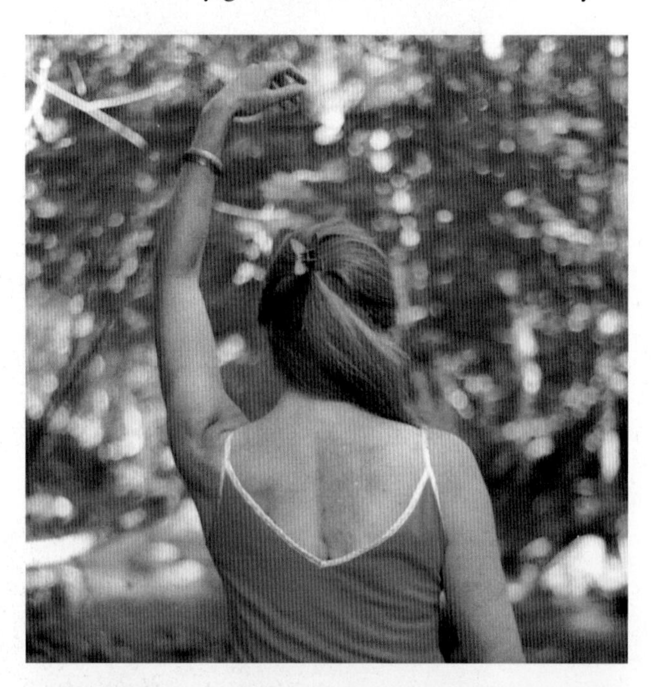

In Honduras and Greece, I saw women combing their hair with their arms raised and relaxed for long periods of time. By practicing Sitting Up *and the* Wrist-Warming Stretch, *and by raising our arms from our upper back, we can enjoy this gesture.*

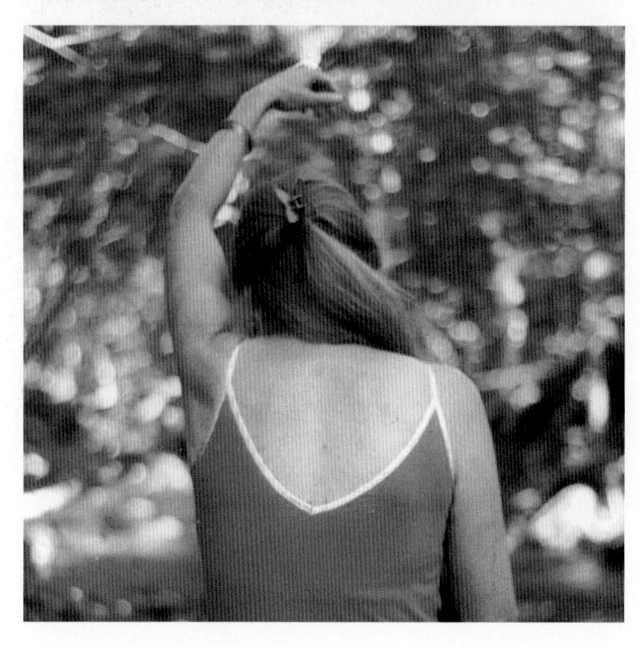

In this position, my pelvis tucks, my back rounds, and my arms tire easily because I raised them from tight shoulder muscles.

This Portuguese woman carrying her bag of potatoes as she does habitually, on her head, exemplifies smooth balance—a straight back, a grounded pelvis, dropped shoulders, and a strong, long neck. She is sturdy and supple.

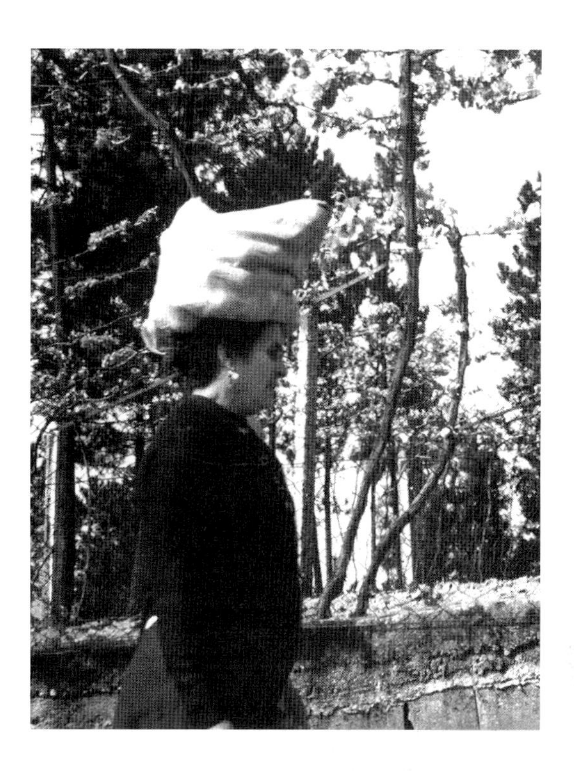

The Honduran man moves with such smooth balance that his pelvis acts as a grounding "seat," steadying his movements. His back remains straight and his movements light.

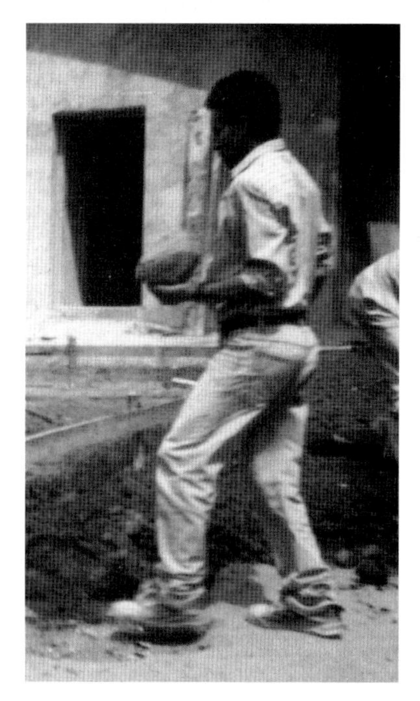

Notice the even groove in the back and the grounded angle of the pelvis of this Greek sculpture (Delphi Museum). His shoulder muscles are relaxed, and his back and buttock muscles are toned. He exudes fluid strength.

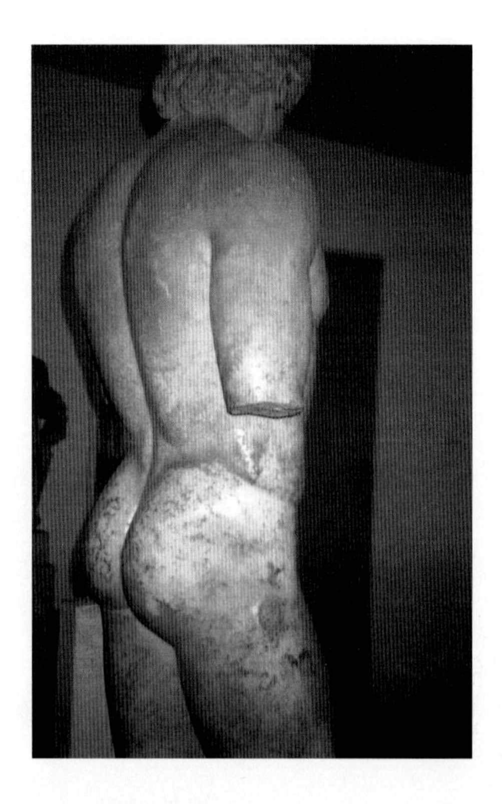

like dance movements, this simple activity brightens our day. A gardener tills and nourishes the soil and then looks forward to the pleasure of seeing plants thrive. We can cultivate our movements by focusing on smooth bodily weight distribution, relaxing our tissues, and looking forward to the pleasure of supple motion. In time, as our activities gently invigorate us, we soften our view of ourselves and of our surroundings.

During my many years of painting everyday life scenes of women and men with limber movements, I disliked my posture, but I did not know what to do about it. I thought of myself as visually sensitive, but only after shifting my body into more centered balance could I *clearly* see fluid muscular functioning in others, as well as in artwork.

Many Greek sculptures portraying harmonious bodily expression, convey a subtle physicality. The principle meaning of the Greek word *paida* is "childish play;" the secondary meaning is "instruction in the training of the body." In *The Greek Way,* Edith Hamilton explains that in ancient Greece, "The truth of poetry and the truth of science were both true."[16]Culture of the mind included culture of the body and soul. For Greeks, exercise meant solitary walks in nature, a balanced diet, intellectual reflection, and a joyful, sensuous appreciation of life and the arts.

In contemporary France, *culture* is used in the expression *culture physique*—physical culture. This expression dignifies physical activity—exercise, sports, movement therapy, and kinesthetics (sense of movement); it places great importance on doing things as naturally as possible and being attentive to health and well-being. Perhaps such emphasis on culturing our body was a reaction to the controlled, "correct" postural model, which developed in highly industrialized countries during the 1920s (see *Setting the Stage, Postural Movements in Highly Industrialized Countries*, p. xvii).

In Honduras, the word *espiritual* (spiritual) is grounded in physical experience. This complimentary word connotes a person with a bright mind, lively movements, poise, and warm feelings. Committing to KENTRO practice is a spirited choice. As we move through our day, our repetitive movements promote expansive expression of ourselves.

I am especially impressed with the KENTRO Body Balance Method. A few of the many benefits I have received from practicing KENTRO movements are:

- my height has increased by three-quarters of an inch
- my sense of well being and self-esteem are enhanced
- my elimination is significantly improved
- I am better able to perform the sports I enjoy
- I get comments of appreciation from strangers on my stunning posture
- I experience less physical fatigue

My patients have also reported significant results.
I prescribe this exemplary method!

—Dianne Rowley, Chiropractor (Costa Rica)

27. Leg Extension

PREPARATION: Stand behind a chair about six inches away from the back of the chair. Practice Elemental Placement.

A. Keep your hips level while you bend slightly forward and place your hands on the back of the chair.
   Keep Grounding yourself, and *relax your belly.*
B. Shift your weight into your right leg and open your left thigh slightly outward, keeping your hips level, and your abdomen relaxed. *Sense expansion in your left hip area and toning in your right buttock.*
C. Keep your hips level and your bellybutton centered with the chair, while you slowly extend your left leg out behind you in increments of one to two inches at a time. Ground your buttocks with each tiny extension. The Leg Extension is complete when your toes lift off the ground. Rest a few seconds in between each small stretch to allow your body to make small readjustments. *Sense extensive stretching and toning through your left buttock and leg.* Stay in this stretch for the duration of one or several yawns.
   Rest and alternate sides. Practice several Leg Extensions at one sitting.

BENEFITS: The *Leg Extension* is an easy way to thoroughly relax, as well as Ground and release your hip/groin/sacroiliac area, while strengthening your pelvis and thighs.

HELPFUL HINTS: Prevent tightening your abdomen, twisting your lower back or pelvis, arching your lower back, or raising one hip higher than the other. Opening your thigh too far outward may strain your lower back. Practice Leg Extension behind your desk or at a dance barre. Practice Pelvic Rock and Pan before Leg Extension.

VARIATIONS: Practice Leg Extension without first rotating your thigh outward before extending it, but then there will be fewer releases of strain. Add Leg Extension to your Walking with a long stride.

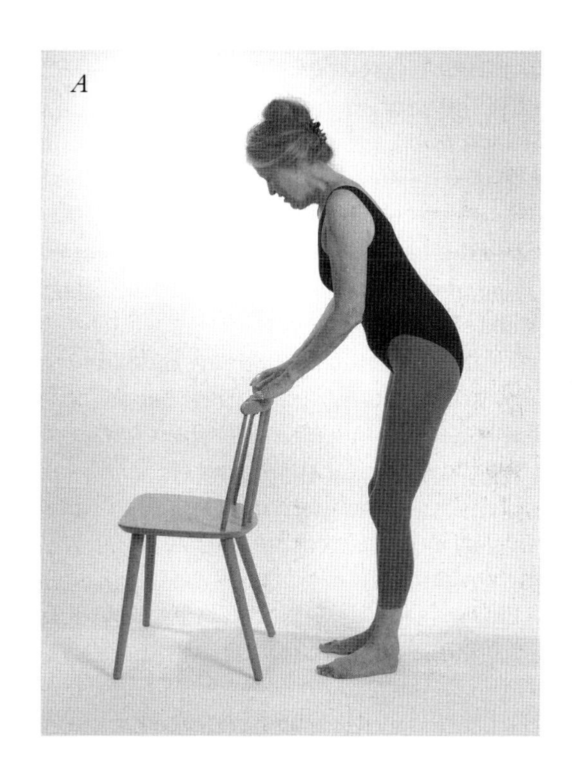

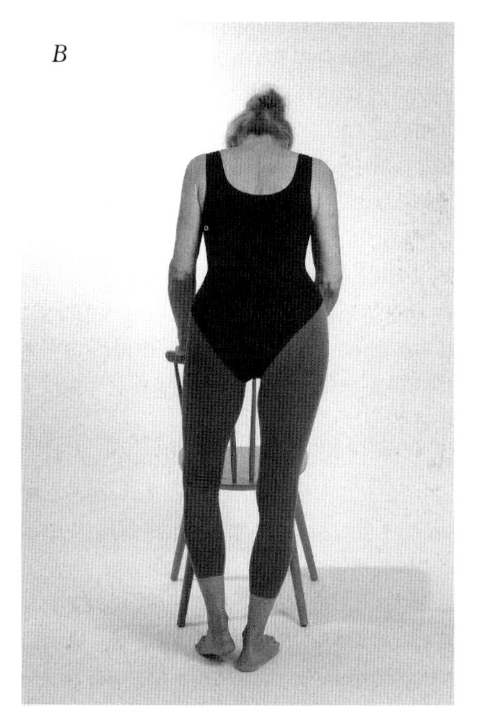

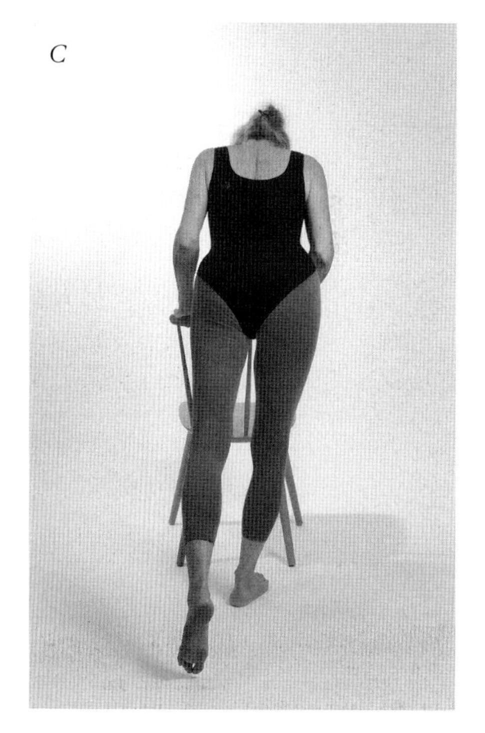

Leg Extension

Love Your Posture

Posture is the process of our body reshaping itself, from moment to moment, during rest or activity. How we feel (pliable or stiff) and move (with suppleness or strain) influences the quality of our everyday lives and how we regard our bearing.

Although we would like to enjoy our posture, we often equate it with a variety of depleting concepts, blaming our distress on congenital spinal weakness, inadequate body shape, repetitive movements, or our lifestyle.

We may strive to convert our movement patterns into a conventional model of "correct" carriage, often over-taxing inflexible shoulder muscles or abdominal muscles, which are not naturally appropriate for *initiating* weightlifting. The tightening of tissues that results from exercising when not in smooth balance may make us feel ill-at-ease in our bodies. After struggling to "stand tall," we may slouch again, hoping to gain some relief from straining into the "right" stance. Attempts to protect ourself from injury may harden the external muscles, while failing to tone the inner muscles. We find that conventional exercise, visualization, weight loss, and other methods for achieving an idealized look or relaxing our bodies do not foster enduring comfort.

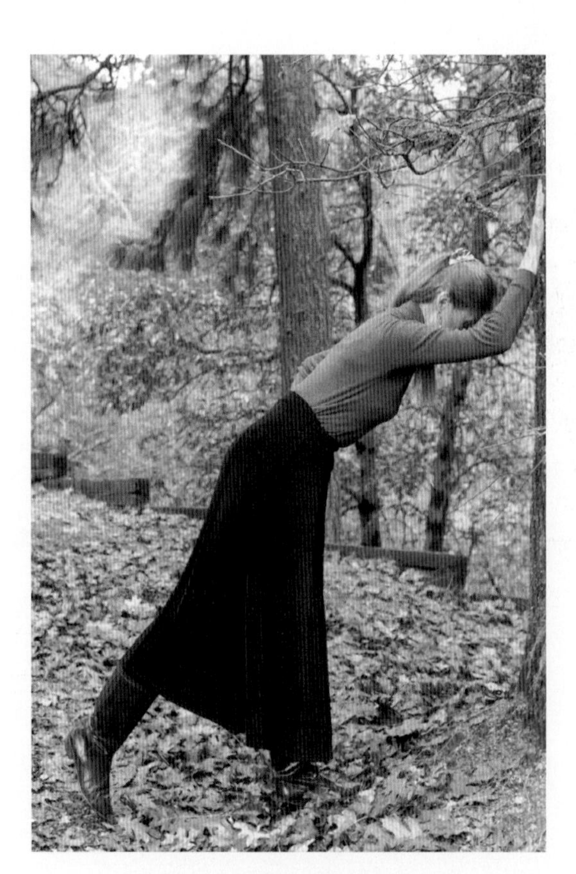

Be practical and practice Leg Extension *anytime, indoors or outdoors.*

Perhaps frustration with our physical expression is actually a signal from the zesty, free spirit within who rejects stressful motion and wishes to express us graciously. Is it really possible to savor our ordinary gestures and experience daily ease? Yes, by letting go of *desiring to change* our physical looks. By viewing our posture as a simple flow of *bodily movement,* centering and balancing movements let our bodies renew us through small shifts in our habitual actions.

KENTRO students have verified that their practice generates suppleness that transforms their physique and reverberates on other levels of their being. Their abdomens gain significant toning and cease sticking out, their rib cages are not raised up so much, their shoulders are not pushed back, and their backs straighten. Likewise, they feel more poised and light-bodied.

Visualizing the body as malleable clay, forming and reforming itself, prepares the way for pleasurable motion. In *Clay and Glazes for the Potter,* Daniel Rhodes explores the plasticity of clay: "Clay, when wet with the proper amount of water, will tend to hold any shape which is given to it."[17] Human beings are close to 70 percent fluid. As with clay, this fluidity generates outstanding elasticity. When it is not wet enough, clay *hardens*. Likewise, we are less mobile when our tissues shorten and tighten. We can extend our range of movement because our bodies are like shapeable clay.

We can be comfortable in our skin when we practice balancing and centering movements with the willingness to let our tissues reshape us into resiliency. By casting a loving eye on our gestures, our routine occupations can strengthen, ease, and delight us.

KENTRO Body Balance gently and profoundly enlivens the body's natural intelligence. Practicing the fun KENTRO exercises has deepened my direct experience of optimal posture and has increased my fluidity and freedom of movement, comfort, and the joy of being. I have naturally integrated KENTRO movements into my daily activities. As a yoga instructor, I find the movements complementary to any yoga practice. I wholeheartedly recommend KENTRO to my family, friends, and yoga students.

—Maureen Claire, Yoga Instructor (Oregon)

28. Between Heaven and Earth

PREPARATION: Stand slightly behind a chair and practice Elemental Placement.

A. With your elbows close to the side of your body, place your hands on top of the chair (with about a foot of space between your hands).
   Combine bending slightly forward with bending your elbows and knees. While you bend forward, keep most of your weight in your heels, Ground your pelvis, let your back straighten, drop your shoulders and chin, level your hips, and center your legs. *Sense a releasing stretch in your buttocks.*

B. Combine straightening your arms from contracted upper back muscles with relaxing your pelvis and straightening your legs, and allow your torso to become slightly more upright (without lifting up your rib cage). Keep most of your weight in your heels.
   Ground your pelvis while your shoulders drop and your arms, back, and knees straighten, and slowly raise up onto your toes. Your pelvis will move closer to the chair. *Sense that the more you relax your pelvis, the more stretching (away from your torso) and release you feel in your buttocks and abdominal muscles; in contrast, sense toning in your upper back and upper arm muscles and lengthening (away from your pelvis) throughout your back.* With your pelvic and back muscles lengthening in two directions, you are in the Between Heaven and Earth stretch. Stay in this stretch for the duration of several yawns and *savor grounding and uplifting feelings in this placement.* Rest and repeat this stretch several times.

BENEFITS: *Between Heaven and Earth* is an essential KENTRO movement because it results in deep relaxation and toning for the pelvic area and strengthens the upper back, upper arm, and leg muscles. This movement is an overall energizing stretch and helps you to feel both grounded and uplifted.

HELPFUL HINTS: The Wrist-Warming Stretch will limber your wrists for Between Heaven and Earth placement. Prevent tightening or tucking your pelvis, arching your lower back, pushing back your buttocks, locking your knees or elbows, or pushing up your shoulders. Practice Between Heaven and Earth for sports, dancing, walking, or lifting. Practice Prayer and Tikanis before Between Heaven and Earth.

VARIATIONS: Practice Between Heaven and Earth by placing your hands on a counter, desk, or massage table. For actively toning your buttocks and thighs, contract your buttocks and stretch your legs as far as you can, until you are on tiptoe.

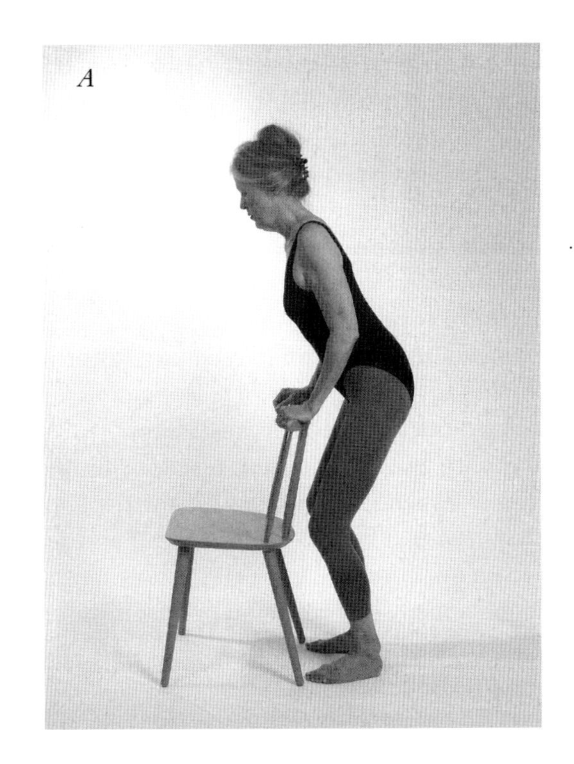

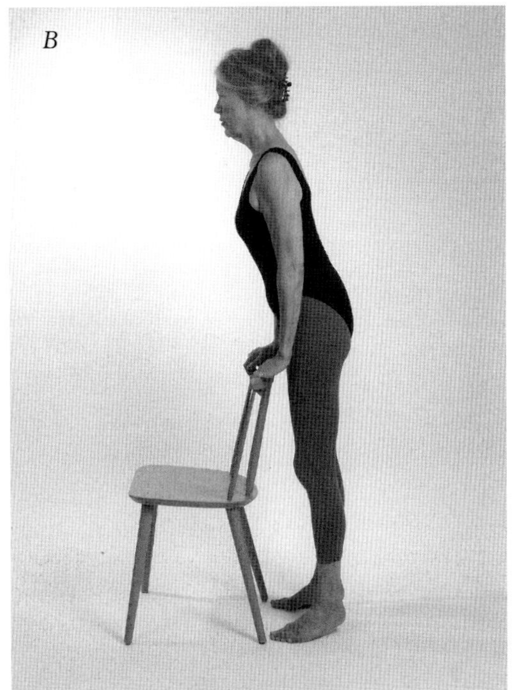

Between Heaven and Earth

Living Between Heaven and Earth

Our bodies can move resiliently by letting our tissues stretch easily in two directions: up and down. From the pelvic center of physical mass, our back muscles extend and straighten while our pelvic muscles expand and lengthen down toward our feet. In the standing position, we are in relaxed uprightness when our leg bones support our pelvis, which in turn allows our pelvic bones to support the torso. Such alignment cultivates a delightful, bi-directional plasticity.

We feel light yet strong in our torso, substantial yet limber in our pelvis. There is a sense of freedom, of our torso reaching toward the sky and our pelvis settling toward the ground. Our physique becomes a metaphor for lightened spirit and grounded soul, connecting our subtle and earthy natures.

We cannot let go of strain or reshape our bodies by force. As we center and balance ourselves, whether standing, bending, sitting, or lying down, bi-directional reshaping *happens on its own.* This feeling of release and renewal is an aesthetic experience emanating from our core. It can be a constant, faithful reminder of our mysterious nature: spirited movement and ensouled body. Because centering and balancing are never mechanical motions, we can easily incorporate this twofold image of ourselves into our KENTRO practice.

KENTRO movements transcend preconceived notions of "correct" posture. After a few years of continuously allowing my pelvis to relax and expand away from my torso to ground myself, I experienced profound physical release. Phrases I had encountered in books on meditation such as: "stretch between heaven and earth," became clear to me. I was likewise able to perceive the truly uplifting, yet grounded, dancing of my main Greek dance teacher, Vassilis Dimitropoulos. When effort is absent, joy is present. We stretch into "living with our feet on the ground and our head in the clouds." We become more sure-footed and our vision can expand.

The dancing of Vassilis (on the left) exemplifies our body's potential for stretching simultaneously in many directions. Practicing the Between Heaven and Earth *movement can harmonize the connections between pelvic, abdominal, and back muscles.*

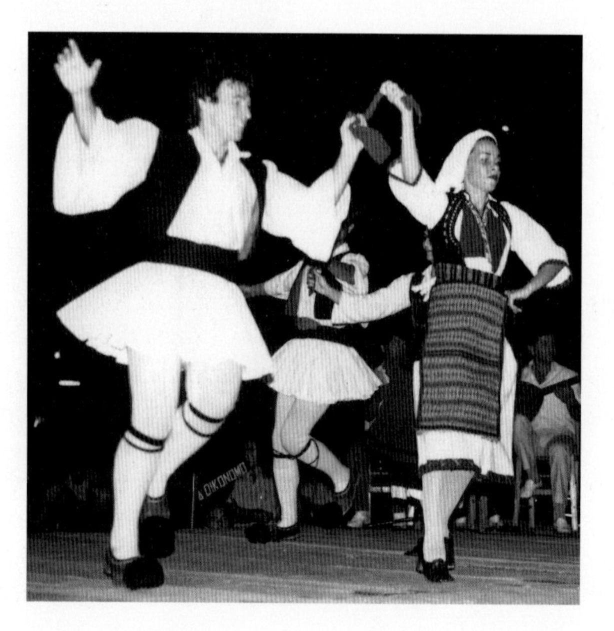

Centering and balancing our movements generates mobility. Physical comfort, stability, and strength occur in rhythm with the frequency of our practice and our individual body histories. With an affectionate view of our bodies, we experience more relaxed thoughts and feel more at home in our activities.

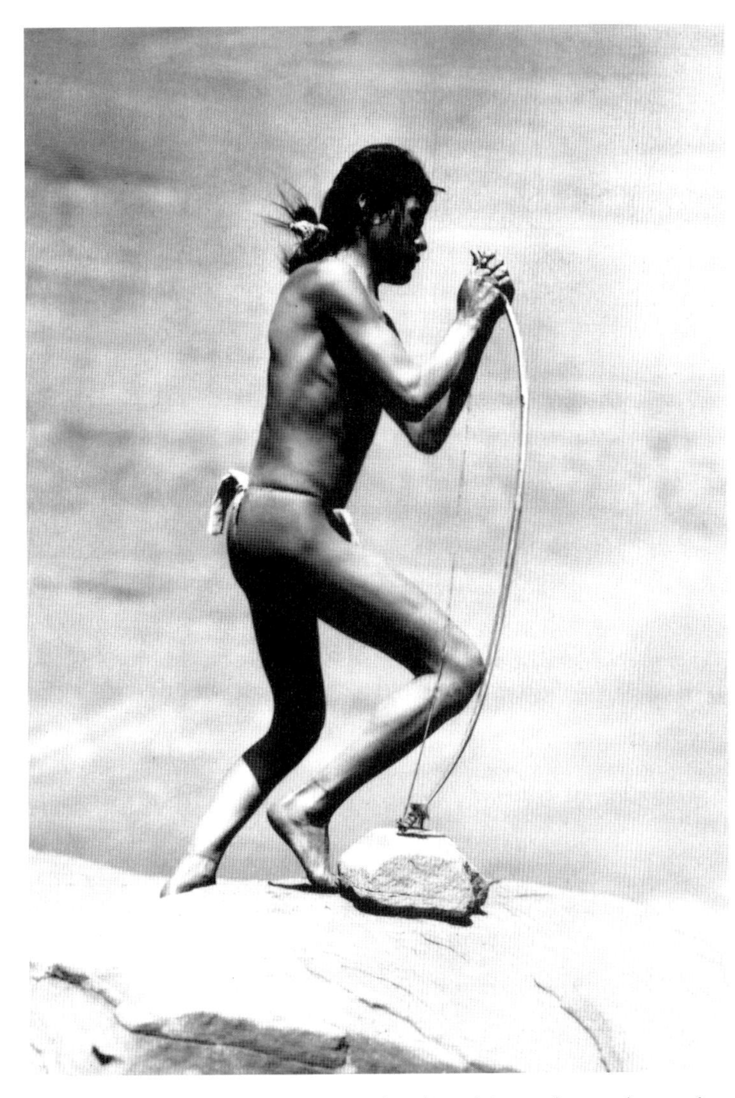

This Navajo Indian moves graciously—his pelvic muscles stretch toward the ground and his back remains straight—while he stretches his bow.

Stretching between heaven and earth moves us into more expansive humanness. When we stand to dance, bend to lift a child, or sit down to type, our naturally expressive bodies extend continuously in two directions. When our torso is spacious and long and our pelvis is fluid and mobile, then our limbs can spread, stretch, and expand us with ease.

And our ordinary activities reflect a quiet contentment.

It is enough for us to *place ourselves* into this process of caring for our inner artist, who can shape our bodies into resilient personal expression. Our movements shift us into the peaceful dynamic that is our nature: stretching between ground and sky.

29. Steer Your Boat

PREPARATION: Stand about six inches behind a chair, practice Elemental Placement, and move into a full Leg Extension (see , p. 176) with your left leg.

A. With your hips level, your bellybutton centered with the chair, and your belly relaxed, contract your left buttock muscles and slowly lift your extended left foot a few inches off the ground. *Sense a "workout" in your left buttock and thigh muscles.* Slowly raise your left leg, letting your torso bend slightly forward. Continue to keep your hips level, your abdomen relaxed, your bellybutton centered, and your back straight. Raise your left leg until you *sense that your left hip will not stay level with your right hip*.

B. Imagine that you had to steer a boat to the right. Contract your left buttock, keep your hips level, and slowly move your left leg six inches to the *left*; imagine resistance from the waves. "Steer" for the duration of a yawn and *sense stretching and toning in your left buttock and thigh muscles.* Move your left leg back in line with your right leg, and set your left foot on the floor to the left of your right foot (with at least four inches between your feet). Rest a moment before continuing to "steer" the boat to the left.

C. Contract your left buttock muscles again and repeat A. You can imagine as much resistance (from the rudder and the waves) as you like while you "steer your boat," as long as your hips stay level. *Sense that the more resistance, the more your pelvic and leg muscles are toned, and your abdominal muscles are stretching and being toned in spaciousness.* Keep contracting your left buttock as you move your left leg slightly toward the *right* as you "steer your boat" to the left. Again, focus on as much resistance as you wish to tone your leg/pelvic muscles. Stay in this stretch for the duration of a yawn.

   Bring your left leg down and set your left foot about four inches away from your right foot. Rest, alternate legs, and again practice the guidelines for "steering" with your right leg. Begin by practicing only two or three sets at a time.

BENEFITS: *Steer Your Boat* provides a thorough, efficient toning of pelvic and leg muscles, providing harmonious strenghtening for all core pelvic muscles and thigh muscles (front, back, lateral).

HELPFUL HINTS: Prevent tucking or sticking out your buttocks, twisting your pelvis or lower back, raising one hip higher than the other hip, arching or rounding your lower back, raising your shoulders, or locking your knees. *Center your bellybutton with the activity.* Practice Steer Your Boat at the office, or dance studio. Practice Pan, Turning, and Leg Extension before Steer Your Boat.

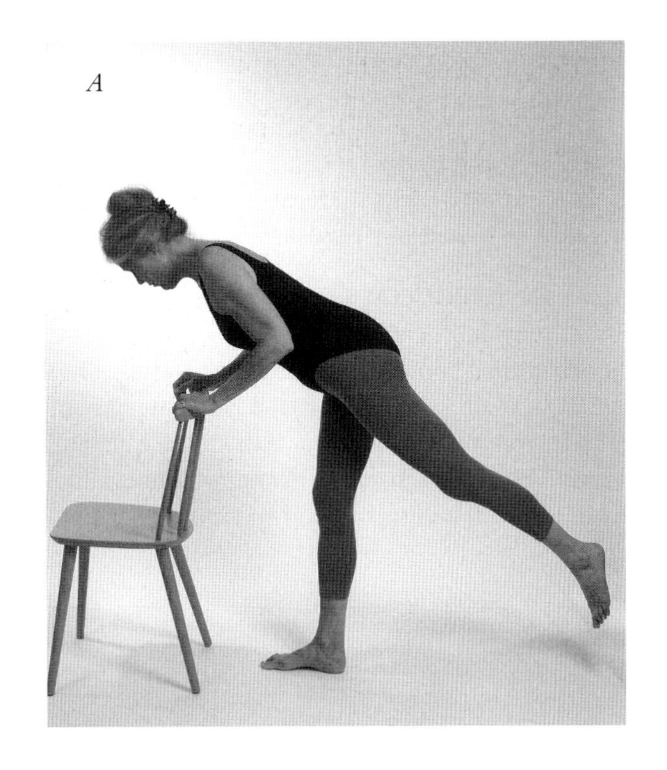

A

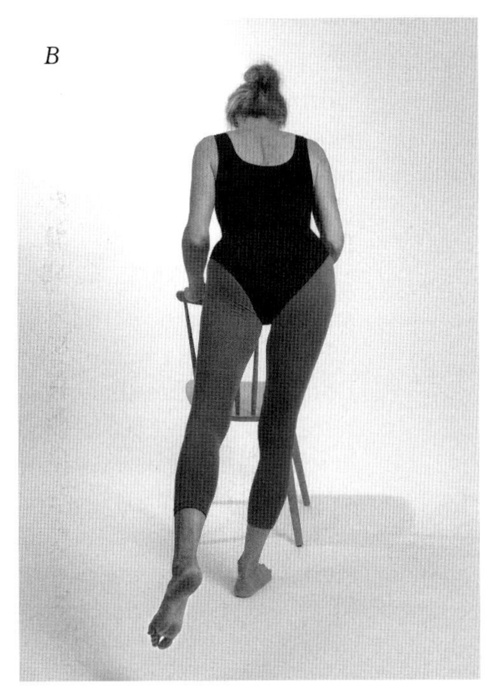

B

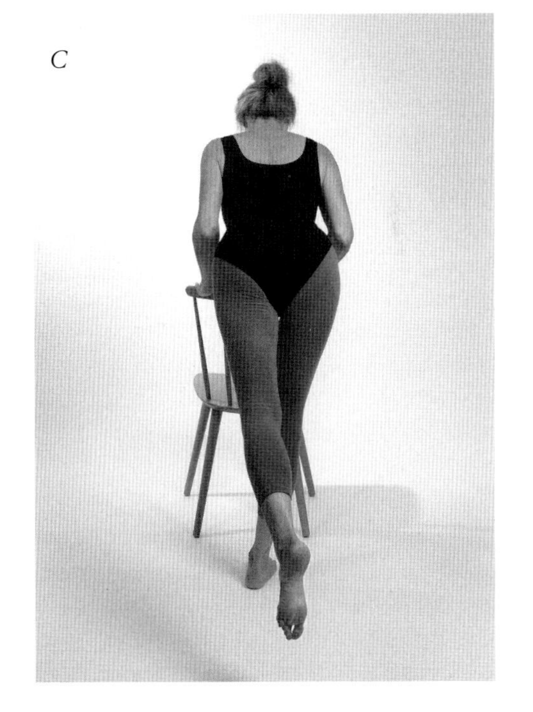

C

Steer Your Boat

VARIATIONS: Try Steer Your Boat by bending your elbows, crossing your forearms, and placing your arms on the top of a counter, with your forehead resting on your hands. Limber your ankles and sacrum by letting the foot of your extended leg "draw" a *horizontally inclined* "figure eight" configuration: a tiny (up and outward turning) circle to the left and, without interruption, delineate a tiny circle to the right.

Stages of Freedom

By practicing KENTRO Body Balance movements, your body will begin to reflect transformations. You cannot categorize these shifts in terms of *beginner, intermediate,* or *advanced.* In the KENTRO approach, you avoid judgments and comparisons with others by focusing on *your feelings*, your *own* stages of letting go, while your body reshapes you into ease. As Hermann Hesse so aptly conveys in several lines of his poem "Stages," renewing and expanding our self spirits our daily living

In all beginnings dwells a magic force
for guarding us and helping us to live.

The cosmic spirit seeks not to restrain us
but lifts us stage by stage to wider spaces
if we accept a home of our own making.

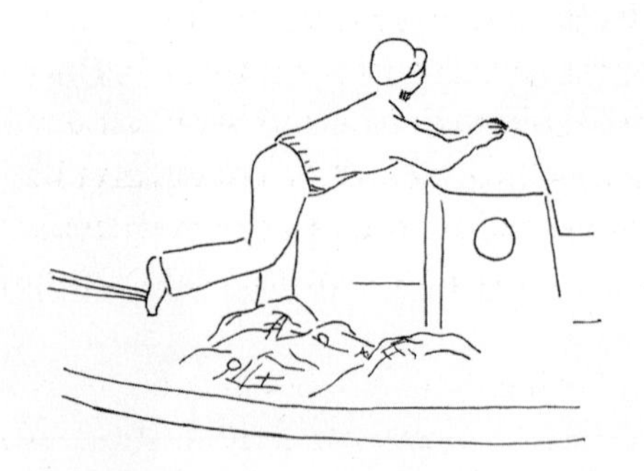

This is a drawing of a Greek man with strong pelvic and leg muscles, which allow him to steer his boat with one foot. He is bending from the hips, and his back straightens easily. This stance is typical of many captains of small boats. Over time, as your tissues become more supple, you will not have to constantly review KENTRO guidelines; you will move spontaneously, with more ease.

In STAGE I, you feel and see dramatic shifts in your body. Because the effectiveness of the simple KENTRO movements may seem astonishing, you are excited but skeptical about the results. You may even feel slightly resistant, since the balancing guidelines and centering feelings are so new and unexpected. Although you are caught off-guard by all the muscular workout sensations, you realize that these aches indicate release of strain because you can sit, garden, or walk all afternoon without your usual back or hip pain. Perhaps you are wary of the unheard of permission to totally relax your body for regaining resiliency, instead of pushing it. Perhaps balancing and centering is still confusing for you, yet you practice KENTRO guidelines because you experience new comfort and stamina during your activities.

By STAGE II, you have assimilated enough images of healthy spines and limber babies and adults to recognize that down-to-earth, comfortable expression is actually widespread. After a few months of practicing the KENTRO method, you recognize that the benefits of your practice transcend conventional exercise or postural "corrections." It still feels unusual at times to think of the slight aches resulting from KENTRO practice as beneficial, even though you ultimately feel more flexible and toned. You may not sense big, continuous changes, or you may become impatient with repeating the simple movements. You may stop your practice because you think you have reached the limit of postural transformation. But having begun KENTRO, you are more aware of how your habitual motion tenses your shoulders, back, pelvis, belly, and neck, and you are able to sense the contrast between muscular tightening and muscular ease. Your back, pelvis, and legs feel more robust whenever you lift an object, and you feel more supple while sitting at the computer. Shifts *are* occurring, only at a quieter, subtler level. Now and then, you experience a significant breakthrough.

At STAGE III, you understand how fruitful it is to integrate centering and balancing movements into your everyday life, because your new mobility is *enduring*. You know that your posture is malleable and the gentle strengthening can continue. You enjoy going within, letting your senses and feelings guide you toward expansive physical expression. You are more willing to practice Elemental Placement and to let your body reshape you because you do not feel as dependent on outside treatment. You experience flow and vitality in your daily occupations.

At this stage, you may feel elated when someone shows interest in the story of your body becoming more elastic. You are eager to place your hands on the troubled areas of your friends and family, showing them how they can perceive the beginnings of smooth balance.

By STAGE IV, you observe that KENTRO movements are more than a practice. They are a way of life—a trustworthy foundation for a refreshing outlook on life, the unexpected result of your dedication to moving with centered balance. You are now in touch with your ability to dissolve limiting beliefs and avoid strained actions. You are more ecologically minded and feel more aware of the connection between the aesthetic, emotional, intellectual, sensuous, and soulful areas of your being. You are truly relaxed in all seats or sofas, and you can stand, sit, or dance for long hours without physical distress.

When you reach this stage, your feelings and gestures become full-bodied through the process of regaining physical resiliency. You sense fluid motion. Now, your body begins to center and balance itself, *without your mental prompting,* just as in the past it automatically overtaxed itself due to stressful movement patterns. And at times, you may feel as though you are a Stage II student again, just beginning—because you are experiencing a more subtle grounding or centering balance, all of which nourish feelings of well-being deep within.

30. Pelvis up the Wall

PREPARATION: Stand with your feet about six inches away from a wall (with your back toward the wall), with a chair just in front of you. Practice Elemental Placement.

A. Relax your shoulders, belly, and pelvis. Level your hips, bend slightly forward (bending your knees), and place your hands on the tiny knob-like ischial tuberosities (the end segment of the pubic bones) located toward the base of your buttocks. Let your hands put upward pressure on the ischials; *sense a beginning of upward stretching in your lower buttocks/hamstring muscles.*

B. Let your hands continue to put upward pressure on the ischials to raise your pelvis up, toward the wall, while you continue to bend forward. *Sense a lengthening in your back and stretching in your hamstrings (back of the thigh).* Some weight may shift toward the front of your feet with the ample lengthening in your hamstring muscles. When you have raised the base of the buttocks as high as possible, "glue" (place) your pelvis onto the wall. Your heels may now be off the ground. Keep on "gluing" your pelvis onto the wall so it does not slide down (and off the wall). *Sense weight shifting into your pelvis.*

C. Take your hands off your buttocks, bring your arms out front, cross your forearms, and place them onto the top of the back of the chair for counterweight: this takes weight off your back and pelvis. *Sense a noticeable stretch in your buttocks and throughout your legs and expansion in your pelvis.* Relax your legs and let weight shift back mostly into your heels as they come down to the ground again. *Sense a letting go in your quadricep (front of your thigh) muscles.* Stay in this extensive stretch only for the duration of several yawns.

BENEFITS: The *Pelvis Up the Wall* movement is particularly relaxing as your pelvic muscles expand and your leg muscles lengthen. As a result, your pelvis regains balanced alignment and your hamstrings become elastic again, without having to undertake extensive stretching to limber your inner thigh muscles. This placement is so effective because there is no effort: your back, torso, and legs are in smooth balance, and the stretch happens at the rhythm of your body's flexibility. *All* thigh muscles stretch harmoniously.

HELPFUL HINTS: Arching your neck or lower back, tucking your pelvis, tightening any muscles, rounding your upper back, or locking your knees takes you out of Pelvis up the Wall. Practice Pelvic Rock and Bending Forward before Pelvis Up the Wall.

VARIATIONS: You can practice Pelvis up the Wall against a tree-trunk or at a dance-barre. This placement is great for keeping your pelvis, back, and legs centered to put on socks, pants, or boots without twisting your back.

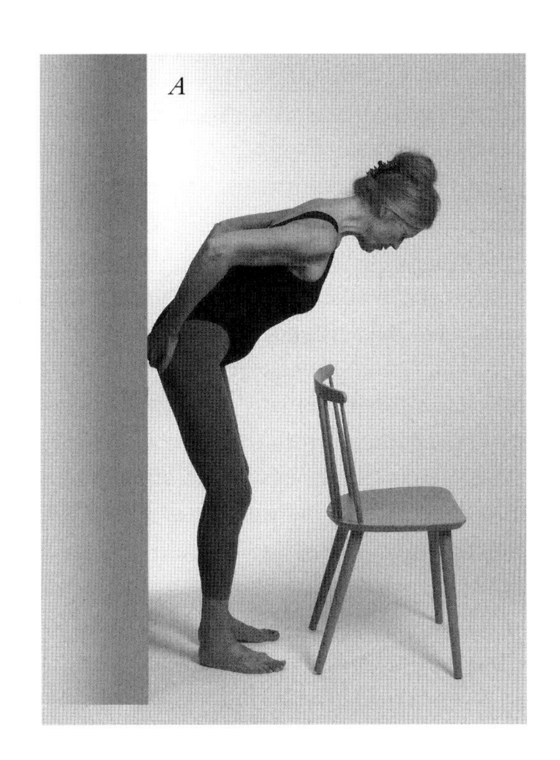

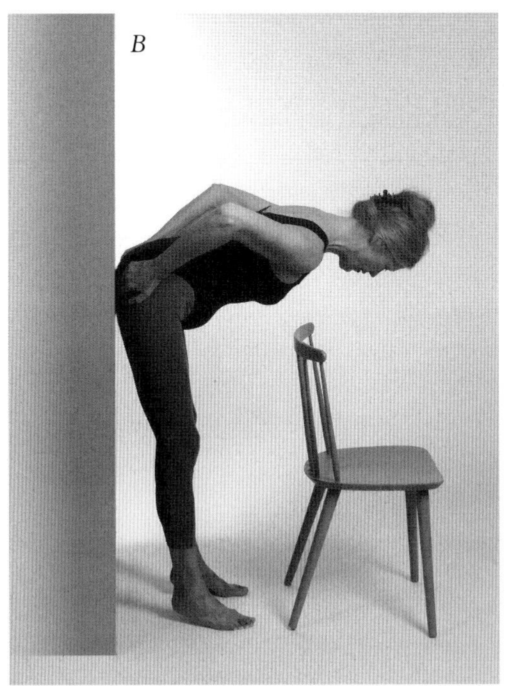

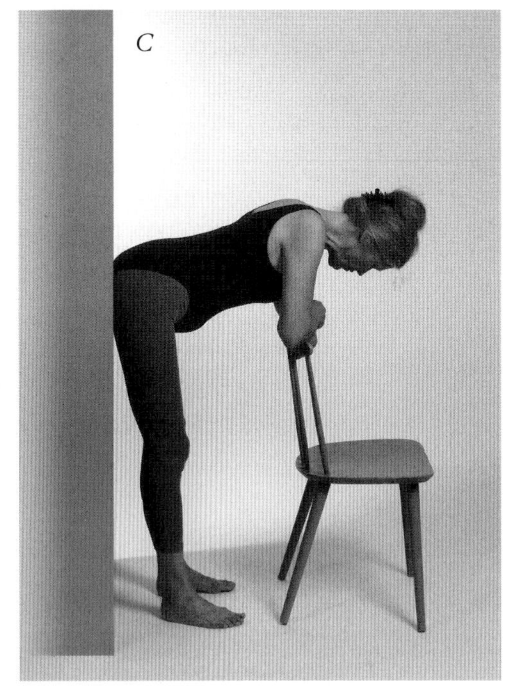

Pelvis up the Wall

Pleasurable Comfort and Ease

When I first started teaching centered balance, I called my classes "Body Alignment and Centering" to describe physical stability and relaxation. I used the image of a palm tree as a logo because palm trees are extremely flexible and the trunk is evocative of a supple human spine. As I deepened my physical reshaping, I wanted to find a new name to describe this process more fully.

I decided the word *balance* was richer and more versatile than *alignment*. Balance evokes images and expressions of proportion, harmony, and equilibrium. Comfortable physical balance can be measured, but balance by itself lacked something. I added the word *body* to *balance* to convey a down-to-earth, palpable physical experience—to fill balance with organic form. However, since my teaching had moved beyond the usual definition of balanced movement and physical well-being, the phrase "body balance" was still inadequate for my purposes. I was searching for a word that would illustrate my particular point of view, which had developed out of personal experience and feedback from students. I knew a compassionate attitude toward our bodies is a more powerful tool for lasting shifts into comfort than just working hard to change our posture through physical balance.

Since my teaching is fundamentally different from conventional back, joint, and neuromuscular therapies and other approaches to postural expression, I wanted a word that would be expansive enough to encompass the program of movements I had developed.

After a year of teaching, I began noticing what a significant influence centering-relaxing thoughts about my body had yielded for me. This process generated an ease that reached out from my creative core, which revealed itself only when I *let go* of stress.

Around the same time, I received a letter from my Greek dance teacher, Vassilis Dimitropoulos, the director of the Center for Hellenic Folk Studies in Athens. On the

This Greek athlete is shown bending slightly backward. Notice his angled pelvis, strong back and buttocks muscles, and broad front. Most of us habitually tuck our pelvis and bend backwards from the "waist," which strains and shortens lower back muscles. This athlete, in contrast, is bending smoothly from the base of the spine, just above the sacrum.

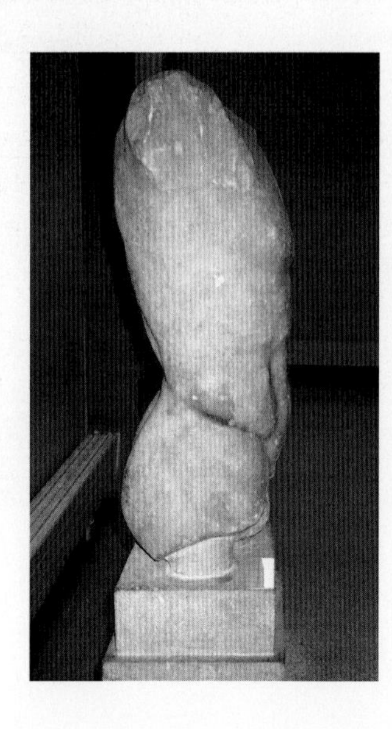

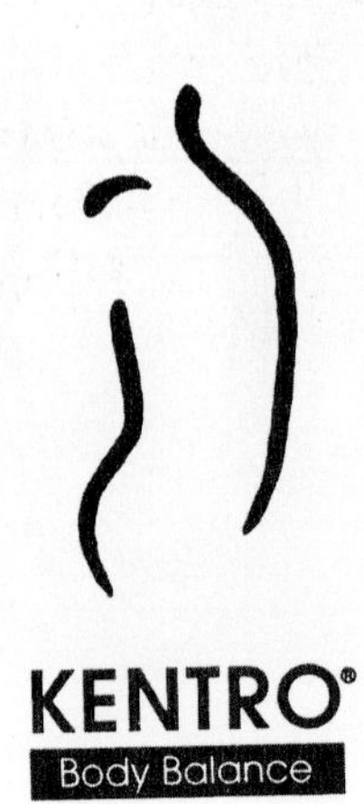

The KENTRO logo suggests anatomical guidelines—an angled pelvis, a straight back, relaxed shoulders, and a broad torso, as well as fluid movement.

envelope, I deciphered some Greek letters. They spelled *kentro*, which means "center" in Greek—an outward location or an inward area of refreshment and repose. It was the word I had been waiting for. I gave it precedence over the phrase "Body Balance." Centering embraces and colors all aspects of our being.

My attention then shifted to creating a new logo that depicted centering as the wellspring of our growth. I did many line-drawings to depict the optimal bone support and elasticity of tissues characteristic of our malleable bodies.

After many months of simplifying and refining endless variations of the logo, I settled on an inspirational image interwoven with the words, "KENTRO Body Balance". The phrase, accompanied by the logo, expresses the idea that centering and balancing our movements can generate a robust resiliency that is native to the divine, earthy artist within us.

The KENTRO exercises are gentle, detailed, make use of the core stabilization systems within the body, and create an environment where complex interactions occur between muscle groups. This is essential for optimal functional movement. I found Angie's ideas on movement fascinating. She states, "Comfort is no longer experienced as passive collapse, but as vibrant ease in the body." I would like to have this phrase put into a poster to hang in all the treatment rooms in our clinic.
—Dean Smith BFA, BScPT Reg. Physiotherapist,
Dip. Manip. P.T., FCAMT (Washington)

31. Swan Neck

PREPARATION: Sit upright on a wedge and practice Elemental Placement.

A. Place the inside of your left hand onto your sternum, with your fingertips spread over the most protruding part of the sternum. Place the fingertips of your right hand onto the protruding joint at the base of your neck (the cervico-thoracic joint), without pushing up your rib cage. Drop your shoulders.

B. Combine slowly stretching your neck out front with upward pressure of your left fingertips on the sternum (as though you are lifting up the sternum). You will *sense a deep stretch in your upper back; it feels as if the sternum "has lifted" toward your throat, which indicates that tight sternal tissues are releasing.*
   Stay in this stretch for the duration of a few yawns and continue.

C. Move back into upright placement of your torso by combining pressure of your right fingertips on the cervico-thoracic joint as your head moves backward and upward (mostly upward) with no pressure of your left fingertips on your sternum. *Sense that as your sternum goes down (on its own), the cervico-thoracic joint does not protrude so much anymore.*

BENEFITS: The *Swan Neck* promotes extensive stretching throughout your neck and torso (thorax). It realigns, releases, and tones your neck and effectively realigns your cervico-thoracic joint and entire rib cage (as tissues regain elasticity). With practice, a "caved in chest" can broaden again, and a "jutting forward" head can become more smoothly balanced.

HELPFUL HINTS: Avoid pushing up your chin or rib cage or pushing back your neck, to avoid strain in your shoulder and neck tissues. Practice Four Directions before Swan Neck.

VARIATIONS: Try placing both hands on your sternum and hanging your head down, which will foster releases in your neck, shoulder, and upper back. In Step C, you can bring your head into smoother alignment by letting your right hand take hold of your hair from the base of your head and, as your right hand pulls up your hair, your head naturally moves back and over your shoulders.

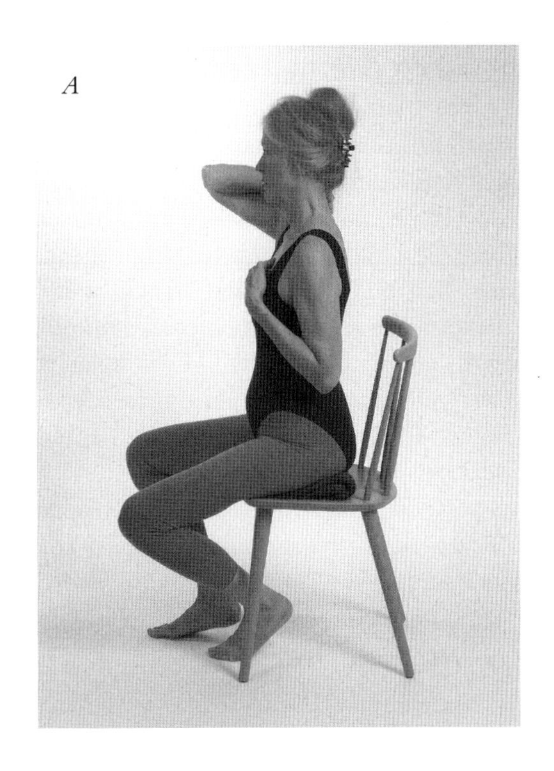

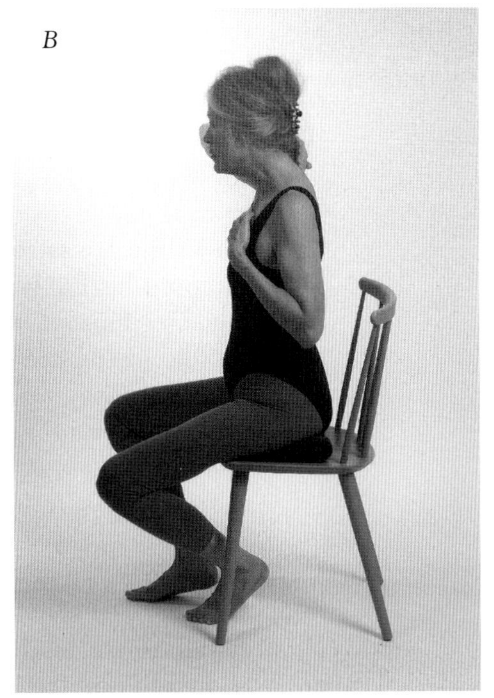

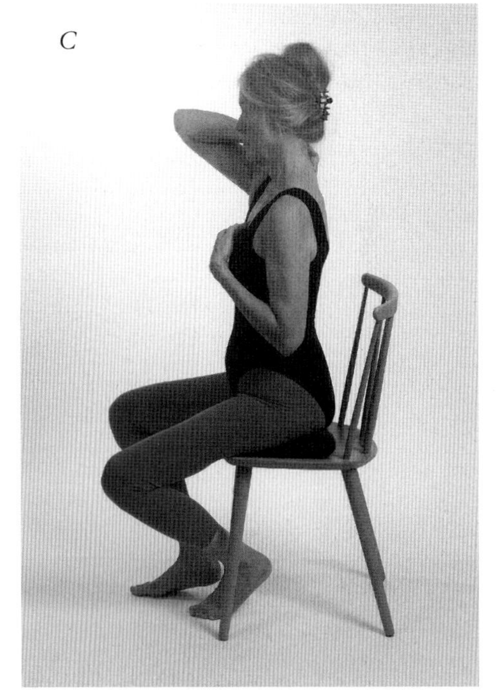

SWAN NECK

Moving from the Inside Out

Shortly before I left France and moved back to the United States, I had the opportunity to teach an American man who had been blind since childhood. My work with John taught me the importance of trusting and developing inner sensing, and the sense of touch. Since he could not *see* KENTRO movements, his first private KENTRO lesson was challenging. I had to search for other means of communication.

When I first met John, I was struck by his relaxed uprightness. He had recently suffered a hip injury and, having received no relief from medical treatments, he wished to study with me. As he already bent in balance from the hips, I felt John's hip would improve with movements that gently stretched his stressed hip as well as his shoulder area. However, I felt disoriented because I could not rely on *my* movements or habitual verbal directions and explanations.

John's patience helped me to slow down, amplify my movements, and experience the subtle benefits of balancing gestures. I adapted centering guidelines to reflect a vocabulary based on sensing and feeling. I closed my eyes while trying out a movement, feeling spaciousness and limbering in my hip and shoulder joints. By placing my hand on John's hand, I helped him feel how much pressure to use on his hip or shoulders. He soon sensed his movements, and his hip and shoulder regained a wide range of motion. He also found it helpful to place one hand on my hip, the other on his hip, as we stretched, shifted our weight, and silently let our bodies relax and release strain.

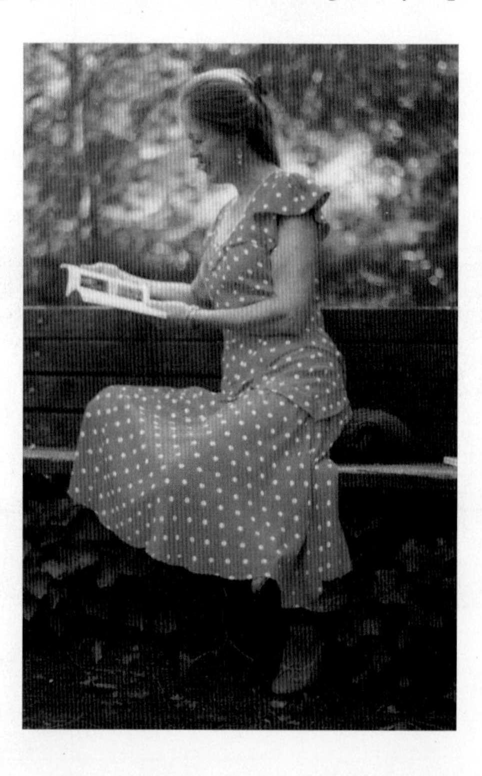

By Sitting up on a thin wedge, we can sense our way into comfortable balance: We let our heads, shoulders, rib cages, and abdomens relax; our pelvises stretch and steady our torsos; and our backs straighten. The Swan Neck *movement realigns the rib cage, broadens the torso, and straightens the neck.*

While I was teaching John, I glimpsed his unconscious habit of balancing himself before an action. He told me he needed to feel solid in his legs and flexible in his pelvis before reaching for a glass or sitting down. He was used to ***moving from the inside out.***

After eight weeks, his hip began functioning smoothly again, and his pelvis and shoulders were more mobile. My teaching had been enriched by John's unique circumstances: I experienced an introduction to our lively sensory system, which I continue to explore, hone, and refine. During my apprenticeship with John, I learned about the complexity of our physiology: the flesh is far more than mechanical muscular function Our sense of movement, time, space, and the quality of our gestures are key ingredients in reshaping ourselves into ease. Our spirited senses can guide us into comfortable action.

Now, in my second year of the KENTRO program, my upper back is more supple and there are new deeper releases in my right hip. Also, at sixty-two, I am able to lift heavy sheet rock for a house renovation and my back stays strong. I am exploring a whole new range of dance possibilities and, at a concert, I felt real free-body dancing. The body dancing itself. This was like a revelation.

—Avram Novick, Chi Gong Instructor and Musician (Oregon)

32. The Executive

PREPARATION: Sit down and place a wedge over the back of your chair.

A. Sit far back on the chair. Place the inside of your left hand (with your thumbs at the base of your rib cage) onto your lower back with upward pressure on your back. *Sense a lengthening in your lower back.* Lift and place the wedge onto the middle of the back of the chair (in line with your upper back) with your right hand.

B Let your left hand slide up your back as you continue stretching your back, without arching your lower back or tightening your abdomen.
Lean back and "glue" your "heart" (upper back) area to the wedge on the back of the chair. Let as much of your body weight as possible shift to the spot (in your upper back) that is glued to the back of the chair. *Sense that your upper back remains stretched*, as weight from your upper back is transferred to the wedge.

C. Your shoulders and rib cage relax downward. Contract your left shoulder blade muscles, detect lengthening in your upper back, and start to raise your left arm/elbow in front, level with your face. *You are bending slightly backward from the small of your back.*

D. Continue contracting your left shoulder blade muscles and raise your left arm above your head. Bend your left elbow slightly outward and place the inside of your left hand on the base of your head to support it. *Sense that you can let the weight of your head drop into your left hand.* Keep contracting your shoulder blade muscles and upper arm muscles, so those muscles support your head.

E. Contract your right shoulder-blade muscles, raise your right arm above your head, bend your right elbow, and place the inside of your right hand over your left hand. Keep your rib cage, chin, and shoulders down. Drop as much weight of your head as possible into your hands. Move your pelvis about an inch closer to the front of your chair to release more weight onto your heart area (where you are "glued" to the chair). *Notice that the more your upper back and upper arm muscles work, the easier it is to release your head (which probably weighs over ten pounds) into your hands.*
At first, you may still "hold on" to your head; but with practice, your *sensing* and *shifting* of weight will increase. Stay in this placement for the duration of a few yawns. Bring your arms down and rest a moment.

BENEFITS: The *Executive* is especially beneficial as a thorough, passive lengthening, straightening stretch that can be felt throughout your upper arms, entire back, and neck. The Executive easily relaxes your upper trapezius shoulder muscles. This movement also helps you sense how to bend backward comfortably, in smooth balance, from the small of your back (fifth or fourth lumbar) instead of from arching your entire lower back (fourth lumbar to first lumbar).

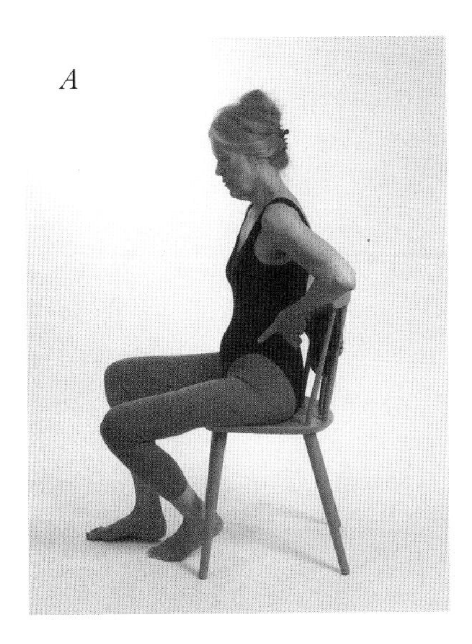

A

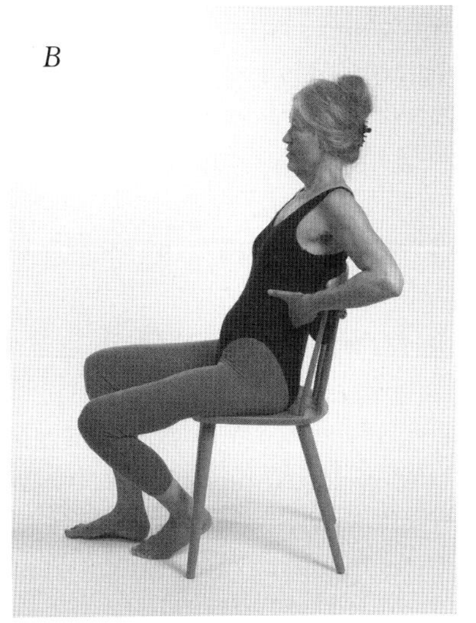

B

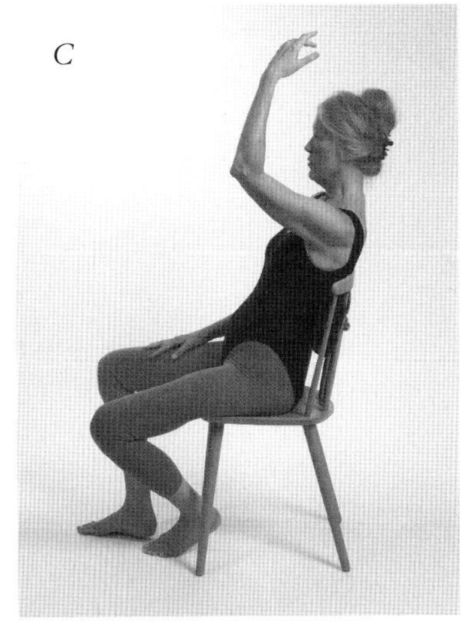

C

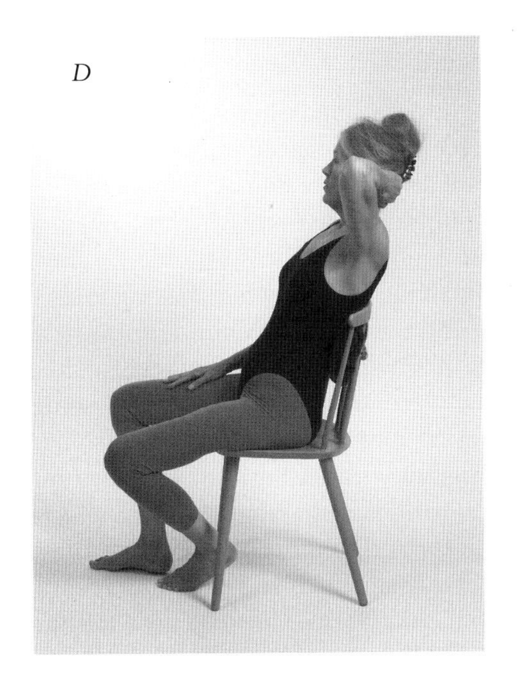

D

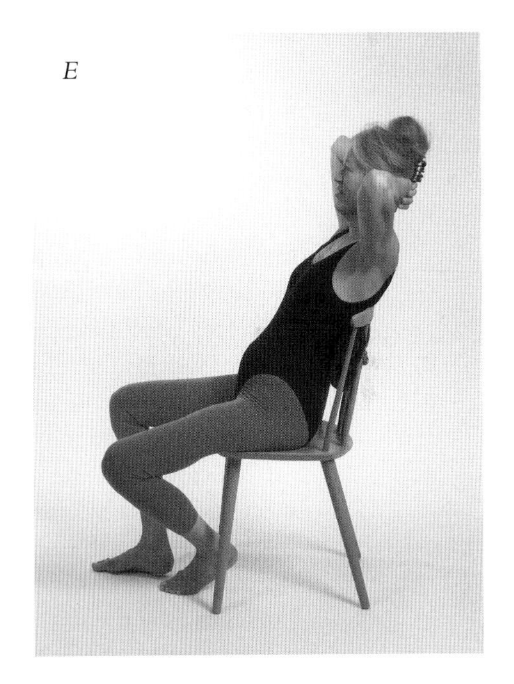

E

THE EXECUTIVE

HELPFUL HINTS: Prevent arching your lower back, tucking your pelvis, raising your shoulders or chin, tightening your abdomen, or upper trapezius muscles (for support). Practice the Executive in bed, and on a sofa. Practice Four Directions before the Executive.

VARIATIONS: Practice the Executive when you are lying down on your back.

Taking a Break from KENTRO

The KENTRO program fosters a playful approach to practicing centering and balancing movements. This leisurely attitude is as important as our practice time. The process of letting our bodies reshape harmoniously is, by its very nature, free of such notions as *should* or *must*. There are no stressful goals, difficult stretches, or external authorities issuing decrees about the quantity or duration of exercises. As we practice the KENTRO guidelines, we simply follow the intimations of our own bodies.

When we feel like taking a break from KENTRO practice, we can do so without anxiety! There are occasions when it is important to simply relax and let our body move as best it can, or when we practice frequently, take off several days to let our body assimilate changes.

When we take a bath, it is next to impossible to sit with a lengthened back and supple pelvic angle. We can forget about balanced motion and have fun massaging our water-softened feet. When we are dancing, we do not have to worry about finding equilibrium and can enjoy moving spontaneously to the rhythm, unless we feel like inviting sensuous centering into our dance movements.

It would be stifling to think about balance while making love. Instead, we can let ourselves be moved by passion and tenderness. While sleeping, it is essential that we receive maximum refreshment. It would interrupt our rest to check if we were continuously lying down in optimal placement. Our common sense tells us we need not practice KENTRO movements every moment.

Most of us begin a new program with enthusiasm and keen interest. Yet we may soon add stress by aiming to "do it right"—making practice a *thing* instead of a *process*. Insidiously, initial interest often turns to obligation (shoulds) and negative judgments ("my posture doesn't look right") that shame us and hamper our natural expression. We can learn to sense and move from our creative core and any time of day, any number of times a day, at a smooth pace suitable for renewal and release.

The centering and balancing movements are most effective when they fit easily into our everyday actions. For example, lifting a casserole or pouring tea relaxes the shoulders, grounds the pelvis, and strengthens the shoulder blade muscles. We can be practical and practice the movements in proportion to our activities.

A student in her second year of KENTRO classes once mentioned that she had not practiced stretches outside of class for two weeks, but she had focused carefully on Walking guidelines during daily walks. As a result, she had experienced grounding and

Whenever I do not practice the KENTRO *guidelines as much as I wish, I integrate centering and balancing movements into my daily life with simple actions like pouring tea. Then I can feel relaxed about taking a break from* KENTRO. *Sitting Back with the* Executive *movement is an effective placement for "lazy" students because this passive placement limbers the upper back and shoulders, and strengthens the back and upper arms. As a result, we can lift things with more ease.*

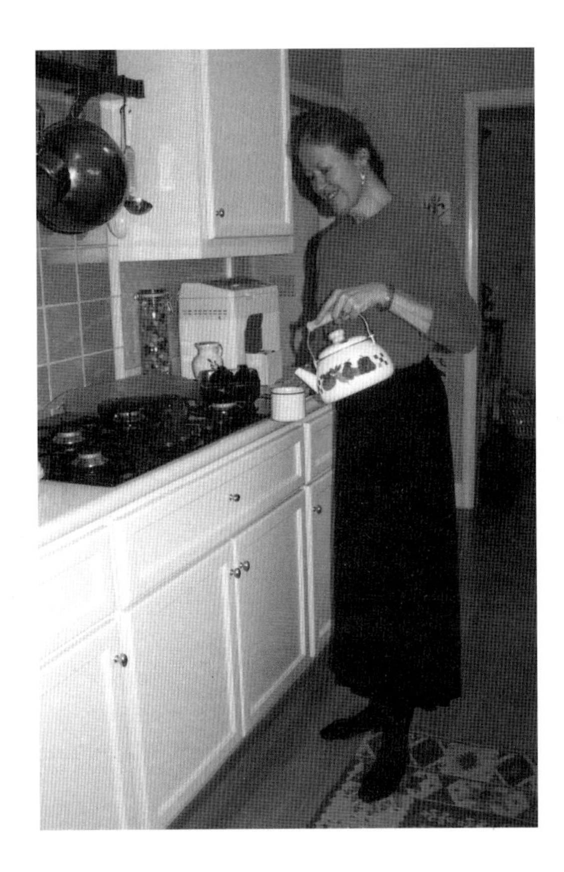

a joyful, new lightness in her walking. The artist within us thrives on our lovely, pliable bodies —the raw material for creative expression in our actions. Smooth motion is more fun than following predetermined rules about postural balance.

By centering our movements, fluid gestures occur quietly, on subtle levels, even when we are not actively practicing specific KENTRO movements. Tolerance and acceptance of our imperfect posture free our bodies to reshape us at propitious times, at our personal rhythm.

33. Belly Dance

PREPARATION: Lie down on your back on a mat or mattress. Practice Elemental Placement.

A. Place the inside of both hands on your innominate (pelvic) bones, spreading your fingers. Keep your hips level.
   Keeping your hips level, relax your back and pelvis, and slowly turn your pelvis to the right by applying forward pressure (toward the ceiling) from the left hand onto your pelvic bones; at the same time, your right hand applies slight backward pressure (toward the mat) to help you turn (see Turning, p. 154) your pelvis without any muscular effort. Remain in this stretch for the duration of a yawn. *Sense gentle lateral stretching in your abdomen and buttocks without* any *muscular tightening.*
   Let your hands turn your pelvis back to its original placement and alternate sides for this relaxing stretch. After a few of these stretches, rest and go on to a more toning stretch, as in B.
B. Place the inside of your left hand onto the left side of your abdomen, and place the inside of your right hand next to your left hand (with your right little finger near your left thumb). Contract the muscles in your bellybutton area and "invite your bellybutton" to stretch to the right, with your hands helping to stretch the bellybutton by pushing it to the right. *Sense toning in your abdomen (especially on the left side) and in both buttocks muscles.*
C. Remain in this powerful stretch for the duration of a yawn. Rest and alternate sides. Expect strong "workout" feelings in your abdomen if you practice more than several Belly Dance series.

BENEFITS: The *Belly Dance* stretch prevents weakening or "pouching-out" of the abdominal muscles because toning occurs throughout the pelvis. Tight tissues will regain elasticity and your pelvis will become more mobile.

HELPFUL HINTS: Prevent tucking your buttocks, shortening (tightening) your belly (which happens when you raise your bellybutton toward your rib cage), lifting up one hip higher than the other, or twisting your pelvis or "waist." If your pelvis feels tight, just practice tiny, hardly perceptible stretches. Over time, as your pelvic tissues become more supple, you will sense obvious Belly Dance stretching. Practice Pelvic Rock, Boat, and Turning before the Belly Dance.

VARIATIONS: Try the Belly Dance when you get up (remaining slightly bent forward for easy Grounding).

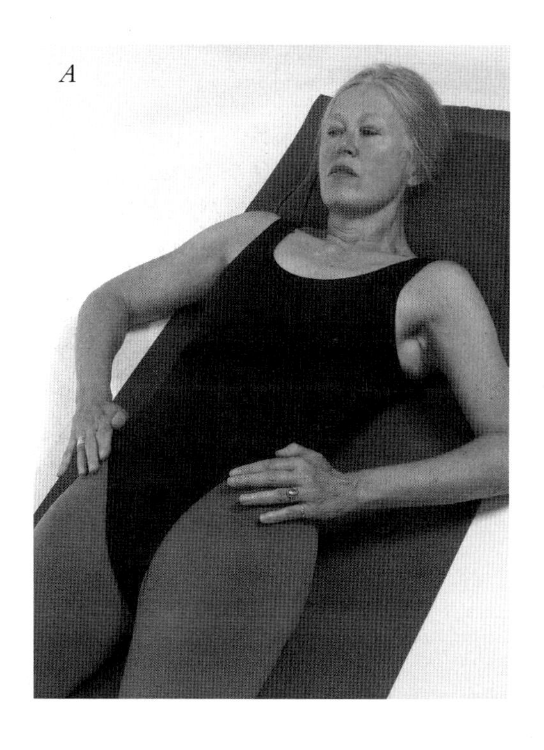

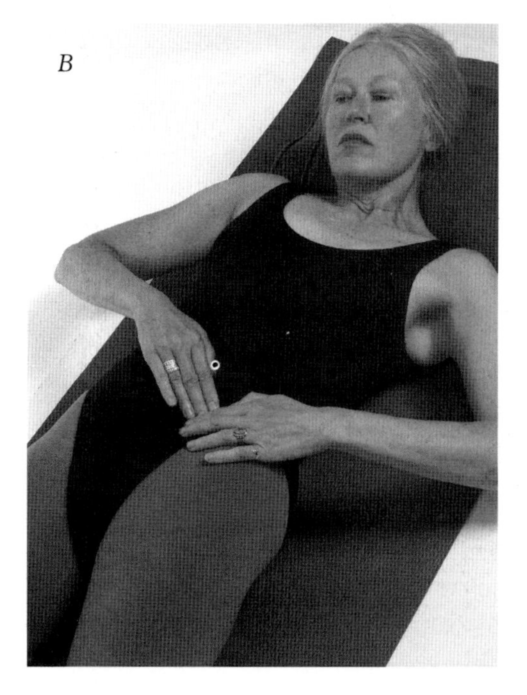

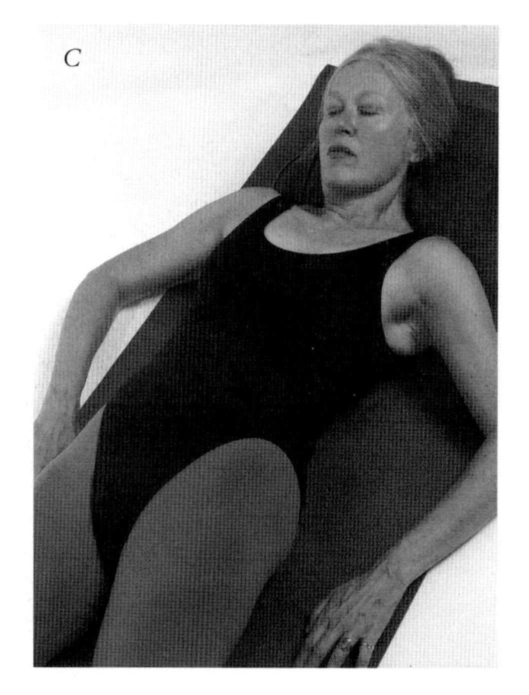

Belly Dance

The Hub of the Wheel

The pelvis is the key area of our bodies for grounding us into freedom of movement in all our activities and rest. To my delight, a dinner conversation at Green Gulch Zen Center in California offered me a metaphor for expanding on the significance of the pelvis. It started when I asked the handsome old man to my right to tell me about himself.

Mr. Wheelwright owned the Green Gulch property and enjoyed living there as a permanent guest of the Zen center. He had not always lived in California. His family had emigrated from England and settled on the East Coast. Following in the tradition of his family, Mr. Wheelwright had built wheels for carts many, many years earlier, before wooden wheels became obsolete, replaced by factory-built wheels. Mr. Wheelwright shared with me some of the secrets of this lost art. He listed the basic ingredients for a durable, strong wheel: great care, patience, and time, from the original selection of the wood to preparing, shaping, and seasoning it, and the particular importance placed on the hub of the wheel. He said that it took three years of skillful work to make the hub, which was the centerpiece, the foundation of the wheel.

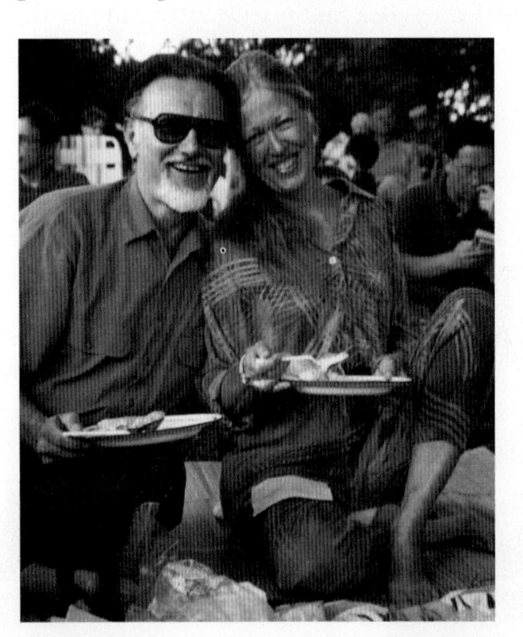

Sitting on a thin wedge enables my pelvis to act as the "hub of the wheel" of my body, allowing me to gain mobility. The Belly Dance *movement can limber and strengthen the abdominal, pelvic, and buttock muscles. In turn, the torso and limbs can become more flexible.*

We sat in soft silence as I absorbed his story. Images welled up inside me of a hub with all its spokes and of a wheel turning, interlaced with the pelvic center of my body, the core of free movement, support, and rest.

I saw a connection between the crafting of wheels—smooth vehicles for motion—and bodily motion. When the hub of a wheel is centered, the span of the spokes is proportional and the wheel functions properly. If the hub is off, the spokes become vulnerable. If our central area for free movement is off—if the pelvis is tucked and tight—it cannot rest optimally on the legs or support the spine. Our extensions (our limbs and trunk) weaken, lose comfortable balance, and compensate through unnecessary muscular effort and holding patterns. In contrast, when our core area is *centered*, other areas of our body can regain suppleness.

From the time I heard Mr. Wheelwright's story, I have been encouraging KENTRO students to practice centering and balancing movements patiently and caringly over several years, so that tightened tissues in the pelvis and in other areas can gradually resolve into increased elasticity. It is helpful to begin as many of our everyday movements as possible from our essential pelvic region: easily bending, turning, and stretching in many directions, as we lift the telephone, buckle the seat belt, and take a stroll.

Students in their first year of practicing KENTRO movements remark that "pulling," stretching sensations in their pelvic muscles are accompanied by feelings of greater support for their torsos and strength in their legs. Rest assured that over a few years' time, strained or injured tissues will expand harmoniously, at the rhythm of your body history and the rate of your centering and balancing practice. You will welcome the spontaneous workout sensations in your pelvis as harbingers of physical grounding—a shaping and reshaping of your core pelvic center—not unlike the crafting of the strong, resilient hub of a wheel.

NOTES

1. The only type of chair in which I do not feel limber and strong is the "cocoon" type—unless I fill it with many wedges, which is impractical, to straighten my back and keep my pelvis elastic.
2. The *anteriorly slanted* pelvis refers to the naturally relaxed pelvic angle, which is relatively more anteriorly slanted when compared to the posterior placement that is caused by tucking the pelvis.
3. *Gray's Anatomy*, 341, 343, 382.
4. *Ibid*, 181.
5. Swami Prabhavananda and Christopher Isherwood, *How to Know God: The Yoga Aphorisms of Patanjali*, Book II, "Yoga and Its Practice" (New York: NAL Penguin, 1953): 110.
6. Swami Hariharananda Aranya, *Yoga Philosophy of Patanjali,* Book II, "On Practice" (Albany: State University of New York Press, 1983): 228.
7. *Ibid*, 228.
8. *Ibid*, 229.
9. *Ibid*.
10. *Ibid*, 230.
11. *Gray's Anatomy*, 354.
12. *Ibid*, 355-356.
13. C. Richard Taylor, Nature, *Freeloading Women* (Vol. 375: May 4,1995): *17* and N. C. Heglund, et. al., Nature, *Energy-saving gait mechanics with head-supported loads* [Vol. 375: May 4, 1995): 52-54.
14. Otto, Pohl. *New York Times*, "Improving the Way Humans Walk the Walk" (Vol. 151: issue 52055, March 12, 2002): F3.
15. *Webster's Dictionary* definition of "beauty."
16. Edith Hamilton, *The Greek Way* (New York: W. W. Norton, 1958): 31.
17. Daniel Rhodes, *Clay and Glazes for the Potter* (Philadelphia: Chilton Book Company, 1973): 10.

PART III

The Evolution of Practice

The body's basic state is pleasure, ease and comfort.

DEEPAK CHOPRA

CHAPTER 10:
Homeplay

YOU CAN ENHANCE your experience of physical resiliency with a variety of *homeplay* projects. Enjoy exploring the suggestions in Section I or Section II.

Section I: Play

Practice the following *homeplay* suggestions with a caring, playful approach to your body, so that you do not give power to someone else's decrees about "fixing" your posture. Your sensibilities will broaden and, in time, you will "feel good inside your own skin."

- BOOKS: If you ever feel confused about certain stretches or exercises, refer to Gray's anatomical descriptions to avoid being sidetracked into "correct" posture that demands exertion and "holding."
- CHILDREN: Observing your child, grandchild, or friend's child at the playground creates exquisite nonverbal communication between the vital, supple movements of the child and your own kinetic sense.
- FAMILY PHOTO ALBUMS: Find some photos of yourself as a resilient small child, and photos of family members (from your grandparents' generation), who have relaxed shoulders and straight backs.
- VIDEOS: Rent videos filmed in countries where a high percentage of people still move comfortably as they rest or work.
- FILMS: Many old-time actors like Charlie Chaplin, Clark Gable, and Vivien Leigh moved with upright ease.
- TELEVISION: Select documentaries that depict limber women and men in archaeological digs, road construction, and farm or factory work.
- MUSIC: Add Samba, Cajun, Indian, or classical music to your movements and stretches.
- WEDGES: Shop for soft, fleece-like fabric or pillows to use as wedges for your sofa, dining-room chairs, and car seat.
- MUSEUMS AND TRAVEL BOOKS: Seek out sculptures and paintings illustrating balanced movement.
- PINUPS: Cut out inspiring images of children, women, and men from travel or parents' magazines and pin up these images on your fridge or paste them into a scrapbook.

- MIRRORS: When you practice *Elemental Placement* standing in profile to a mirror, you probably *think* that your torso is exaggeratedly far out front and your pelvis too far back, but your reflection in the mirror shows that you are actually upright.
- SPREAD COMFORT: Practice *Elemental Placement* before you move into your tai chi, yoga, sports, or dance sequence.
- SHARE YOUR EASE: When you are with your family or friends and feel an urge to share the *Shoulder Roll* or *Gliding* with them, touch them gently, and avoid pushing their bodies into a specific "look."
- CHORE TO PLEASURE: When you wash dishes or vacuum, affirm that you will *play* this activity. Integrate as many centering and balancing movements as possible into your gestures. Add powerful images of yourself moving like a dancer or as a limber Aikido master.
- CELEBRATION: When you experience new suppleness, celebrate yourself!

Section II: Movement Notes

Treat yourself to an attractive notebook. Your notes will intimately mirror your progressive shifts into centered balance.

A. Write short notes (for example "smooth walking", "I feel younger") at least once a week for a few minutes.

B. Write down words you associated with posture/movement and contrast them with words that describe KENTRO guidelines. For example:

LIMITING MOVEMENT/POSTURE	EXPANSIVE MOVEMENT/POSTURE
hold	release
maintain	let go
control	joy
change	shift
should	compassion
correct	resilient
goal	process

C. Write down a memory of *feeling joy* in your movements. "When I was twelve years old and used to run through the town park I felt bouncy and strong!"

D. If you are inclined to journal, write down experiences generated by your Kentro practice, connecting you with your body and feelings on a deeper level. For example, one of my students, Joaquin Lopez (actor and singer), wrote the following: *I allow myself to sink into my body comfortably. Being in my body allows me to be in my flesh. To be me.*

Your *homeplay* will stimulate you and pamper your body. Embellish your KENTRO practice with explorations of your own.

CHAPTER 11:

Combining Kentro Movements

WHENEVER YOU WISH to prevent or alleviate distress in any of the four key areas of your body, consult the list below for a summary of KENTRO movements that focus on each of these areas. You will then have a good sense of how to "mix and match" the movements. *Every* KENTRO *movement will benefit surrounding areas and will reverberate through your whole body: when you practice the* Four Directions *you may experience a release (and hear a "pop") in your neck.* Always start with Elemental Placement.

Movements for the Four Key Areas:

1. Pelvis/Hips

- PELVIS: Grounding, Bending Forward, Boat, Prayer, Walking, Pelvic Rock, Farmer's Rest, Turning, Arms Hug the Wall, Gliding, Between Heaven and Earth, Pelvis Up the Wall, Belly Dance.
- HIPS: Grounding, Little Moon, Bending Forward, Leg Rotation, Boat, Walking, Pelvic Rock, Pan, Turning, Gliding, Leg Extension, Between Heaven and Earth, Pelvis Up the Wall, Steer Your Boat, Belly Dance.

2. Legs/Feet

- LEGS: Grounding, Little Moon, Bending Forward, Leg Rotation, Arms Hug the Wall, Walking, Pan, Gliding, Leg Extension, Pelvis Up the Wall, Steer Your Boat.
- FEET: Grounding, Little Moon, Walking, Pan, Gliding, Leg Extension, Between Heaven and Earth, Pelvis Up the Wall, Steer Your Boat.

3. Back/Shoulders/Hands

- LOWER BACK: Grounding, Shoulder Roll, Bending Forward, Prayer, Arms Hug the Wall, Lying Down, Heart Stretch Lying Down, Pelvic Rock. Farmer's Rest, Croissant, Between Heaven and Earth, Pelvis Up the Wall.
- UPPER BACK: Shoulder Roll, Goose Neck, Tikanis, Lifting, Prayer, Arms Hug the Wall, Heart Stretch Lying Down, Carrying, Looking for Elbow Room, Farmer's Rest, Four Directions, Croissant, Between Heaven and Earth, Swan Neck, Executive.

- SHOULDERS: Shoulder Roll, Goose Neck, Tikanis, Prayer, Arms Hug the Wall, Looking for Elbow Room, Four Directions, Swan Neck, Executive.
- HANDS: Shoulder Roll, Tikanis, Looking for Elbow Room, Wrist-Warming Stretch.

4. Neck/Head

- NECK: Shoulder Roll, Goose Neck, Tikanis, Looking for Elbow Room, Farmer's Rest, Between Heaven and Earth, Swan Neck, Executive.
- HEAD: Shoulder Roll, Goose Neck, Tikanis, Prayer, Lying Down, Looking for Elbow Room, Farmer's Rest, Between Heaven and Earth, Swan Neck, Executive.

❁ ❁ ❁

You will find it infinitely satisfying to sense which Kentro movements are appropriate for ease in various actions. The more you become familiar with movements that are beneficial for the following twelve situations, the more you will be able to discern movements that are particularly helpful for other activities. Always start with *Elemental Placement*.

1. Gardening

Grounding, Little Moon, Shoulder Roll, Bending Forward, Tikanis, Lifting, Prayer, Heart Stretch, Lying Down, Carrying, Pelvic Rock, Farmer's Rest, Turning, Gliding, Pelvis Up the Wall [see Gardening Figs. on p. 212].

2. Preparing a Meal

Grounding, Shoulder Roll, Bending Forward, Tikanis, Lifting, Pelvic Rock, Looking for Elbow Room, Pan, Turning, Gliding, Croissant, Wrist-Warming Stretch.

3. Meditating

Grounding, Little Moon, Shoulder Roll, Goose Neck, Sitting Up, Sitting Back, Tikanis, Leg Rotation, Prayer, Pelvic Rock, Looking for Elbow Room, Four Directions, Between Heaven and Earth, Pelvis Up the Wall, Swan Neck.

4. Sitting at a Computer

Grounding, Shoulder Roll, Goose Neck, Bending Forward, Sitting Up, Sitting Back, Tikanis, Leg Rotation, Pelvic Rock, Looking for Elbow Room, Farmer's Rest, Turning, Four Directions, Croissant, Wrist-Warming Stretch, Swan Neck, Executive [see Sitting at a Computer Figs. p. 213].

5. Dancing

Grounding, Little Moon, Shoulder Roll, Goose Neck, Bending, Tikanis, Leg Rotation, Prayer, Arms Hug the Wall, Heart Stretch Lying Down, Walking, Pelvic Rock, Looking for Elbow Room, Pan, Farmer's Rest, Turning, Four Directions, Gliding, Leg Extension, Between Heaven and Earth, Pelvis Up the Wall, Steer Your Boat, Swan Neck, Belly Dance.

6. Yoga pose: Vhirabadrasana II (Similar to KENTRO Steer Your Boat)

Grounding, Little Moon, Shoulder Roll, Bending Forward, Tikanis, Leg Rotation, Prayer, Arms Hug the Wall, Pelvic Rock, Pan, Turning, Four Directions, Gliding, Leg Extension, Between Heaven and Earth, Pelvis Up the Wall, Steer Your Boat, Belly Dance.

7. Auto Care and Driving

Grounding, Little Moon, Shoulder Roll, Goose Neck, Sitting Back, Tikanis, Leg Rotation, Arms Hug the Wall, Pelvic Rock, Looking for Elbow Room, Turning, Four Directions, Wrist-Warming Stretch, Swan Neck, Executive [see Figs. 11.9–, 11.13, p. 214]

8. Mothers with Babies

Grounding, Shoulder Roll, Bending Forward, Tikanis, Boat, Lifting, Prayer, Carrying, Pelvic Rock, Turning, Gliding, Croissant, Between Heaven and Earth, Belly Dance.

9. Weight lifting

Grounding, Shoulder Roll, Bending Forward, Tikanis, Leg Rotation, Boat, Lifting, Arms Hug (and "push") the Wall, Heart Stretch Lying Down, Carrying, Pelvic Rock, Looking for Elbow Room, Turning, Four Directions, Gliding, Croissant, Wrist-Warming Stretch, Between Heaven and Earth, Swan Neck, Belly Dance.

10. Giving a Massage

Grounding, Little Moon, Shoulder Roll, Bending Forward, Tikanis, Lifting, Prayer, Arms Hug (and "push") the Wall, Heart Stretch Lying Down, Pelvic Rock, Looking for Elbow Room, Turning, Four Directions, Gliding, Croissant, Wrist-Warming Stretch, Between Heaven and Earth, Swan Neck [see Massage Figs., p. 215].

11. Post-Surgical Rehabilitation

Grounding, Little Moon, Shoulder Roll, Bending Forward, Sitting Back, Tikanis, Prayer, Lying Down, Heart Stretch Lying Down (gently!), Pelvic Rock, Looking for Elbow Room, Farmer's Rest, Four Directions.

12. Hiking

Grounding, Little Moon, Shoulder Roll, Bending Forward, Tikanis, Lifting, Leg Rotation, Prayer, Arms Hug the Wall, Heart Stretch Lying Down, Walking, Carrying, Pelvic Rock, Turning, Gliding, Leg Extension, Between Heaven and Earth, Pelvis Up the Wall, Steer Your Boat.

❁ ❁ ❁

The KENTRO Body Balance method can be especially beneficial to those whose occupations involve repetitive movements, such as chiropractors, musicians, osteopaths, dentists, gardeners, surgeons, practitioners of yoga and martial arts, dance instructors, computer users, and sports practitioners, as well as massage therapists and nurses. The KENTRO movements help prevent injuries that are caused by lack of joint flexibility; strained, over-stretched/shortened muscles, nerves, and other tissues; or by repeatedly pushing the body into injurious positions and actions.

By balancing and centering our movements, we can regain suppleness and tone *during* our activities. Movements that were once tiring and distressing can become comfortable and pleasureable.

(Left). Grounding, Bending Forward, Pelvic Rock

(Right). Grounding, Bending Forward, Pelvic Rock, Turning

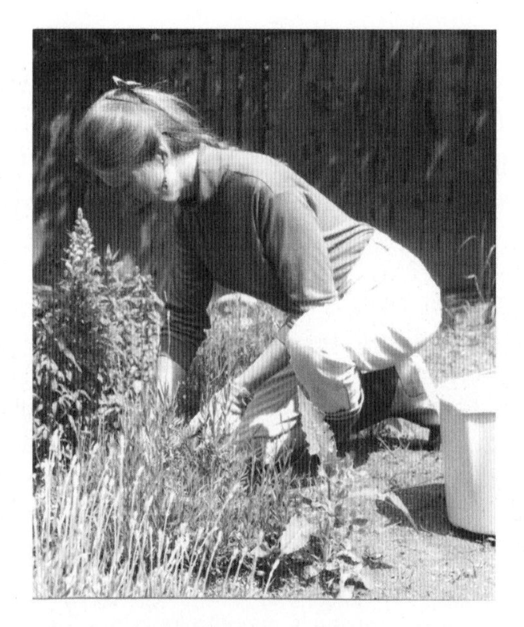

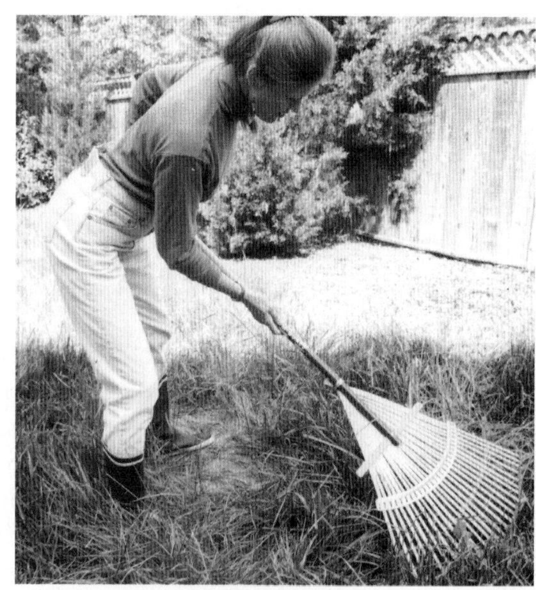

(Left). Grounding, Bending Forward, Pelvic Rock, Tikanis

(Right). Grounding, Bending Forward, Pelvic Rock, Tikanis, Lifting, Shoulder Roll, Gliding

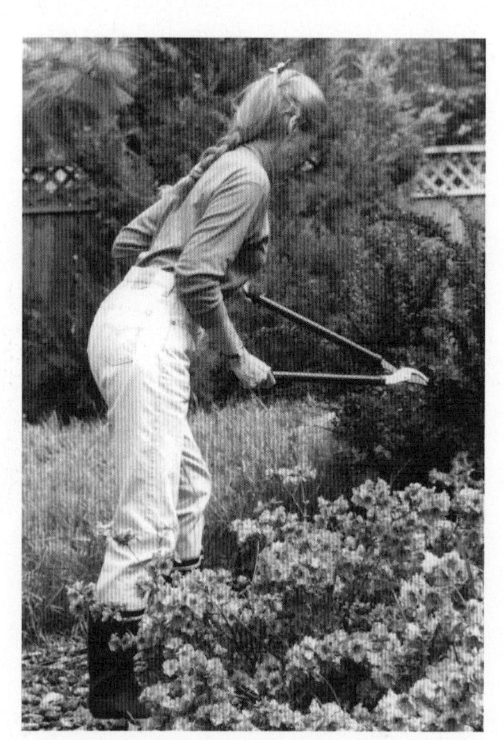

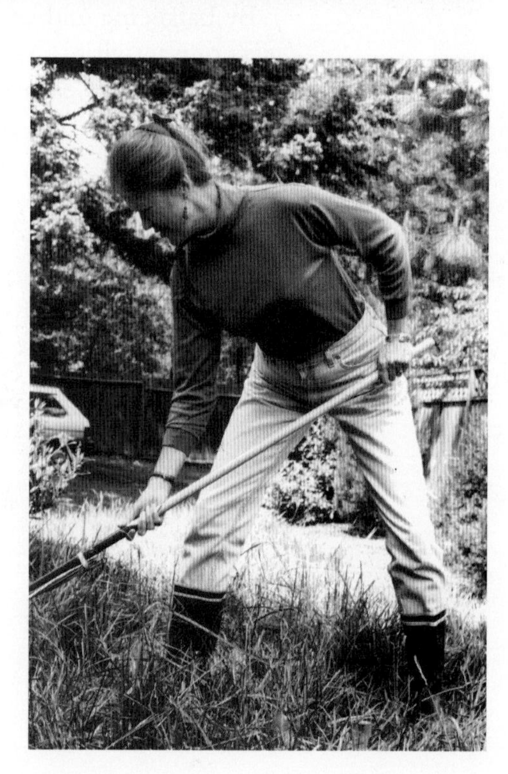

GARDENING

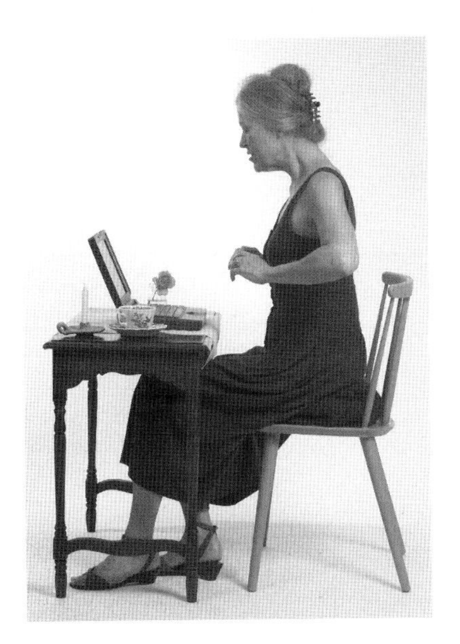

Sitting Up, Looking for Elbow Room

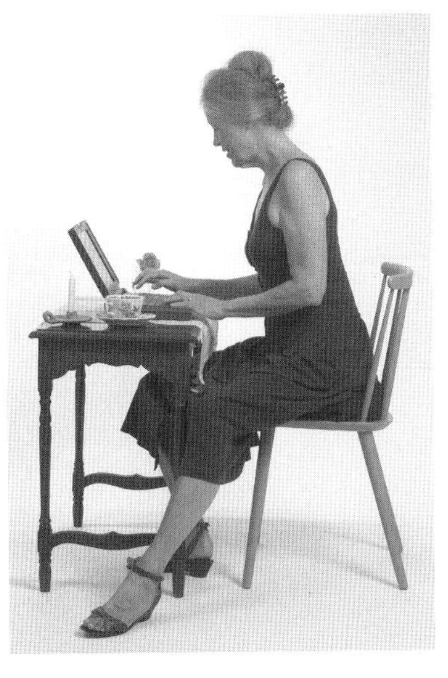

Grounding, Bending Forward, Leg Rotation

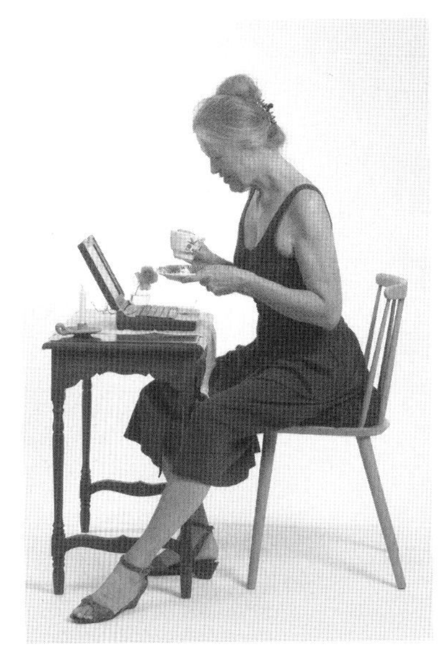

Bending Forward, Turning, Pelvic Rock, Goose Neck

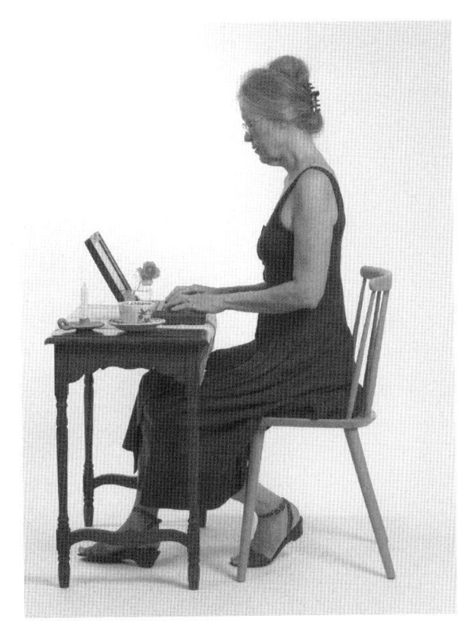

Grounding, Sitting Up, Goose Neck

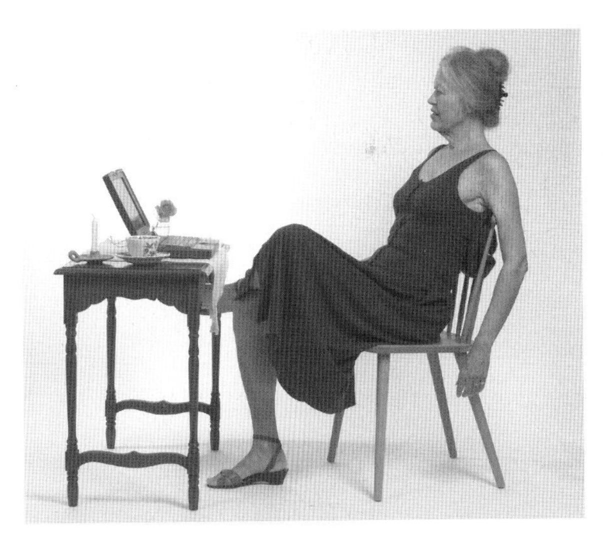

Shoulder Roll, Sitting Back, Leg Rotation

SITTING AT A COMPUTER

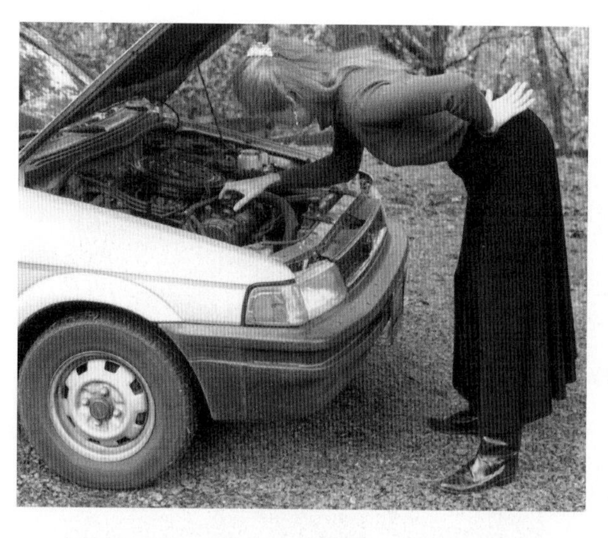

Comfort: Grounding, Goose Neck, Bending Forward

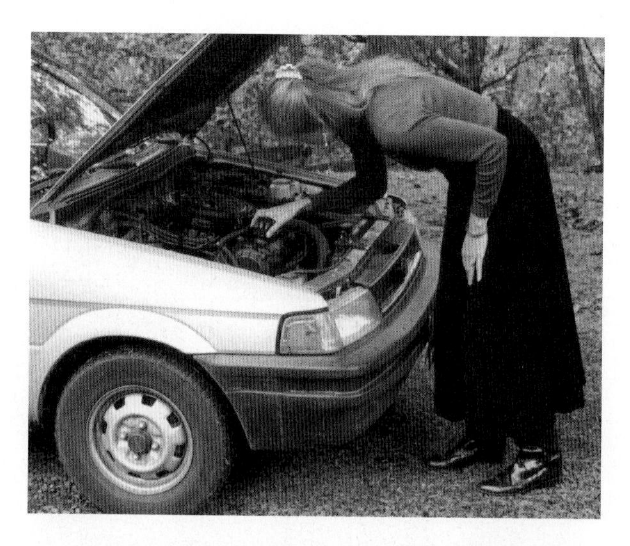

Discomfort: A tucked pelvis and rounded back, strained shoulders and poor leg alignment.

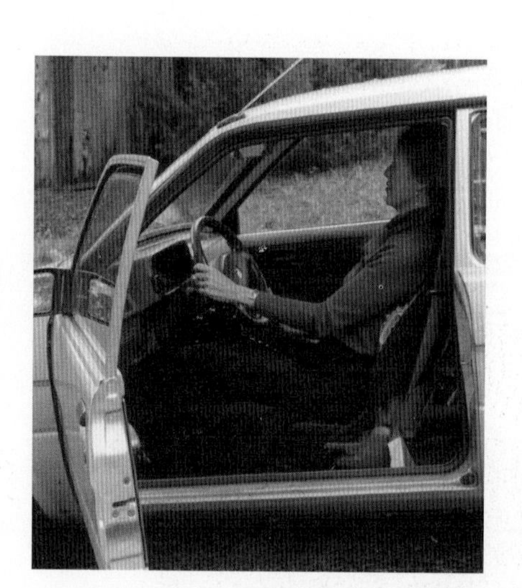

Comfort: Sitting Back, Tikanis, Leg Rotation

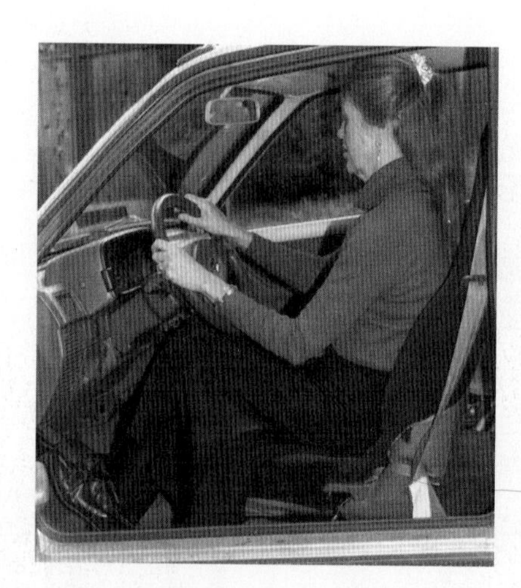

Discomfort: A tucked pelvis and rounded back, the head too far out front, and strained shoulders.

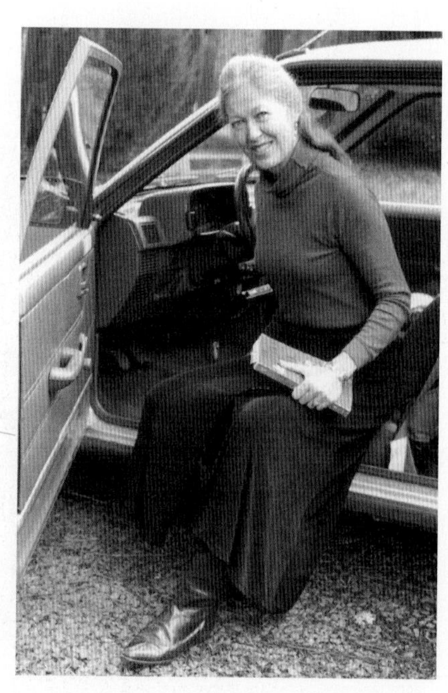

Comfort: Leg Rotation, Turning

AUTO CARE AND DRIVING

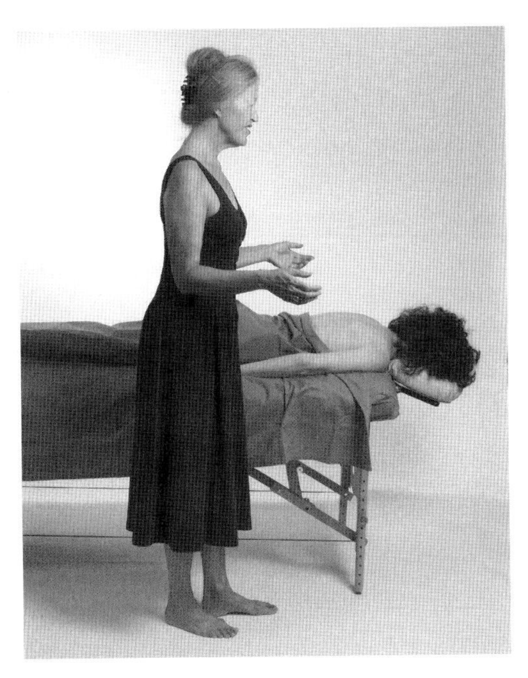

Grounding, Tikanis

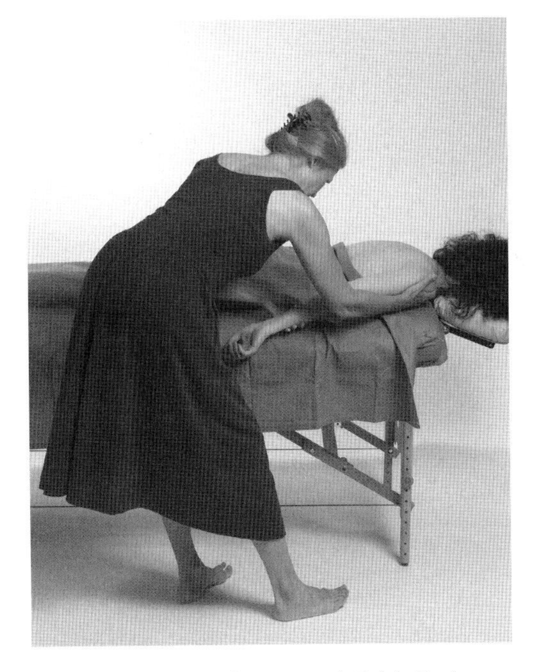

Grounding, Bending Forward, Pelvic Rock, Between Heaven and Earth

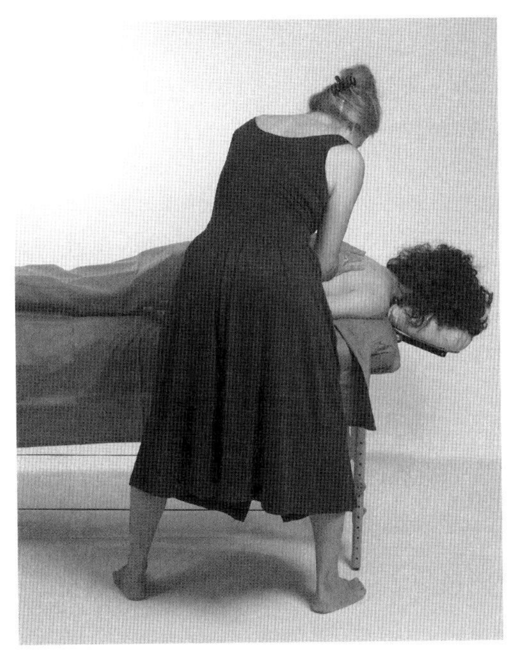

Grounding, Bending Forward, Pelvic Rock, Turning, Gliding, Croissant

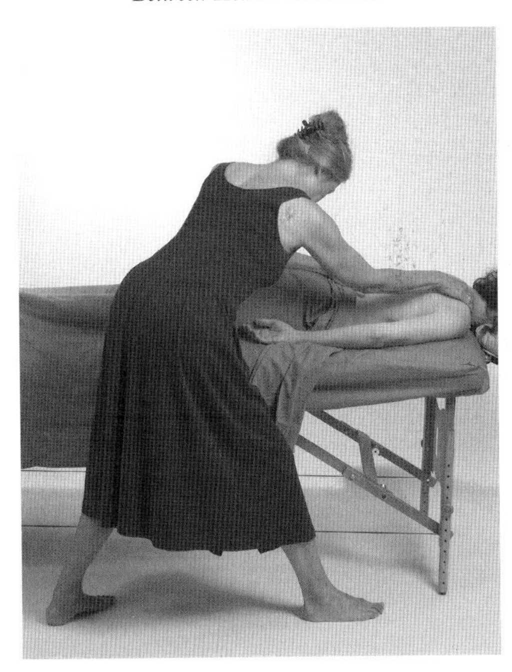

Grounding, Bending Forward, Lifting, Pelvic Rock, Gliding

GIVING A MASSAGE

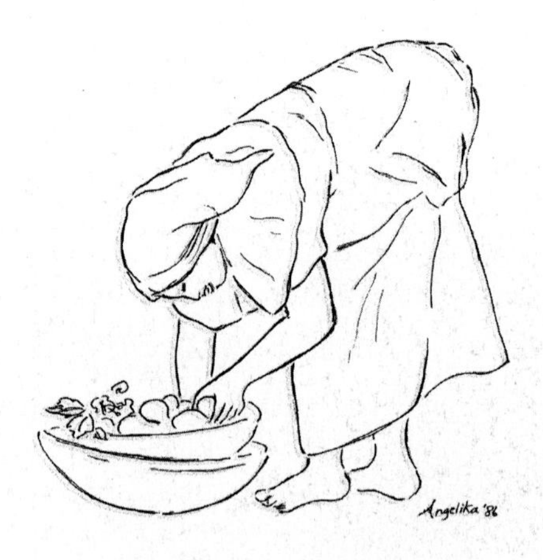

Epilogue

We can feel at home in our bodies
by sensing comfort, by feeling ease
as we move through the day
with zest
in intimate connection
with our activities
and our rest.

Ordinary actions
can ground us
each day —
as typing, lifting children
and preparing a meal
feel like play.

As a tree is sacred
so are our senses.
We can relish moving
to our heart's delight.
This is our nature
ever bright.

APPENDIX

A Physical Therapist's Revelation

The KENTRO Approach to Optimal Posture

By Martha Plescia, PT

I CLEARLY REMEMBER my first meeting with Angelika Thusius in 1990. In the moment before I met her, I made an effort to stand up straight: I tucked my buttocks under slightly, pulled in my stomach, lifted my chest, and squared my shoulders. I wanted to demonstrate to her that I already knew good posture. After all, as a physical therapist I had been instructing people to stand and sit up straight for years. I was skeptical that Angelika had much to offer me, but she had been highly recommended, and I was curious.

Immediately after we exchanged greetings, Angelika asked me to place my fingertips at the creases between my thighs and abdomen (I was still standing), and then she guided my legs slightly backward into a more vertical alignment. I felt tension of the muscles and ligaments under my fingertips ease. Next, she instructed me to relax my buttocks and back, and I was surprised to realize that they had been tense. As I consciously relaxed them, my torso seemed to relax and lengthen. When she pointed out that balanced posture should not require effort, I knew that I had just experienced the truth of that. It was a revelatory moment for me, as exciting as it was humbling.

I soon learned how the concepts of balanced posture apply not only to standing but also to all positions and movements of daily activities. The concepts I learned from Angelika have been invaluable to me. Within weeks of beginning to realign my body under her instruction, I felt that I was moving in a more relaxed and lengthened way. I sensed clearly that I was more soundly supported by my legs and pelvis and that I was more stable. The chronic ache I had had in my lower back whenever I stood for long was gone. In the years since, my postural habits have continued to improve, and with that has come a shift in my self-perception, a strengthening of my self-esteem.

In my efforts to pass along the concepts of KENTRO† Body Balance to others, I began writing about it in 1997. In the following summary, I describe the differences between the KENTRO model and the conventional model of optimal standing posture, and I also present indirect evidence that seems to support the proposal that the KENTRO model is the more balanced. I believe that scientific studies will eventually offer further validation of its optimal balance, but meanwhile, I hope that many people, with the help of Angelika's book, will experience the truth of it themselves.

† For simplicity in communication, I use the term "KENTRO" (Greek for "center") as the name for the form of posture that Angelika describes, although she uses the term only in reference to the guidelines she developed for teaching people to balance their bodies.

The KENTRO Model

For optimal posture, the center of mass of each area of the body should be as vertically aligned as possible with the center of the weight-bearing joints below them.[1] Such posture applies minimal stress to the joints and requires minimal muscular activity to maintain.[2] The weight-bearing joints include the vertebral, sacroiliac, hip, knee, and ankle joints. With this in mind, compare the two models of standing posture presented in Figures A.1 and A.2.

The conventional model of optimal posture (Fig. A1) gives the impression of being straight and slim because the buttocks are slightly tucked and this narrows and straightens the silhouette of the body. However, when the buttocks are tucked, the pelvis moves forward and the legs slant. The hip joints end up slightly in front of the axis of gravity (the vertical line going through the body's center of mass), and the ankle joints are well behind it. The spine, too, is not well aligned with the axis of gravity, so it tends to collapse, increasing its curves. Although the silhouette of the body may appear to be straight, the spine is not, and the weight-bearing joints of the body are not well aligned with the axis of gravity.

Because it is not a balanced posture, effort is required to hold it and joints are stressed. The rib cage is lifted to straighten the upper back and keep the head over the center of gravity. This lifting of the rib cage over-arches and compresses the lower thoracic vertebrae. The shoulders have to be held back because the increased curve of the upper back tends to push them forward. The abdomen is held in because the tucking of the buttocks shortens the abdomen and makes it prone to sticking out. The holding of the abdominal muscles hinders normal diaphragmatic breathing, creating the potential for other problems.

With the KENTRO model of optimal posture (Fig. A.2), the pelvis is

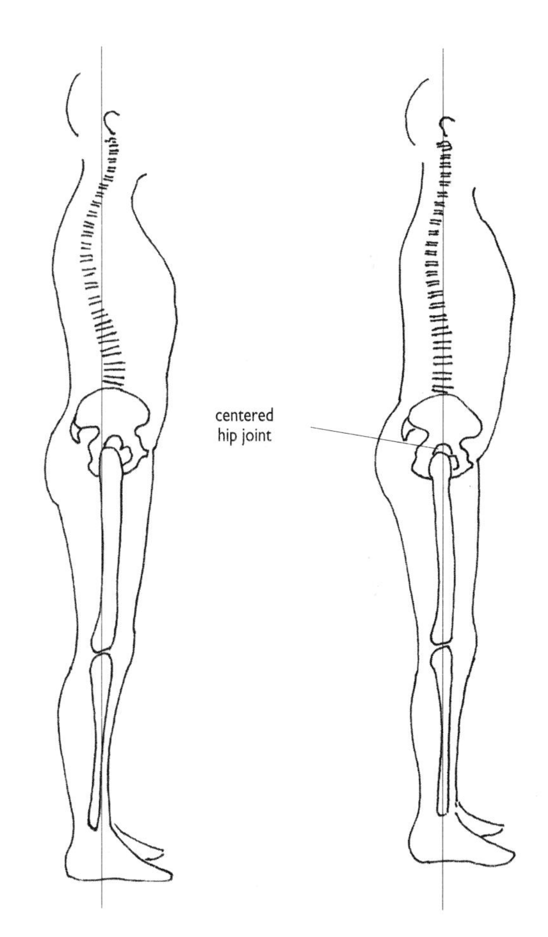

Fig. A1–A.2. Models of optimal posture

A.1 (left), the conventional model. A.2 (right), the KENTRO model. Notice the alignment of the plumb line with the center of the head and with the vertebrae and the joints and bones of the legs. The vertebrae, joints, and bones of the legs are in better alignmentfor weight-bearing in the KENTRO model than in the conventional model.

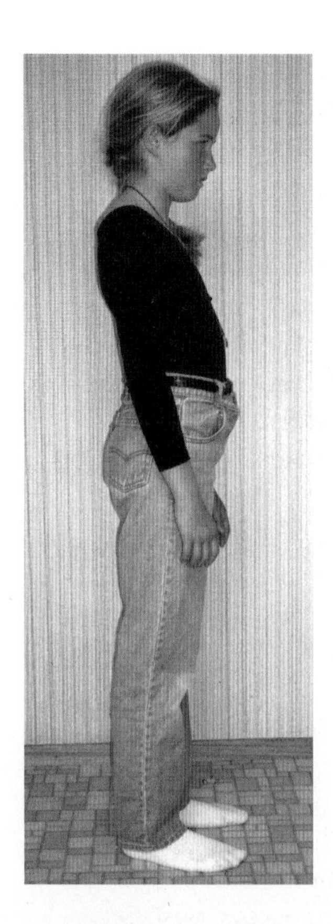

Fig. A.3. The model demonstrates excessive anterior (forward) rotation of pelvis. This is not *advocated in the* KENTRO *model of optimal posture.*

farther back and more "anteriorly rotated" —that is, the top is rotated more forward, the bottom more backward. This allows the legs to become more vertical, which in turn aligns the hip, knee, and ankle joints with the axis of gravity. The more anteriorly rotated position of the pelvis combined with the more vertical legs fully preserves the natural lumbosacral arch, which is crucial for the verticality of the lumbar spine above and its excellent alignment with the axis of gravity. With the entire spine relatively straight, the center of the head is easily in line with the axis of gravity, and the shoulders are naturally farther back and down.

This posture eliminates much of the muscle holding and joint stresses throughout the body which are prevalent in less balanced postures. Furthermore, since the spine is in a stable position, it is capable of maximum weight-bearing.

The differences in pelvic position and leg alignment between the KENTRO model and the conventional model may appear to be subtle, but they are crucial for spinal alignment. *Any* flattening of an individual's natural lumbosacral arch, due to even slight tucking of the pelvis and slanting forward of the legs, prevents balanced alignment of the spine above it.

Note again in the conventional model of optimal posture (Fig. A.1) that the lower legs slant slightly forward, the back slants slightly back, and the approximate centers of the head, hip joints, and ankle joints are not quite vertically aligned. Since this posture is not optimally aligned and, therefore, requires effort to maintain, people lose it as soon as their attention wanders. They tend to shift their hips farther forward and slump until the ligaments of their hips and spines arrest movement. All around us we see the rounded backs and forward heads and shoulders of people who have been tucking their buttocks and shifting pelvises forward to "rest on ligaments" most of their lives. In contrast, posture that is well balanced is easy to maintain without conscious effort or holding. (See *Setting the Stage: Postural Movement in Highly Industrialized Countries,* p. xvii).

It is important to understand that the KENTRO model of posture does not advocate an excessive anterior rotation of the pelvis. It seeks the normal mid-range position of all joints involved. An excessive anterior pelvic rotation (Fig. A3) would cause an exaggerated mid-lumbar lordosis (arching). People who tend to stand with this excessive mid-lumbar lordosis are often advised to tuck the buttocks and pull in the stomach. Although these actions do flatten the excessive mid-lumbar arch, they also flatten the natural lumbo-sacral arch below it, pulling the entire spine above it out of natural alignment. Thusius's KENTRO guidelines for balanced posture demonstrate the appropriate way to improve the posture. (See *A Passionate View of Physiology,* p. 10).

Most very young children move with balanced posture. After about the age of three, many of them lose it, perhaps because most of them are beginning to emulate the postures of older people around them. Some people do retain the posture of their childhood into adulthood. This balanced posture is seen in many traditional cultures (for example, in South America and Africa) and in pockets of industrialized societies (for example, in Portugal, Greece, England, Ireland, Italy, and Spain). These people move with significant lumbosacral arches, straighter spines, open chests and relaxed yet toned abdominals and buttocks. This, Thusius says, is an effortless, balanced posture which is the birthright of all people. (See *Setting the Stage,* p. xvii.)

Why do people of some cultures generally maintain the posture of their early childhood when others do not? Thusius does not believe that their spines are inherently different. Certainly, genetics play a role in the way we are all aligned and move, but she proposes that our perceptions (conscious or not) of what postures appear to be attractive or normal and the movement habits we fall into are the greater influence.

Thusius points to a shift in aesthetics (i.e. fashion) that has occurred over the last several decades in heavily industrialized societies as evidence that altered perceptions of what posture looks best has been a major cause of widespread postural changes. In the United States and Europe prior to World War I, a more anteriorly rotated pelvis and a straighter back and more forward torso were fashionable and more common. (See *Setting the Stage,* p. xvii.) In fact, fashions amplified the buttocks with bustles and the bust with full bodices. With World War I, the "lean modern look" became fashionable. The buttocks were slightly tucked under, the legs went forward, and the torso tended to collapse slightly backward. From this posture evolved an exaggerated version, "the debutante slouch:" the legs were very slanted, the buttocks very tucked, and the spine collapsed. This posture, which is widely considered to look "sexy," is still commonly seen in advertisements today.

Changes in posture have been so widespread that medical as well as popular views and definitions of normal posture have also altered. Thusius has observed that as fashions regarding posture changed, so did medical textbook depictions of normal posture. What is typical posture, however, does not mean that it is optimal. In short, fashion has not only contributed to the unbalanced postures prevalent today, but it has also influenced the conventional medical model of optimal posture.

The amount of prolonged sitting required of us in industrialized countries (from first-grade on or earlier) is frequently cited as a primary cause of poor posture. But how much is the *way* we sit a greater factor, and how much has fashion influenced that? Sitting with the pelvis posteriorly rotated—which is almost inevitable in all the chairs designed with bottoms that slope down in the back—flattens the lumbo-sacral arch and causes the spine to collapse. Trying to sit with a straight spine while the pelvis is forced by the chair into this posterior rotation, takes constant muscle effort. Sitting at the edge of these chairs improves pelvic alignment somewhat (since it places the pelvis in a more anterior position), but the edge of the chair may put excessive pressure on the back of the thighs. Sitting with a small wedge under the buttocks helps maintain the more anterior pelvic position for effortless sitting with an optimally balanced spine. (See Movement 6: *Sitting Up* , p. 72 and Vignette 6: *Keep Your Furniture., p. 74)*

Excellent alignment of the spine is extremely important when we bend forward, especially when bending while lifting, because the compressive forces on the vertebral discs are considerable. The more the vertebrae are kept in optimal alignment, the better the discs and joints can handle the forces. Here again, the relationship of the pelvis

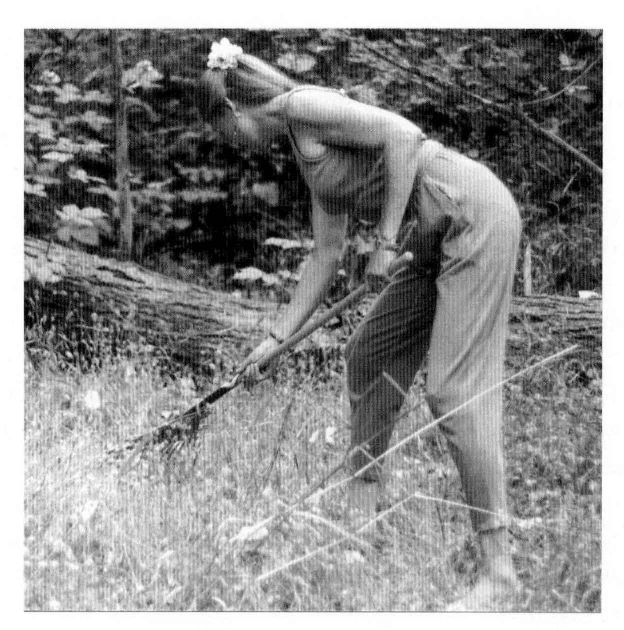

Fig.A.4. Keeping the spine well-aligned by bending the hips and knees protects the spine.

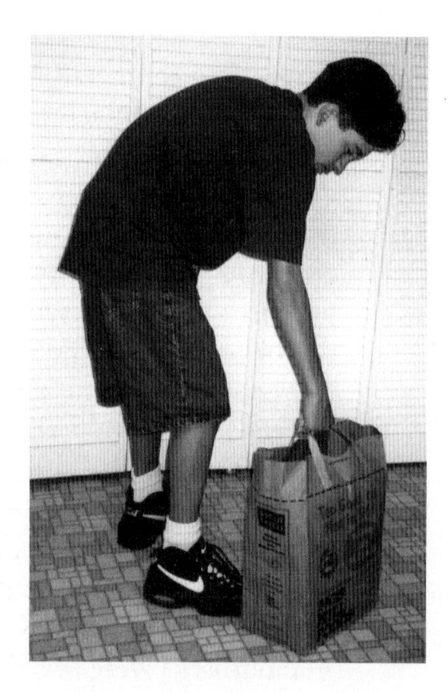

Fig. A.5. Bending in the spine instead of bending the hips and knees makes the spine vulnerable to injury.

to the spine is critical: the normal (neutral) lumbosacral angle must be preserved in order for the spine to have optimal alignment. This requires bending only at the hips and knees, not in the back (Fig.A4). Yet curling the spine from the shoulder level down appears to be the most common way of bending in our society (Fig. A5).

Rounding the back over-stretches back ligaments and muscles, denies the back muscles a chance to do the work they need to do to remain strong, and wedges the vertebral discs between the vertebrae, accelerating disc degeneration. In addition, the forward bending of the back causes the neck to bend backward (compressing structures) and the shoulders to slide forward (contributing to shoulder impingement).

Moving in an imbalanced way—for example, lifting with a rounded spine—often causes a sudden injury. The relationship of the imbalanced movement to the injury is clear. Cause and effect are not as clear, however, when people move out of balance for years before they develop the painful consequences. Tissues of the body adapt to habitually poor posture: some tissues shorten and others lengthen and weaken.[3] As adaptations accumulate, structures such as joints are stressed and put out of proper alignment. However, it is not until tissues reach the limits of their adaptability that symptoms appear—gradually or suddenly—perhaps in the neck, shoulder, jaw, or knee. While people may think that they are random victims of spinal or hip arthritis, shoulder impingement, TMJ or patellar syndrome, plantar fascitis, tennis elbow, headaches, carpal tunnel syndrome, and so on, their habitually poor posture may have been the root cause.

Most people would like to have good posture (unless they think that slouching looks sexy). Even if they don't know that good postural habits help prevent myriad muscular-skeletal problems, they want to look better. Yet they tend to think it is hopeless because their bodies won't straighten even when they try, or they think that their slouch has been genetically predetermined, or that it is an inevitable part of aging. They don't realize that just as their bodies were misshapen by poor postural habits, they can gradually be realigned and reshaped through postural improvement.

Angelika Thusius has demonstrated on herself and hundreds of clients that, with specific stretches[††] and with a conscious commitment to practice moving in balance throughout each day, the body's prior adaptation to unbalanced posture can be largely corrected. Stretches such as those that she teaches are a crucial component of the reshaping process but, as Thusius emphasizes, they cannot by themselves result in well-balanced posture. Tissues are shaped according to how they are used; therefore, a commitment to practice moving in balance day after day is of utmost importance. It takes time and patience for lasting changes to take place. Various manual therapies (e.g. myofascial release, CranioSacral therapy, and visceral manipulation) can often facilitate the reshaping process, but they, too, cannot succeed without the concurrent, sustained practice of moving in balance.

To move in balance, one has to know what balanced posture is. Thusius does not ask her clients to imitate any outward model of posture, not even the Kentro model described here. Rather, she teaches them to sense their bodies—to know where there is tension or compression, where there is relaxation and freedom, where there is support or not. Finally, they come to know what optimal posture and movement *feels* like: relaxed, supported, unstressed—balanced!

Implications for Physical Therapists

An instructor in a course for physical therapists asked our group rhetorically, "What is ideal posture?" Immediately she added, "You *nev*er see it." Most of us in the room laughed as we tried to sit up straighter. She briefly showed a slide depicting conventionally accepted optimal standing posture, explained what landmarks on the body should line up with each other (they didn't quite), and went on. I had seen this and similar pictures of "ideal posture" many times before and had never questioned them.

I believe that we in the physical therapy profession do need to question this conventional model of optimal posture. Is Angelika Thusius correct in asserting that it is not well balanced and that it takes too much effort to maintain? Is the model she presents, with its more anteriorly rotated pelvis, more angled sacrum, greater lumbosacral arch, and more vertical legs and spine, optimally balanced over the weight-bearing joints? Does it require less effort to maintain?

[††] Thusius teaches clients to do stretches in a manner that is far more gentle than how they are usually taught. As people who have experienced the effects of various light-touch therapies know, very gentle specific forces (grams or ounces) applied to tight tissues can elicit (possibly through neurological reflex mechanisms) relaxation responses that are at least as complete and long-lasting as any obtained through more forceful methods.

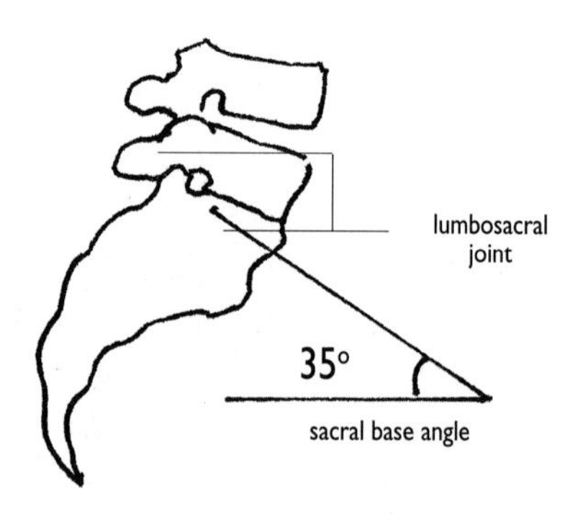

Fig. A.6. Sacral base angle of 35 degrees. This much of an angle at the sacral base corresponds to a significantly slanted sacrum, as in the KENTRO *model of optimal posture. A smaller sacral base angle—which corresponds to the more vertical sacrum observed in conventional models of optimal posture—increases the likelihood of osteoarthritis at the lumbosacral joint.*

There is no explicit research, to my knowledge, regarding what is optimal pelvic placement in standing posture. However, I believe the following information lends credibility to the KENTRO model.

One research study examining the clinical relevance of the lumbosacral angle found that a sacral base angle of less than 35 degrees (Fig. A.6) predisposes people to osteoarthritis at the lumbosacral joint.[4] However, it has been stated in medical literature that a sacral base angle of 30 degrees is optimal.[5] This implies that what has been called optimal posture actually predisposes people to osteoarthirits at the lumbosacral joint. The KENTRO model of optimal posture, with its more slanted sacrum and greater sacral base angle, would not.

Angelika Thusius studied for decades the postures of people of various cultures and nationalities and observed unique and consistent characteristics of posture among those known to have remarkably low incidence of back pain. The posture of these people appeared to be exceptionally balanced and relaxed, similar to the posture she observed in very young children. It was the posture of these adults and very young children that led to her understanding of balanced posture.

Women of certain African tribes were found to have very low energy expenditures compared to control groups when carrying loads of up to 70 percent of their body weight.[6] Their load-carrying efficiency was attributed by the authors of the study to their efficient use of the body as a pendulum. Their posture, though not mentioned, must surely be a factor: they could not carry these loads with the ease and energy-efficiency with which they do unless their bodies were optimally aligned for weight-bearing. Indeed, pictures in a *New York Times* article about the study did have a picture that depicted a woman carrying heavy loads in the unique posture that Thusius describes as optimally balanced.[7] Also, Thusius has long observed that those populations of people who traditionally carry large loads supported on their heads have this same posture.

The very structure of the pelvic bones seems to indicate that they are meant to bear weight in the more anteriorly rotated position described in the Kentro model of posture. Weight from the trunk is transferred through the pelvis to the legs by way of the sacroiliac and hip joints. The thickest part of each hip socket—the part one would think is designed to bear the most weight—is more vertically aligned with the sacroiliac

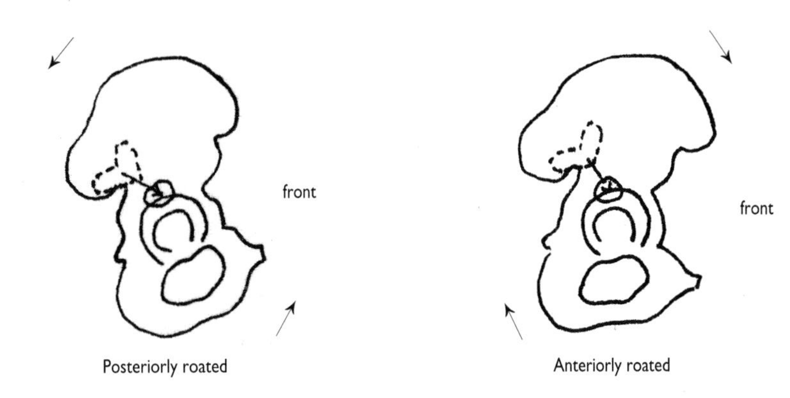

Fig. A7. Posteriorily rotated pelvic bone (left) typical in the conventional model of optimal posture. In contrast, the more anterirorly rotated pelvic bone (right) as in the KENTRO model. The sacroiliac joint (indicated with dotted boomerang shape since it is on the other side of the bone) and the thickest part of the hip socket (marked with solid oval)—which seems meant for the most weight-bearing—are better aligned with the axis of gravity (vertical alignment) in the KENTRO model (right) than in the conventional model (left).

joint above it when the pelvis is more anteriorly rotated than when it is more posteriorly rotated (Figs. A.7).

Clearly, more scientific research is needed to clarify what optimal posture is. The research is unlikely to happen as long as conventional concepts are accepted as definitive. Since physical therapists are daily witnesses to the damaging effects of poor postural habits and since we are in an excellent position to teach postural improvement, I hope we will seriously question the commonly accepted concepts of optimal posture and help test the new ones. Angelika Thusius's KENTRO concepts, in particular, are very deserving of our attention.

NOTES

1. M. A. MacConnaill and J. V. Basmajian, *Muscles and Movements* (New York, Robert E. Krieger Publishing Co., 1977): 217
2. Ibid: 216 and D. J. Magee, *Orthopedic Physical Assessment* (Philadelphia, WB Saunders Company, 1992): 579
3. S. Sahrman, Diagnosis and Treatment of Movement Impairment Syndrome (USA: Mosby, 2002): 15.
4. R. O. Kissling, M. F. Waldis, and A. Tschopp, "Is the geometry of the lumbosacral transition clinically relevant? *Journal of Manual and Manipulative Therapy* 2 (3, 1994): 102-111.
5. J. Owen and A. Middleeditch, *Functional Anatomy of the Spine* (Oxford, Butterworth-Heinemann Ltd. 1991): 295 and C. Kesner and L. A. Colby, *Therapeutic Exercise*. Second edition. (FA Davis Company, 1990).
6. N. C. Heglund, et. al., "Energy-saving gait mechanics with head-supported loads" *Nature*: vol. 375, May 4 (1995): 52-54.
7. *New York Times* (March 12, 2002): page F3.

Selected Reading List

Bender, Sue. *Everyday Sacred.* San Francisco: HarperSanFrancisco, 1995.

Bloom, William. *The Endorphin Effect.* London: Judy Piatlus Limited, 2001.

Cameron, Julia. *The Artist's Way*. New York: Jeremy P. Tarcher/Putnam Books, 1992.

Chopra, Deepak. *Ageless Body, Timeless Mind.* New York: Harmony Books, 1992.

Dalai Lama and Cutler, C. *The Art of Happiness.* New York: Riverhead Books, 1998.

Diamond, Irene and Orenstein, Gloria Feman. *Reweaving the World, The Emergence of Eco-feminism*. San Francisco: Sierra Club Books, 1990.

Dossey, Larry, *Reinventing Medicine.* San Francisco: HarperSanFrancisco, 1999.

Graf von Duickheim. Karlfried. *Hara*. London: George Allen and Unwin LTD., 1962.

Gray, Henry. *Gray's Anatomy.* New York: Bounty Books, 1977.

Gray, John. *How to Get What You Want and Want What You Have.* New York: Perennial, HarperCollins, 2000.

Johnson, Robert A. *Ecstasy*. San Francisco: HarperSanFrancisco, 1987.

Lambert, Susan. *Matisse-Lithographs.* London: Her Majesty's Stationary Office, 1981.

Mehl-Madrona, Lewis. *Coyote Medicine.* New York: Fireside Books, 1997.

Moore, Thomas. *Care of the Soul*. New York: HarperCollins, 1992.

Northrup, Christine. *Women's Body, Women's Wisdom*. New York: Bantam Books, 2002.

O'Donohue, John. *ANAM CARA*. New York: HarperCollins, 1997.

Page, Christine R. *Frontiers of Health.* Essex: C.W. Daniel Company Limited, 1992.

Pearsall, Paul. *The Pleasure Prescription.* Alameda, Calif.: Hunter House, 1996.

Pert, Candace B. *Molecules of Emotion.* New York: Scribner, 1997.

Rubenfeld, Ilana. *The Listening Hand*. The Rubenfeld Synergy Method®. New York: Bantam Books, 2001.

Stern, Anthony. *Everything Starts from Prayer.* Ashland, Ore: White Cloud Press, 1998.

Stevens, John. *The Shambhala Guide to Aikido.* Boston: Shambhala Publications, 1996.

Weil, Andrew. *Spontaneous Healing.* New York: Fawcett Columbine Book, 1995.

Whyte, David. *The Heart Aroused.* New York: A Currency Book, Doubleday, 1994.

ACKNOWLEDGEMENTS

I AM FORTUNATE THAT MY MENTORS, Gela Meyer (Honduras), Sheila Healey, Galea Parsons, and Rosaline Badmin (England) continually gave me their support for bringing my vision to fruition with this book. Bouquets of appreciation to all the students who have gifted me with their invaluable responses to practicing KENTRO movements. Special thanks to Martha Plescia, who, over many years, generously perused the physiologically oriented chapters. I am grateful to the following people who, in various roles, participated in the creation of this book: Jenny Simmons, Tomaseen Foley, Nancy Hackleman, Melissa Michaels, Gabrielle Leslie, Judith Sanford, Beth Hoffman, Cheryl Turner, Tish McFadden, Darrelle Cavan, Patricia Khun, Rosemary Maitland, Chinook Dimitre and family, Marion Moore, Linda Thomas, Diane Mathews, Lori Quick, Raina Sanderson, and Christy Collins.

Thanks to my editor at RiverWood Books, Steven Scholl, for encouraging my writing and focusing on excellence for the book. My publisher, Gary Kliewer, skillfully brought it all together.

My deepest gratitude is to my husband, Darwin, for his patience and kindness, and for being my grounding force.

Index

Index, continued

Photography credits

Photos and illustrations not credited below are from Angelika Thusius.

Preface:
p x. Bottom left, Kevin Peer. Bottom right, Suzanne Arms.

Introduction:
p. xvi. Maja Zürcher

Part I:
p. 8, Kim Carrol
p. 12, Fig. 3.6, Janet Michaelis
p. 17, Fig. 3.23, Kim Carrol
p. 19, Fig. 3.24, Carrie Reitman
p. 24, Toubis
p. 26, Cyril Maitland
p. 27, top right, Eric Crystal
p. 32, top, Stella Karas

Part II:
p. 56, Vassilis Liappas
p. 64, Vassilis Liappas
p. 68, c. 1940, Library of Congress
p. 70, top right, Vassilis Liappas
p. 74, bottom left, Ashland Christian Fellowship; bottom right, Robert Frost
p. 75, c. 1893, Library of Congress
p. 79, left, Vassilis Liappas; right, Library of Congress
p. 80, top left and right, Kim Carrol; middle left and right, Suzanne Arms; bottom, Cyril Maitland
p. 81, Robert Frost
p. 84, far right, Carrie Reitman
p. 89, Kim Carrol
p. 92, Janet Michaelis
p. 98, Figs. 9.3, 9.4, Kim Carrol; Figs. 9.5, 9.6, Giuseppe Saitta
p. 108, Robert Frost
p. 130, top middle and right, Kim Carrol
p. 134, Elise Miller
p. 136, Kim Carrol
p. 140, Francoise
p. 144, Kim Carrol
p. 152, Cyril Maitland
p. 161, Robert Frost
p. 168, Maja Zürcher
p. 172, Kim Carrol
p. 173, top, Marilyn Benioff; bottom, Ashland Christian Fellowship

p. 178, Kim Carrol
p. 183, Library of Congress
p. 194, Kim Carrol
p. 199, Claire Sponheim
p. 212, Kim Carrol
p. 213, Robert Frost
p. 214, Kim Carrol
p. 215, Robert Frost

Appendix
p. 220, Fig. A.3, Martha Plescia
p. 222, top left, Fig. A.4, Tomaseen Foley, top right, Fig. A.5, Martha Plescia